"Wow! Hope is alive!! I have just finished reading *Healing Schizophrenia* and I loved it, from the title to the last paragraph. This book is exquisitely sensitive while also being boldly adventuresome. It presents a balanced picture of the multi-faceted aspects of treatment and care of persons diagnosed with schizophrenia while also opening up a wealth of possibilities that challenge the current treatment paradigm. Boldly confronts the reader with the possibility that psychosis is more than a physical brain disease and that psychosocial and psychospiritual aspects of the person need to be taken into account. I found this book to be the most comprehensive and easiest to read research on the role and effects – both positive and negative – of medication in the treatment of schizophrenia. Goes beyond medication and encourages the use of complementary therapies such as counselling. The view of schizophrenia presented has the possibility of offering hope to all who read the book, especially to diagnosed persons and their families. I would love to see *Healing Schizophrenia* become prescribed reading for all psychiatrist intern and mental health professionals."

Sister Rosalind Cairns
Director, Mental Health Chaplaincy
Healthcare Chaplaincy Council of Victoria

"*Healing Schizophrenia* is essential reading for social workers who are working with people who are on medications to treat mental illness. The holistic approach considers the body, mind and soul, and notions of healing and recovery from schizophrenia that are consistent with post-modern social work theory and practice. This is an extremely thoughtful and well-researched book which provides useful practical information and self-help guidelines. It will prove an extremely useful resource as it provides detailed information about uses of particular medications and likely side effects. Given the huge impact that medication has on a person's health and wellbeing, social workers cannot afford to ignore this aspect of assessment and intervention. This book is the first of its kind and the author is to be congratulated for his valuable contribution to holistic approaches in mental health. *Healing Schizophrenia* is highly recommended for social work education as well as for users of mental health services."

Jennifer Martin, PhD
Associate Professor in Social Work
RMIT University, Melbourne

HEALING
SCHIZOPHRENIA
USING MEDICATION WISELY

JOHN WATKINS

MICHELLE ANDERSON PUBLISHING
MELBOURNE • LONDON

THE INFORMATION IN THIS book is based on the author's personal research and opinions and is intended to assist readers in their journey of healing and recovery. It is provided for educational purposes only and cannot replace competent medical diagnosis and treatment. People with a psychiatric condition are advised to seek assistance from appropriately qualified mental health professionals. Anyone already receiving medical treatment should consult with the prescribing doctor before altering and/or stopping such treatment. The author and publisher specifically disclaim responsibility for any adverse consequences which may result from use of the information contained herein.

Published in Australia 2006 by
Michelle Anderson Publishing Pty Ltd
email: mapubl@bigpond.net.au
www.michelleandersonpublishing.com

Copyright John Watkins 2006

Cover design: Deborah Snibson Modern Art Production Group

National Library Cataloguing-in-Publication data

Watkins, John,
Healing schizophrenia : using medication wisely.

Bibliography.
Includes index.
ISBN 0 85572 376 9.

1. Mental illness - Alternative treatment.
2. Schizophrenia - Treatment. 3. Holistic Medicine.
I. Title

616.898069

"This is a book that offers many answers about the treatment of schizophrenia. It presents a long-needed almanac on schizophrenia and the mental health field and strives to give accurate and balanced accounts of key viewpoints as well as supporting evidence from a range of stakeholders in various debates. This should make *Healing Schizophrenia* singularly helpful and probably quite different to other books on schizophrenia treatment and related mental health topics. The quality and comprehensiveness of the information is compelling. Drawing on a wide range of informants and sources the author makes painstaking efforts to navigate through many issues with balance and objectivity in a field where even people with genuinely held beliefs all too often find themselves caught up in controversy. This book could play a definite role in building new bridges between the stakeholders in debates in the mental health field. *Healing Schizophrenia* is a clearly written knowledge resource which would be useful to any person with a genuine desire to deepen their understanding of what the author has referred to in the book's subtitle as 'Using Medication Wisely'."

Allan Pinches
Consumer Consultant in Mental Health

"Thank you so much for giving me the opportunity to read your book. I think *Healing Schizophrenia* will be a great reference for mental health professionals and carers and consumers. You have given hope to those of us who thought there was none. You have filled a gap in literature on schizophrenia: medical books are too technical while many lay books on the subject are too 'alternative' and don't provide enough information on medication. Although I found it hard going in parts, *Healing Schizophrenia* was nevertheless inspiring, reassuring, thought-provoking, and informative."

Sian Morgan
Consumer

"*Healing Schizophrenia* has surprised, frustrated, and lifted me. The surprise was the sound of the author's voice – intense, but considerate of readers like me with many of the terms used which he did explain. The frustration arose not just because of the truths he was very carefully revealing about the medications and about the mental health system in general, but because in the process of digesting this new (to me) information and its importance, I continually found past frustrations and gut-wrenching memories from seven or eight years ago coming back to reproach me for questions I too easily stopped seeking answers for then (when my daughter Sian was first diagnosed). I was lifted by much of the analysis of treatment and the practical, healthy, and even inspiring alternatives, e.g. the Soteria Project, gave me hope. It is strange that such simple information is not usually dispensed along with the medication. Thank you for giving me an opportunity to update my knowledge on schizophrenia. This book *needs* to become a best-seller."

Angela Morgan
Carer

"*Healing Schizophrenia* differs from any other book I have read on the subject. The author is not daunted by complexity: he does not take sides in the great mind-brain debate in psychiatry and values the evidence of personal experience as much as he does that of science. His focus on neuroleptic medications for schizophrenia exposes the uncomfortable truth that these treatments can be as damaging as they are helpful. He argues that these drugs are overused and that they should be prescribed with more caution, in lower dosages, and always in combination with psychosocial approaches that harness the wisdom gained from personal experience. *Healing Schizophrenia* stands out as a highly readable and useful resource for service-users, professionals, and others who want to ensure neuroleptics help recovery rather than hindering it."

Mary O'Hagan
Former mental health service user;
Commissioner, Mental Health Commission New Zealand

Medicines will be well used when the doctor understands their nature, what man is, what life is, and what constitution and health are. Know these well and you will know their opposites; you will then know how to devise a remedy.

Leonardo da Vinci

To Fiona, whose love, sanity and patience
have been a blessing to me.

Contents

Introduction

THIS BOOK PROVIDES INFORMATION of great importance to anyone involved with the use of neuroleptic medications, whether as patient, prescriber or carer. Now commonly referred to as *anti-psychotic* drugs, and once known as *major tranquillisers*, these powerful medications are routinely given to people diagnosed with schizophrenia or other types of psychotic disorder. Among the questions most often asked about these widely used drugs are the following:

- What do neuroleptic drugs actually do?
- What do neuroleptic drugs *not* do?
- How can neuroleptic treatment help?
- Are there people who do *not* benefit from neuroleptic treatment?
- What side effects do neuroleptics have?
- Can these side effects be avoided?
- How long should neuroleptic treatment be continued?
- Can it be safely stopped?

- How is it possible to maximise the potential benefits of neuroleptic treatment while at the same time minimising the possible risks?
- Are neuroleptic drugs the only effective form of treatment for schizophrenia?

It is impossible to give definitive answers to these questions since a great deal depends on the treated person's specific circumstances. These include highly individual characteristics such as age, gender, physical health, genetic and biochemical constitution, social circumstances, the kind of symptoms experienced, and type of drug (or combination of drugs) being taken. Nonetheless, readers can be assured they will find much in this book that is relevant to their own situation. *Particular emphasis has been given to providing information in a simple and clear form so that it can be put to immediate practical use.*

Before proceeding I would like to state that this has been a very difficult book to write. Powerful feelings have welled up all the way through, ever more so as it neared completion. Many times I have felt quite overwhelmed by the task of trying to understand and make sense of the vast amounts of complex and highly technical information it has been necessary to gather, examine, and evaluate. Many times, too, I found myself wishing I had chosen a simpler topic. I have frequently thought how much easier it would be to simply ignore certain issues or turn away from some of the more difficult questions. I am pleased I did not succumb to these temptations. I have no doubt that the information, ideas and practical suggestions which form the substance of this book are far more comprehensive – and more truthful – than they may have been if I had chosen to shy away from the more challenging issues. I am confident that readers who are prepared to make a similar effort will find they are more than amply rewarded.

Adding to the difficulty of writing about an inherently complex subject has been the often contradictory nature of much of the available information. Who do you believe when many highly regarded "experts", all of whom appear to be equally well-qualified, so often seem to be saying quite different things? Some of these discrepancies are doubtless due to the fact that those involved in intensive research into psychiatric medications are rarely practicing mental health clinicians. They therefore lack the regular hands-on experience that affords true insight into how people in the real world actually respond to various kinds of treatment. On the other hand, very few clinicians are directly involved in carrying out research on the drugs they routinely prescribe. Differences of opinion can become even more pronounced when one takes into account the views of those whose expertise is based, not on professional qualifications or academic research, but personal experience. Although people who have taken neuroleptic drugs often have a great deal to say about this subject, their views and opinions are rarely given the attention they deserve. Another vexing issue has been the question of how best to respond to the many glowing claims made about the ever-expanding range of psychiatric medications when concerns are now often expressed about the impartiality of the research upon which some of these claims are based.

The anticipated response of readers has been a further powerful influence. Like all authors I have wondered about how this or that individual or group may react to the often challenging, and at times controversial, nature of what I have said. These concerns have meant that much of the writing was done in the company of a host of disembodied voices: those of psychiatrists and other mental health clinicians, "consumers" (people who take neuroleptic drugs), "carers" (relatives of such people), support workers, and lay readers, including the friends, colleagues, or employers of individuals diagnosed with schizophrenia. While I would like to think that anyone interested in the therapeutic use of neuroleptics would be prepared to give this book open-minded consideration, previous experience suggests this is unlikely to occur. In fact, if the response to my earlier books is any guide, certain people are likely to find aspects of what is said here quite discomforting. Some will choose to deal with their anxiety by means of avoidance and denial. I anticipate similar reactions to what I have said, or sometimes merely implied, about the nature of "mental illness", schizophrenia in particular. A predictable consequence of such reactions is that neuroleptic and other psychiatric medications will continue to be misused. Indeed, it is my firm belief that such misuse is *inevitable* so long as drugs are seen as the only truly important aspect of treatment, as is increasingly the case with schizophrenia and many other psychiatric conditions.

I expect that, while many people who have taken neuroleptic medications will find much in this book that is helpful and affirming, others may well be highly critical. Indeed, I fully expect that some who adamantly oppose the use of psychiatric medication will accuse me of selling out, simply because I have acknowledged its possible value for some people – assuming, of course, that it is used properly. One of the reasons some people are highly critical of medication is that their own experiences with it, and perhaps with psychiatry generally, have been predominantly negative. While I feel great sympathy for such people, I would remind them that care needs to be exercised when making generalisations on the basis of personal experience: for every horror story about medication (and psychiatry) there are others far more positive. I am also very mindful of the anguish experienced by many carers who have watched with growing feelings of helplessness and despair, as a cherished family member has become increasingly absorbed in an alien world and gradually slipped away. The promise of a simple remedy, one that would restore the former self and make everything all right again, is so tantalising! And yet nagging doubts remain: Is a chemical imbalance *really* all that is going on? Is medication, however effective, *really* all that is needed? Is it realistic to think that simply taking a few pills will free a sensitive, troubled soul from complex, often long-standing, social, psychological, and spiritual problems and concerns?

In an era in which unfettered access to information of every kind is seen as an inalienable right, it may come as something of a surprise to learn that it is actually extremely difficult to get to the truth about neuroleptics and other widely-used psychiatric medications. This is partly due to the inherent complexity of the subject. As a result of this, there are many legitimate differences of opinion as well as contrasting ways of interpreting the bewildering masses of data generated by clinical experience and pharmacological research. At least as important is the fact that the mental health field has evolved into a conglomerate of lucrative industries. Among these, powerful vested interests compete, protecting their individual territories by aggressively promoting their own views above those of others. The biomedical paradigm within which mainstream psychiatry now operates has come to exert tremendous influence. So much so, in fact, that few people even question the wisdom of relying almost exclusively on powerful drugs, which are often administered automatically once a diagnosis such as schizophrenia is given. Indeed, if certain recent trends catch on, "pre-emptive treatment" could soon become a common practice, with troubled individuals being given potent drugs even *before* a psychiatric diagnosis has been formally applied.

In such a climate it is good to be reminded that, while proponents of biomedical psychiatry have acquired a near-monopoly over conventional views about how best to treat mental illness, a range of contrasting opinions exist which deserve thoughtful consideration. For example, though it is now widely accepted that most people who receive a diagnosis of schizophrenia will require long-term medication to ensure their stability, authoritative clinical research has clearly established that a significant proportion of such persons can do well *without* routine medication. On the other hand, it is also well known that some people do poorly despite strict compliance with prescribed treatment regimes. These thought-provoking facts raise many important questions about the proper role of psychiatric drugs and about the nature of the conditions they are used to treat.

While neuroleptics have played a decisive role in the evolution of the psychiatric treatment of psychosis, and will doubtless continue to do so well into the foreseeable future, the fact that they have become the predominant treatment modality is a cause of concern to many thoughtful people. These drugs and the mind-set that accompanies them have come to define everyday clinical practice so completely that few people realise there are a host of contentious issues surrounding their use. How best to use these drugs — indeed, whether to use them at all — are questions no one involved with schizophrenia can afford to avoid.

It should be emphasised that it is *not* the aim of this book to suggest that neuroleptic drugs are somehow bad or that they do not have a potentially useful role to play in treating schizophrenia and other psychotic conditions. Rather, its purpose is to encourage readers to think more carefully about the way these and other psychiatric drugs are used and to offer some scientifically credible suggestions as to how they might be employed more effectively. It aims, in particular, to contribute to the development of a holistic approach, in which medication represents but *one* component of comprehensive treatment. Far from encouraging non-compliance, it is the author's sincere belief that, by providing truthful information about what neuroleptic drugs do — and what they do not and cannot do — and by describing how it is possible to use them in the context of a holistic approach, some people who would otherwise refuse prescribed medication may actually become less resistant to this aspect of treatment.

A wealth of information has been provided with these aims in mind. *Chapter One* briefly describes the historical origins of neuroleptic treatment before addressing the difficult question of how these drugs work. This is followed by a detailed discussion of an issue at least as important as that dealt with in the opening chapter, namely the various side effects of neuroleptic medications. A comprehensive overview of the drugs referred to as *atypical neuroleptics*, the most recent innovation in schizophrenia treatment, is provided in *Chapter Three*. One of the main themes of this book – how neuroleptic drugs can be used in the overall context of a holistic approach to schizophrenia – forms the subject matter of *Chapter Four*. *Chapter Five* discusses innovative research carried out in the 1970s, which clearly demonstrated the feasibility of treating acute psychosis without neuroleptic medication or with only minimal amounts of it. Open-minded readers will doubtless find the ideas outlined in this section extremely thought provoking. Some may even find them inspiring.

The difficult question of how long neuroleptic treatment should be continued is discussed in detail in *Chapter Six* and *Chapter Seven*. The research outlined will certainly challenge those committed to the view that most diagnosed people will require large doses of maintenance medication indefinitely. "Using Medication Wisely" is the self-explanatory title of *Chapter Eight*. Considerable experience has shown that the five principles it outlines provide a reliable basis for safe and effective medication use. A range of individualised strategies are described in *Chapter Nine*. Clinical research suggests these may represent feasible alternatives to continuous, high-dose neuroleptic treatment for many people. *Chapter Ten* is specifically intended for those who wish to reduce or even completely stop their medication. While it is not the author's intention to encourage anyone to refuse prescribed treatment, it is a fact that a substantial number of people will choose to do so at some time – often without telling anyone. The guidelines outlined in this chapter are based on the principles of risk-minimisation, and are intended to reduce the likelihood that medication reduction and/or cessation will result in undesirable consequences.

Chapter Eleven is a late addition. During the long period of researching and writing *Healing Schizophrenia*, my attention was repeatedly drawn to information that struck me as far too important not to include. Specifically, this chapter discusses the extent to which vested commercial interests – particularly, but not exclusively, the pharmaceutical industry – have come to exert a powerful influence over basic mental health research, education, and clinical practice. I imagine that many readers will find it unsettling to learn about the various behind-the-scenes forces that influence how psychiatric drugs are now tested, promoted and used. While the issues discussed are certainly controversial, the views expressed are based upon factual information from a wide range of authoritative and highly credible sources. I will be pleased if what I have written makes a small contribution to breaking the conspiracy of silence that has long surrounded these matters.

A personal reflection on the nature of healing forms the essence of the final chapter, "The Most Powerful Drug There Is". Here a critical eye is cast over the way research into the mode of action of neuroleptic drugs has led to the formulation of theories which emphasise the notion that schizophrenia is primarily the result of some kind of malfunction in the diagnosed person's brain, an idea which translates into the now frequently made claim that neuroleptics rectify the "chemical imbalance" that is said to be the underlying cause of psychotic symptoms. Within this paradigm the recent advent of atypical neuroleptics has been hailed as a breakthrough which represents a major step toward the eventual development of a pharmaceutical cure for schizophrenia. With the brave new world of molecular psychiatry fast approaching, the need has never been more urgent to contrast contemporary approaches to psychiatric treatment with more traditional ideas about health and healing. In this context it is especially important to ask whether the use of modern drugs can be compatible with therapies whose aim extends beyond symptom control to encompass the broader objective of "healing the soul" – the literal meaning of the word "psychiatry".

Appendix A contains information about optimal dosage ranges of some commonly used neuroleptics, while *Appendix B* outlines a range of practical strategies for preventing or minimising medication side effects.

A willingness to ask questions and look beyond the surface of things is required of anyone who wishes to gain a deeper understanding of the proper role of neuroleptic drugs. A fair degree of humility is also necessary. While researching this book, I was surprised at the number of times I had to acknowledge my own ignorance. Despite having been involved in the mental health field for more than twenty-five years, time and again I found myself thinking "I didn't know that" as I came across some new facts or discovered a different way of looking at those already familiar. I was also reminded that it can take a long time for new information to become widely known and accepted, and that many years may pass before novel ideas gradually find their way into everyday clinical practice. Substantially longer delays can be anticipated in the case of ideas which challenge the medical, psychiatric or economic status quo. It is good to remember, too, that today's innovative idea or apparently radical suggestion may well be taken for granted tomorrow.

Chapter One

THE CHEMISTRY OF TRANQUILLITY

Dialectical views of the potential of pharmacology: medication, in the wrong hands, as thief of the self; medication, in the right hands, as restorer of the self.

Peter Kramer[1]

CONTEMPORARY PSYCHIATRIC TREATMENT OF schizophrenia and other psychotic conditions is now firmly centred on the use of a group of drugs known collectively as *neuroleptics* or *major tranquillisers*. Neuroleptics in turn belong to a much larger group of chemical substances that are referred to as *psychoactive drugs* since they have their principal effects on the mind, particularly on key aspects of mental functioning such as mood and emotions, thinking, and perception. Other major classes of psychoactive drugs include *anxiolytics* (anxiety reducing), anti-depressants, mood stabilisers, and sedative-hypnotics (sleep inducing). *Psychopharmacology* is the scientific study of the effects of psychoactive drugs and the clinical application of such knowledge for therapeutic purposes. The psychoactive drugs routinely used in psychiatry are referred to as *psychotherapeutic medications* since they are administered with the intention of bringing about various desirable changes in the treated person's psychological and emotional state (e.g. elevating and/or stabilising mood, reducing anxiety, ameliorating distressing thoughts and perceptions).

Neuroleptics are often referred to as *anti-psychotic* because of their reputed ability to reduce or eliminate psychotic symptoms, such as hallucinations and delusions. However, there is, in fact, considerable uncertainty about what these drugs do and how they work. Furthermore, feelings and opinions surrounding their use are extremely varied and often highly polarised. Many see them as a veritable godsend, perhaps none more so than those who have experienced or witnessed at first hand the profound transformation these drugs can sometimes bring about in a treated individual's behaviour and thinking. Relatives of diagnosed people are often especially grateful for drugs which may have allowed a level of functioning that otherwise seemed impossible. Understandably, many families enthusiastically endorse the use of such medication, with some even living in fear of the possibility that a diagnosed relative will stop taking it, only to "go off the rails" once more. By contrast, there are those who consider neuroleptic drugs an unmitigated evil: powerful and dangerous "zombie potions" used indiscriminately and insensitively to impose the mind-numbing "chemical straitjacket" into which psychiatry's unwilling victims are coerced and entrapped. Such people may even accuse those who prescribe the drugs of being corrupt and venal drug push-ers who surreptitiously foist their toxic wares on vulnerable and unsuspecting people in the guise of legitimate psychi-atric treatment or therapy.[2]

Inevitably, the truth lies somewhere between these extremes. Like other medical drugs (and such social drugs as alcohol) neuroleptics are a two-edged sword, a power-ful tool that can produce great benefits when used with wisdom and skill, but which are capable of causing harm if used unwisely or inappropriately. Irish psychiatrist Dr David Healy, formerly the secretary of the British Asso-ciation for Psychopharmacology and an international authority on the therapeutic use of psychotropic drugs, acknowledges that, while it is certainly possible for neuro-leptic medications to be abused, they also have the potential to be highly beneficial:

> It must be stressed ... that despite what has often amounted to misuse of these drugs for the purposes of control, there is a benign use of neuroleptics that should not be lost sight of ... *These drugs are immensely useful — when used properly.* Their proper use depends greatly on a close cooperation between taker and prescriber. The takers need to learn what particular neuroleptics can do for them — how best to use them — but also their limitations — what they do not do. A failure to recognise the limitations of neuroleptics has led in the past, and still leads now, to many prescribers prescribing doses that actually make conditions worse or to takers self-medicating with doses that aggravate their conditions.[3]

As a first step in developing a balanced and informed attitude toward neuroleptics it may be helpful to take a closer look at what this group of drugs actually do. To this end it is instructive to briefly consider the history of neuroleptics, starting with the first of their kind, chlorpromazine.*

The Chemistry of Tranquillity

In 1952 researchers seeking an effective pre-anaesthetic sedative which would help protect surgical patients against post-operative shock, observed that the drug chlorpromazine (Largactil)‡ seemed to induce a peculiarly nonchalant attitude. This was described at the time as resembling a kind of "artificial hibernation". It was soon suggested that this drug might play a useful role in the treatment of disturbed psychiatric patients and experiments were subsequently carried out to test this idea. The first British report describing the results of these tests appeared in the *Journal of Mental Science* in 1954. Induction of a profound

---

* It should be pointed out that while chlorpromazine was indeed the first *synthetic* drug to be employed as an "anti-psychotic" medication, it was not, in fact, the first substance to be used for this purpose. The earliest known effective treatment for schizophrenia was actually a herb, Indian snakeroot (*Rauwolfia serpentina*), used in India over two thousand years ago to treat a variety of mental disorders. See Bhatara, V. et al. (1997) 'Rauwolfia Serpentina: The First Herbal Antipsychotic'. *American Journal of Psychiatry*, Vol. 154, No. 7.

‡ Most prescription drugs have a *generic name*, based on their chemical composition, and one or more *brand names*, used by the manufacturer to distinguish their own brand of this particular product from those of other manufacturers. When medical drugs are referred to in this book, the generic name is given first followed by one or more common Australian brand names in brackets. Thus, Largactil is one of a number of available brands of the neuroleptic drug, chlorpromazine.

state of "psychic indifference" was identified as being one of chlorpromazine's most notable effects:

This is perhaps the characteristic psychiatric response to chlorpromazine. Patients responding well to the drug have developed an attitude of indifference both to their surroundings and their symptoms best summarised by the current phrase "couldn't care less". As a result one has observed a loss of subjective anxiety and of distress arising from tension feelings; a reduction in the abnormal behavioural responses to hallucinatory experiences and a loss of interest in them; a lessening of conviction in delusional concepts; and a lessening of preoccupation with obsessional and hypochondriacal ruminations ... In the presence of the fully developed response ... the patient lies quietly in bed, staring ahead, unoccupied and showing little or no interest in what is going on around him. He answers questions readily and to the point, but offers little, if any, spontaneous conversation. Questioning reveals that he is fully aware of his circumstances but that the distress they may formerly have caused him has gone.[4]

The first North American report on the effects of chlorpromazine noted similar responses. Significantly, while all persons given this drug were observed to become emotionally indifferent, these pioneering researchers commented that, "We have not observed a direct influence of the drug on delusional systems or hallucinatory phenomena."[5] Because chlorpromazine's principal effect is to induce a state a calmness resembling tranquillity, it and similar drugs soon came to be called "tranquillisers", a practice maintained for many years. It is noteworthy that what were thought at the time to be quite exceptional therapeutic results were obtained with dosages of chlorpromazine that would come to be considered extremely low, perhaps even sub-therapeutic, by later standards. Thus, while in the early 1950s chlorpromazine dosages of 50-100 mg per day were usual, it had become common during recent decades for people to receive total daily dosages of 800-1000 mg or even far more. This fact raises a number of important questions which will be considered later.

Within a short time chlorpromazine was being used widely in mental hospitals throughout Europe and the USA, resulting in a remarkable change in the behaviour of many once intractably disturbed psychiatric patients. Clearly, a major revolution was at hand, one which would soon lead to a search for more drugs with therapeutically useful effects. Before long a number of compounds had been identified which proved to be even more potent than chlorpromazine. Soon a large and constantly growing range of neuroleptic drugs were in common use throughout the world. Thus began the era of modern psychopharmacology.

A Neuroleptic Smorgasbord

For convenience the neuroleptic era is often divided into two phases. For reasons that will become clear later, drugs commonly used between the 1950s and the early 1990s are now often called *conventional, classic,* or *typical* neuroleptics. Since clozapine (Clozaril) was introduced in 1990, a growing number of neuroleptics referred to as *second-generation, novel,* or *atypical* have become available. Routine use of many of the earlier drugs has now largely been superseded by the more recently introduced atypical neuroleptics.

(a) Conventional or Typical Neuroleptics

The most frequently used typical neuroleptics include those classed as either *low potency* or *high potency*. The low potency neuroleptics tend to be given in relatively large doses (ranging from a few hundred milligrams up to a thousand milligrams or more), while the high potency drugs are effective when administered in much smaller amounts (from a low of a few milligrams to a high of several tens of milligrams). The most commonly prescribed low potency conventional neuroleptics include:

- chlorpromazine (Largactil)
- thioridazine (Melleril)

Commonly prescribed high potency conventional neuroleptics include:

- haloperidol (Serenace)
- pericyazine (Neulactil)
- pimozide (Orap)
- thiothixene (Navane)
- trifluoperazine (Stelazine)
- zuclopenthixol dihydrochloride (Clopixol)

Conventional neuroleptics are usually given orally in the form of tablets or syrup, although some can also be given by injection. Some can be administered in the form of long-acting intramuscular injections (see below).

See Appendix A for information regarding optimal dosage ranges of some of the most commonly prescribed neuroleptic drugs, both conventional and atypical.

(b) Depot Neuroleptics

Partly as a response to the issue of medication non-compliance, a range of long-acting injectable neuroleptics have gradually been developed. These preparations are often referred to as *depot* neuroleptics, since they are formulated in such a way that, once injected, they provide a store in the body from which the active drug is slowly released over a period of several weeks to a few months. Depot injections are typically given at intervals of 2 to 4 weeks. The most frequently prescribed depot neuroleptics in current use include:

- flupenthixol decanoate (Fluanxol)
- fluphenazine decanoate (Modecate)
- haloperidol decanoate (Haldol)
- zuclopenthixol decanoate (Clopixol Depot)

Note: Zuclopenthixol acetate (Clopixol-Acuphase) is a short-acting (1 to 3 days) neuroleptic sometimes used in the early treatment of acute psychosis. Although it is given as an intramuscular injection it is only effective for a few days and is therefore not considered a true depot. Acuphase treatment is limited to a maximum of four injections that are generally administered 2-3 days apart. Midazolam (Hypnovel) is another short-acting injectable drug sometimes used to help calm people experiencing acute psychotic excitement. It is *not* a neuroleptic, however, but a member of the benzodiazepine family (this group of anxiety-reducing drugs are discussed in *Chapter Nine*).

(c) Novel or Atypical Neuroleptics

Clozapine (Clozaril) was the first of the second-generation or atypical neuroleptics to be introduced into regular use. A number of other drugs with similar properties soon followed and are now used widely. Currently available atypical neuroleptics include:

- aripiprazole (Abilify)
- amisulpride (Solian)
- clozapine (Clozaril)
- olanzapine (Zyprexa)
- quetiapine (Seroquel)
- risperidone (Risperdal)

These drugs now tend to be used in preference to the earlier conventional neuroleptics. The main reason for this is that they are reputed to have fewer deleterious side effects than the older drugs. It is also believed that some people who have failed to benefit despite prolonged treatment with conventional neuroleptics may respond somewhat better to clozapine. *The effects and side effects of atypical neuroleptics are discussed in detail in Chapter Three.*

Note: In Australia, no atypical neuroleptics were available in the form of long-acting depot injections until very recently. However, in 2003 a long-acting form of risperidone, marketed under the brand name Risperdal Consta, was approved by regulatory authorities. Unlike earlier depot preparations, which begin to take effect almost immediately, there is a time lag of approximately three weeks, from the time of first injection, before Risperdal Consta reaches a therapeutically effective level. Use of this and other long-acting atypical medications, yet to be introduced, is likely to become increasingly common.

However, at the time of writing most people on depot treatment are still receiving conventional neuroleptics, a fact which has a number of important consequences (see *Chapter Two*).

Are Neuroleptic Drugs "Anti-Psychotic"?

As the range of available tranquillising drugs grew and they began to be widely used, efforts were made to determine more precisely what effects they have on those who take them. Thus, research was conducted in 1964 under the auspices of the US National Institute of Mental Health (NIMH) to determine the impact of neuroleptic drugs on 24 target symptoms of schizophrenia.[6] The top four symptoms, in which either marked or moderate response to these medications occurred, were found to be, in descending order:

- Combativeness (74% of patients)
- Hyperactivity (73% of patients)
- Tension (71% of patients)
- Hostility (67% of patients)

Next in order were hallucinations (58% of patients), then negativism (58%), and delusions (48%). Further analysis of this research revealed that only slightly more than 30% of patients reported experiencing a *marked* reduction in hallucinations while only 21% experienced a *marked* reduction in delusional thinking.

A considerable body of subsequent clinical research has confirmed the relatively limited effectiveness of neuroleptic drugs on delusions and hallucinations. For example, a study carried out in 1988 found that a substantial proportion of diagnosed people were still experiencing psychotic symptoms when discharged from hospital, despite having received quite large doses of neuroleptic drugs. The patients in this particular study were discharged on mean medication doses equivalent to 920 mg of chlorpromazine yet 31.4% were still experiencing hallucinations (compared to 78.1% experiencing them when admitted) and 51.0% still had persistent delusions (93.8% at admission).[7] Interestingly, these researchers also noted there was an overall increase in the severity of what are referred to as *negative* symptoms, between admission and discharge. These include social withdrawal, loss of motivation, and anhedonia (inability to experience pleasure). A recent review published in the *American Journal of Psychiatry* analysed data obtained from the US Food and Drug Administration (FDA) database on trials of neuroleptic drugs. It found that the average level of symptom reduction was 16.6% with the newer atypical medications, and 17.3% with the older drugs, leading the reviewers to state that, on average, people treated with these medications only tend to experience "a modest reduction in symptoms".[8]

These and other findings suggest that, rather than being specifically "anti-psychotic" in the sense of having a direct ameliorative effect on *positive* psychotic symptoms such as delusions and hallucinations, the primary effect of neuroleptics is to reduce tension, agitation and irritability.[9] Indeed, until growing concerns about side effects led to their use being restricted to the treatment of more severe kinds of mental disturbance such as psychosis, neuroleptics were regularly given to people experiencing a wide variety of psychological problems. These included anxiety, nervousness, insomnia, and other varieties of relatively minor emotional distress.*

As explained above, neuroleptics help to induce a state of calmness by damping and muting a person's emotional responses to both their surroundings and their inner experiences – including their symptoms. They do this whether or not the person concerned is diagnosed with schizophrenia or some other type of psychiatric disorder, or even if they are mentally well. For this reason neuroleptics of one sort or another are given, as a matter of course, to all agitated, hyperactive, over-stimulated and aggressive psychiatric patients on admission, e.g. they are the drugs of choice in the initial management of acute manic excitement.

In the early 1960s researchers established that neuroleptics selectively attach themselves (bind) to neuronal receptors in certain parts of the brain, thereby blocking the activity of one of the key neurotransmitters, dopamine ("neuroleptic" literally means "to clasp the neuron"). It was subsequently found that classic neuroleptics have a particular affinity for the so-called dopamine D2 receptors located in the brain's limbic system. Dr David Healy has described the therapeutic consequences of such neuroleptic-induced *dopamine blockade* as follows:

---

* It is worth noting that a number of neuroleptic drugs are still widely used to treat common *non-psychiatric* medical conditions. These include anti-emetic medications (used to prevent and treat nausea and vomiting) such as prochlorperazine (Stemetil) and metoclopramide (Maxolon) and anti-histamines such as promethazine (Phenergan) used to alleviate allergy symptoms. Characteristic neuroleptic side effects are generally not a problem if very low dosages of these drugs are used though they may occur with larger ones. Some individuals who are extremely sensitive to the effects of neuroleptics have been known to experience distressing side effects even on very small doses of these commonly prescribed drugs.

What binding to D2 receptors does is to produce a feeling of indifference, a sense of being shielded from stress, a "who cares" feeling that many people under stress find immensely useful. Neuroleptics are also called "major tranquillisers" for this reason. But the tranquillisation they produce is not like the wave of calm relaxation that Librium, Valium, and alcohol bring about … It is much more a case of finding oneself not getting worked up than finding oneself tranquillised down … they produce a feeling of detachment – of being less bothered by what had formerly been bothering … more able to focus on tasks that need doing, less in a daydream, not distracted by internal dialogues, strange thoughts, or intrusive imagery.[10]

Despite the fact that they are primarily *non-specific calming agents,* neuroleptics have been heavily promoted as being specifically "anti-psychotic" or even "anti-schizophrenic" drugs. Indeed, they are commonly given to people who see or hear things others do not (hallucinations) or who entertain unrealistic or irrational beliefs (delusions). While neuroleptics *do* sometimes help to eradicate or at least ameliorate such symptoms, David Healy has pointed out that often their effect is simply to make the voices or delusional preoccupations less problematic as a result of the fact that the drugs tend to dampen the treated person's reaction to them:

To observers, it often appears that some days or weeks after claiming to hear voices or after coming out with some strange ideas, people who take neuroleptics begin to behave more "normally", as though the voices and the ideas have cleared up. It is this clearing up that has led to the impression that neuroleptics are anti-schizophrenic. More often than not, however, sensitive questioning reveals that the hallucinations or delusions have not entirely disappeared. It is more usual that takers of neuroleptics still have their voices or some of their ideas but they are less worried by them.[11]

The fact that people who take neuroleptic drugs often feel less troubled by voices and other previously disturbing experiences means that they are less likely to talk about them, thereby giving rise to the possibly misleading impression that these experiences have stopped. (It is worth noting that diagnosed people may also have various *other* reasons for concealing the fact that they are still experiencing symptoms, e.g. to expedite their discharge from hospital, to avoid the shame and stigma that comes with being perceived by others as "mad", or to avoid being given even more medication.) It is actually very difficult to find out precisely how many people who may *appear* to be symptom-free are actually not. However, when Professor Ian Falloon conducted careful interviews with diagnosed people in their own homes after they had been treated for an acute schizophrenic episode, he found that 92% of those with significant negative symptoms were also experiencing hallucinations, delusions, or thought disorder.[12] Professor Falloon pointed out that many of these people only disclosed their symptoms when systematically questioned in their own homes, and that they had been consistently described as free of any psychotic symptoms at their aftercare clinics.

Treatment Resistant Patients or Patient Resistant Treatment?

The belief that neuroleptic drugs are specifically anti-psychotic has led to the notion that diagnosed people who do not become completely symptom free on adequate doses of these medications are manifesting a greater or lesser degree of what has come to be called *treatment resistance*. Many people diagnosed with schizophrenia continue to experience symptoms of some kind (referred to as *residual symptoms*). This fact has motivated treating professionals and researchers to do a number of things in an attempt to overcome this perceived problem. Although these endeavours have been well intended, they have sometimes had unfortunate consequences. For example, as part of an effort to eradicate their symptoms *completely*, many people have been given ever-increasing quantities of neuroleptic drugs that in some cases have been increased to massive amounts (known as "heroic" doses) which have then been continued for years on end. This sometimes still occurs despite good evidence that, for most people, large doses of neuroleptics are no more effective than much smaller ones, and can only lead to problematic side effects. Furthermore, diagnosed people still sometimes find themselves being given two (or even more) different neuroleptics simultaneously, despite clear evidence that there is no pharmacological justification for such combinations. As with high doses generally, such "neuroleptic cocktails" significantly increase the risk of deleterious side effects (some of which may be resistant to treatment). For a long time it was common practice to routinely give other kinds of drugs to counteract the side effects caused by excessive doses or combinations of neuroleptics. It is now known that commonly used "side-effect tablets" have various side effects of their own which may interfere with neuroleptic treatment (see *Appendix B)*.

As well as encouraging what is known as *psychiatric polypharmacy*, the erroneous belief that neuroleptic drugs are specifically effective against psychotic symptoms has for several decades had the effect of discouraging mental health professionals from investigating *non-drug strategies* for dealing with disturbing experiences. This still occurs even though a growing body of research has belatedly confirmed that many diagnosed people can learn to stop or control voices and other distressing experiences quite effectively, using a range of non-pharmaceutical techniques.[13] Despite repeated confirmation of the potential usefulness of these innovative approaches, very little effort has yet been made to teach them to diagnosed people on a large scale.

Nor has the relatively low level of effectiveness of "antipsychotic" drugs led to a general reappraisal of what is called the *dopamine hypothesis* which holds that schizophrenia symptoms like hallucinations and delusions are caused by excess dopamine activity in certain parts of the brain. Such a reappraisal certainly *should* have occurred, given that it is now well known that, although substantial blockade of dopamine receptors is achieved almost *immediately* after a conventional neuroleptic is administered, amelioration of psychotic symptoms often takes weeks or months to occur – if it happens at all. Researchers have found that dopamine blockade is just as complete in those who do *not* respond to neuroleptic treatment as it is in those who do.[14] In short, if excessive dopamine activity – a chemical imbalance – was really the fundamental cause of schizophrenia symptoms, there should be no such thing as "treatment resistance". In an article published in the *British Journal of Psychiatry* in 1991, David Healy commented:

> While an initial study suggested that there were abnormalities in the dopamine system of individuals with schizophrenia, more recent studies have suggested that there are no apparent abnormalities in the dopamine system, or of the D2 receptor in particular, in schizophrenia. These findings led one of the principal advocates of the dopamine hypothesis, Arvid Carlsson, to conclude that the dopamine hypothesis of schizophrenia is no longer tenable.[15]

That the chemical imbalance hypothesis has not only survived but is spoken about by many people as though it were an established *fact* suggests that, rather than being simply a theory, this idea has achieved the status of a dogma in certain quarters.

The growing realisation that neuroleptics are not as effective as was originally hoped has galvanised the search for more effective drugs, particularly ones which might benefit the relatively large proportion of diagnosed people deemed to be treatment resistant (it has been estimated that over 25% of people treated with the older neuroleptics continue to experience a significant level of symptoms).[16] These efforts have recently resulted in the advent of a range of atypical neuroleptics (*Chapter Three*). While it is too early to say what might happen in the long-term, these drugs have already had a very significant impact. While they have not overcome the problem of treatment resistance they have proven to be helpful to a proportion of people who respond minimally or not at all to treatment with the older drugs. Most importantly, they appear to have fewer of the debilitating neurological side effects which have long bedevilled therapeutic use of the original neuroleptics, especially when they are administered in large doses.

The systematic search for more effective neuroleptics continues apace and will undoubtedly lead to the introduction of many new drugs in coming years. While these are likely to offer certain benefits, particularly in terms of being "cleaner" (i.e. having fewer debilitating side effects), it is important to remember that whatever their potential value may be, there are very real limits to what neuroleptics – or indeed *any* psychiatric drugs – can realistically be expected to do.

A Neuroleptic Shield

Many observers have noted that people diagnosed with schizophrenia are often extremely sensitive. Indeed, some researchers believe that a distinguishing characteristic of such persons is that they are endowed with an *exquisitely sensitive* nervous system.[17] There is little doubt that, from a very early age, many such persons appear to possess a remarkable sensitivity to both sensory and emotional stimuli. As well as contributing to their original predisposition to psychosis, persistent uncompensated hypersensitivity may render a person susceptible to experiencing further psychotic episodes, especially if they are exposed to excessive stress (this susceptibility is now often referred to as the diagnosed person's *vulnerability* to relapse). While a host of influences might contribute to the development of hypersensitivity, it is possible that genetic factors may play some part. The following statement from the highly regarded psychiatric reference, *Comprehensive Textbook of Psychiatry,* alludes to such a possibility:

All schizophrenics are, at least originally, more sensitive than the average person. It is likely that the increased sensitivity and heightened responsiveness to sensory and emotional stimulation is present in schizophrenics from an early age, possibly from birth. Schizophrenia may be characterised by a genetic hypersensitivity that leaves the patient vulnerable to an overwhelming onslaught of stimuli from without and within.[18]

The ability of neuroleptic drugs to induce a state of psychic indifference can make them extremely useful in certain circumstances, especially if a person's difficulties are directly related to their constitutional hypersensitivity. Professor Luc Ciompi, an internationally renowned authority on schizophrenia, has recently surmised that rather than having a direct effect on a diagnosed person's perceptions and thought processes, neuroleptics may actually have their primary impact on the *emotional* level. This results from the fact that they tend to dampen activity in certain parts of the brain's limbic system, whose functions include modulation and control of mood and motivation.[19] In Professor Ciompi's opinion, one potentially beneficial consequence of such limbic modulation is that neuroleptics can act as *general buffers* which help protect hypersensitive individuals from the potentially destructive impact of stressful stimulation:

As for medication, and the neuroleptics in particular, the view developed here does not question their potential usefulness, either in acute [psychotic] conditions or as preventive measures against relapses. Their ability to reduce sensitivity to stress and the vehemence of emotions, and thus to act as an effective "brake" in cases of psychotic "runaway" suggests their main function is as general buffers.[20]

The stress-buffering effect of neuroleptics makes them potentially beneficial in at least two important ways. Firstly, by helping to calm people who are anxious, bewildered, and frightened – feelings that often become very intense during a psychotic upheaval – they can exert a significant *therapeutic* effect. In this regard neuroleptics have been likened to non-specific fire hoses that help cool the brain temporarily while the "fever" of acute psychosis subsides. David Healy points out that, "neuroleptics immediately induce an ataractic state or state of psychic indifference", adding that, "several weeks in such a state is conducive to recovery."[21] Furthermore, to the extent that they can help hypersensitive individuals avoid becoming too emotionally worked up in the first place, these drugs reduce the likelihood that they will again tip over into a psychotic state, i.e. experience relapse. Thus, in addition to their therapeutic action, neuroleptic drugs can also exert a valuable *prophylactic* effect. Professor Manfred Bleuler (son of the pioneer Swiss psychiatrist who coined the term "schizophrenia" in 1911, and also recognised as one of the world's foremost authorities on schizophrenia) describes the potentially beneficial effects of neuroleptics thus:

Neuroleptics act by changing the activity or the sensitivity of definite neurological systems. The therapeutic consequence consists mainly in *calming agitation* and *diminishing the sensitivity to stimulation* both by psychodynamic experience and by experience from the outer world. For these reasons, neuroleptics are of great value in many schizophrenic conditions.[22]

Especially when they are feeling tired, stressed, or over-stimulated, people diagnosed with schizophrenia sometimes find it difficult to attend to, sort, and correctly process information from inner and outer sources. At such times they may find themselves becoming increasingly susceptible to distraction by irrelevant stimuli (e.g. background noises) and have trouble remaining focused on specific tasks, i.e. a tendency to mentally wander off due to a reduced ability to concentrate on and selectively attend to one thing at a time. One man described his own experience of these kinds of difficulties as follows:

> Everything seems to grip my attention ... I am speaking to you just now but I can hear noises going on next door and in the corridor. I find it difficult to shut these out and it makes it more difficult for me to concentrate on what I am saying to you. Often the silliest little things that are going on seem to interest me. That's not even true; they don't interest me but I find myself attending to them and wasting a lot of time this way.[23]

Researchers have found that, for at least some diagnosed people, the arousal-reducing effect of neuroleptic drugs may have a beneficial effect on information processing efficiency by helping to reduce distractability and improve sustained attention.[24] (It is very important to note, however, that neuroleptics can sometimes have a deleterious effect on various aspects of cognitive functioning, an issue discussed in *Chapter Two.*)

Alleviating Mental Dis-Ease

A range of evidence supports the view that *anything* which helps a diagnosed person feel calmer and less hyper-stimulated can have substantial therapeutic benefits. It has been noted, for example, that even highly aroused acutely psychotic individuals may begin to settle very soon after entering a quiet, low-stimulus environment. Indeed, in such circumstances psychotic symptoms sometimes begin to diminish *without any other specific treatment.** Professor Ciompi's research has confirmed the old idea that, more than anything else, disturbed persons are in need of "asylum" in the original sense of a sanctuary and place of refuge and safety (scientific research supportive of these views is discussed in detail in *Chapter Five*). On the basis of his own findings and those of other researchers, Professor Ciompi has concluded that "Drug therapy can become unnecessary even for acute schizophrenics if other conditions for therapy are particularly favourable."[25] In Ciompi's view a warm, emotionally supportive environment is especially desirable for those experiencing acute psychotic turmoil:

> In contrast to the usually tense and bewildering admission wards, a therapeutic setting as relaxing, secure, and supportive as possible would be indicated ... for highly agitated and frightened psychotic patients. This seems

---

* In reflecting on what life was like in the old-style mental hospitals prior to the advent of neuroleptic drugs, Australian psychiatrist John Cawte has noted that "A shared cup of tea was the major tranquilliser in 1952". See Cawte, J. (1998) *The Last of the Lunatics*. Melbourne: Melbourne University Press, p.64

to be confirmed by current Scandinavian research on therapeutic environments as well as by our own experiences ... In the warm, open, supportive and relaxed emotional atmosphere of a small and stimulus-protected open house ... highly psychotic patients quite often improve or even recover within days or weeks, with no or only minimal neuroleptic medication.[26]

That the effectiveness of neuroleptic medications is largely related to the fact that they act as *non-specific calming agents* is further supported by research carried out by a group of highly regarded psychopharmacologists and published in the *American Journal of Psychiatry* in 1989. This study compared the therapeutic effectiveness of neuroleptics with non-neuroleptic sedatives (such as Valium-type drugs) and placebo treatment on people experiencing a psychotic episode or an acute exacerbation of their psychotic symptoms. Somewhat to their surprise, these researchers noted that the *same* overall degree of improvement occurred during treatment with all of the agents tested. The authors summarised their observations thus:

In studies in which neuroleptics were compared to active non-neuroleptic sedative agents, both treatments produced similar symptomatic improvement in the first days, and perhaps weeks, of treatment. The proper interpretation of these findings is not clear. *Perhaps the early effects of anti-psychotic drugs are non-specific and largely the same as those of sedative agents.* The success of placebo treatment suggests that early improvements may be largely due to the non-specific effects of hospitalisation or other clinical interventions apart from the specific therapeutic effects of prescribed pharmaceutical agents ... These findings also suggest the need for further studies designed to compare the acute response to treatment with neuroleptics and the response to treatment with non-neuroleptic sedative agents.[27]

The potential therapeutic use of various drugs belonging to the benzodiazepine family (e.g. Valium) is discussed extensively in *Chapter Nine.*

Aspirin For The Soul

Even though they do not have a specific and direct anti-psychotic effect as such, use of neuroleptic drugs may nevertheless result in an amelioration of psychotic symptoms such as hallucinations and delusions. This may come about *indirectly* as a result of the fact that these drugs can help reduce the intensity of the underlying emotional tensions and unresolved psychological conflicts that provide the fertile ground in which the seeds of such symptoms germinate, take root, and flourish. For example, hostile attacking "voices" (auditory hallucinations) are less likely to occur, and will generally be less vociferous, when the powerful feelings of self-condemnation or even self-hatred from which such experiences often evolve, have been muted by drugs. Likewise, as the deep-seated feelings of fear, resentment, and self-criticism, upon which persecutory delusions are often founded, begin to lose their potency and force, these once firmly held beliefs will also often begin to fade considerably. (This interpretation of the "anti-psychotic" effect of neuroleptics helps explain the time lag mentioned earlier, between the onset of dopamine blockade and the amelioration of psychotic symptoms.) It is worth noting, furthermore, that even if symptoms do *not* disappear completely, the state of psychic indifference induced by the neuroleptics often means that any remaining symptoms cause considerably less distress than they would have otherwise. Symptoms which are less emotionally charged are invariably far easier to ignore.

For obvious reasons, drugs which help reduce anxiety and emotional distress (whether or not such feelings are directly related to symptoms) are highly sought after and, as long as they are used wisely and with skill, can be extremely beneficial. It is vital to remember, however, that the most neuroleptic treatment of schizophrenia can do is to provide *symptomatic relief.* As desirable as this may be at times, it does not get to the root of the problem. Relying too heavily on drugs to suppress delusions and hallucinations risks turning attention away from the psychological origins of these symptoms. It also tends to discourage efforts to address deeper personal issues (such as the devastatingly low self-esteem which may have given rise to persecuting voices or compensatory grandiose delusions). Once a diagnosis has been made and a course of treatment commenced, it is increasingly common for any further discussion between patient and prescriber to focus almost exclusively on the effects and side effects of the drugs.

A real danger exists that medication might come to be seen by *everyone* concerned as a panacea for any and every problem the diagnosed person happens to experience, perhaps even as an all-purpose psycho-analgesic, a kind of "aspirin for the soul". An ineffective drug regime or one causing disabling side effects is clearly unacceptable.

Nevertheless, it is possible for people to feel *too* comfortable on their medication, and to be lulled into a false sense of security and an attitude of emotional complacency which may inhibit their motivation to do the work required to foster growth, healing, and recovery. As Peter Chadwick explains, the fundamental nature of many of the basic aspects of recovery, such as re-building impaired self-esteem or re-establishing a sense of meaning and purpose in life, make them a *necessary* complement to medication:

> Nobody who becomes seriously mentally ill has high self-esteem. If ex-patients' self-esteem is not strengthened by the peers and professionals they work with, they will always remain vulnerable, no matter what medication they take and no matter what case-management or relapse-preventative strategies are assembled.[28]

In order to reduce the likelihood of falling into a state of medication-induced complacency, diagnosed people must remember that while effective neuroleptic treatment may help to open up a range of possibilities, making use of these opportunities is something only they can do.

Psychic Indifference: A Two-Edged Sword

The characteristic effect of neuroleptic drugs – induction of a state of psychic indifference – gives them the potential to both help and harm. To the extent that they calm agitation and reduce tension these drugs can help hyper-alert and over-stimulated people regain their emotional equilibrium and re-connect with ordinary reality. With the cooling of their fevered minds, diagnosed people can begin to feel more comfortable in themselves and, as a consequence, be able to think more calmly and clearly. As they start feeling less threatened and overwhelmed, they may also become more inclined to remain open to others and more receptive to hearing what they have to say. By reducing the intensity of experience and dampening down the spiralling energies that drive an emotional chain-reaction, the timely administration of neuroleptic medication to someone who is beginning to "spin out" may help to abort an incipient psychotic episode. (Simply being in a quiet, supportive, low-stress environment for a short while may sometimes have a similar effect.) Furthermore, on-going administration of neuroleptics – referred to as *maintenance treatment* – can substantially reduce the likelihood of relapse for those susceptible to experiencing further psychotic episodes.

There is little doubt that many diagnosed individuals have found neuroleptic drugs to be extremely helpful tools in their quest to maintain emotional and psychological stability. One of Dr John Nelson's clients gave the following description of the beneficial effects he experienced on these medications:

Man, I was really out of it before you gave me this medicine ... I couldn't get rid of the nutty idea that I should kill my child because I thought he was possessed by the devil. Now the voices leave me alone so that I can sleep and think my own thoughts. My wife is giving me another chance, and my boss has let me come back to work. I feel like a regular person again instead of another screwball on a mission to save the world. I can live with the side effects a lot easier than I could live with those crazy thoughts and feelings.[29]

It is unlikely that there is any kind of pharmaceutical treatment which, while conferring a range of benefits, does not at the same time entail at least the possibility of causing some problems. Regarding the useful stress-buffering effect of neuroleptic drugs, Professor Ciompi has recently observed that, "Although this function may certainly be advantageous in some situations, it may be superfluous or even harmful in others."[30] Thus, while a *moderate* reduction in a diagnosed person's sensitivity to stimulation via the induction of a mild degree of psychic indifference may be highly beneficial at times, *excessive* desensitisation, or desensitisation that is not desired, can lead to various problems. Though relatively minor in many cases, such problems may be far more serious in others. Hints that neuroleptic drugs have the potential to cause problems as a result of their *main* effects (to say nothing of their various possible "side effects") have been evident since the early 1950s when the drugs were originally introduced to psychiatry. The following anecdote from the first British medical report on the effects of chlorpromazine (Largactil) illustrates one possible outcome of a neuroleptic-induced attitude of profound emotional indifference:

> One woman patient who prior to treatment had been in a state of agitation and tension as the result of severe external stress had lost her agitation and tension within thirty-six hours of the first injection and was lying quietly in bed, immobile for long periods but fully conscious. Whereas formerly any discussion of her troubles had precipitated tears and a restless agitation that subsided only after abreactive screaming bouts, she was now able to discuss the situation calmly, and

contrasted her previous behaviour with her present inability to feel any distress at all. "I don't think you could make me cry now whatever you said to me" was her own description.[31]

It is instructive to reflect on the fact that neuroleptics as a class were once widely known as *ataractic* drugs, a name derived from the ancient Greek word, *ataraxia*, meaning impassiveness. The Oxford Dictionary defines "impassive" thus: deficient in or incapable of feeling or emotion, undisturbed by passion, serene, without sensation, not subject to suffering. As suggested earlier, there is sometimes a rather fine line between a sufficient degree of drug-induced impassiveness to be therapeutically beneficial, and a degree which may be debilitating or even disabling. In some instances neuroleptics may enhance tranquillity by dampening anxiety and agitation, but at the cost of inhibiting a diagnosed person's capacity to experience *normal* feelings. Mark Vonnegut has provided a graphic account of what this can be like:

On *Thorazine* [chlorpromazine] everything's a bore. Not a bore, exactly. Boredom implies impatience. You can read comic books and *Reader's Digest* forever. You can tolerate talking to jerks forever. Babble, babble, babble. The weather is dull, the flowers are dull, nothing's very impressive. Muzak, Bach, Beatles, Lolly and the Yum-Yums, the Rolling Stones. It doesn't make any difference. When I did manage to get excited about some things, interested in some things, it still didn't have the same old zing to it. I knew that Dostoyevsky was more interesting than comic books, or, more accurately, I remembered that he had been. I cared about what happened ... but it was more remembering caring than really caring.[32]

Excessively prolonged use of neuroleptic drugs at high doses – or even very small doses in the case of those who are unusually susceptible to their effects – can result in the dulling of a person's sensory and emotional sensitivity. Dr Nelson lists the following characteristic features of what has been referred to as the *zombie effect* of neuroleptics: inattentiveness to one's surroundings, loss or muting of spontaneity and creativity, diminished ability to think abstractly, emotional numbing, indifference to the future, clouding of consciousness.[33] With skilful treatment it is generally possible to avoid or minimise problems such as these. It is important to understand, however, that neuroleptics can have a range of quite *subtle* effects which, though mild, may nevertheless have significant detrimental consequences for the affected person's quality of life and psychological recovery. One woman gave the following poignant description of the advantages and disadvantages of neuroleptic treatment:

The pills only subtract, never add anything. They close in my life from both sides and make me less aware. When I'm having those weird feelings or falling apart, that's okay, but they keep me from tuning in to good things, too. They cloud up my thinking and my senses like a smoke screen between me and the world. When I take them I feel less of a person, less than all I am.[34]

As skilled clinicians and experienced psychiatric clients know, the art of using medication wisely involves finding ways to make use of its potentially beneficial effects while at the same time doing everything possible to minimise the detrimental effects it can also have. Those who wish to master this art require a thorough knowledge of the many side effects, both gross and subtle, that are known to be associated with the therapeutic use of neuroleptic drugs.

Chapter Two

SIDE EFFECTS OF NEUROLEPTIC MEDICATIONS

The problem of "side effects" is not only a physical but a metaphysical problem: a question of how much we can summon one world without summoning others.

Oliver Sacks[35]

HAVING A GOOD UNDERSTANDING of the wide range of possible neuroleptic side effects is important for a number of reasons. First and foremost, it is impossible for anyone to make intelligent decisions about medical treatment, or give truly *informed* consent, if they lack adequate information about both the potential beneficial effects and the possible adverse effects of the various drugs they have been advised to take. Furthermore, failure to recognise medication side effects, should they occur, significantly reduces the likelihood that they will be dealt with in an adequate way. In order to avoid, or at least minimise, the many possible adverse effects of neuroleptic treatment, it is essential to know just what those effects might be.

As surprising as it may seem, it is actually quite difficult to obtain reliable estimates of the frequency of the various side effects of neuroleptic drugs. In individual cases much depends on the way in which information is elicited. Researchers have found that reports of side effects are least frequent when investigators rely on patients' spontaneous complaints. General questions (e.g. "How do you feel?") tend to elicit a little more information, while specific questions (e.g. "Does this medication ever make your mouth feel dry?") often reveal the presence of side effects that would otherwise have gone unreported.[36] For reasons mentioned below (and discussed in detail in *Chapter Eleven*) there is little doubt that the incidence of many neuroleptic side effects has for a long time tended to be systematically under-estimated.

It is not uncommon for effective treatment of schizophrenia to be compromised as a direct result of a failure to properly manage issues related to the adverse effects of medication. One obvious way this occurs is when diagnosed people who are troubled by side effects "vote with their feet" and simply refuse to take the drugs that have been prescribed for them, or else take them in smaller amounts or less often than recommended. While such understandable non-compliance may prevent or alleviate troublesome side effects it could also mean that the individuals concerned are deprived of some of the potential benefits of neuroleptic treatment, such as the calming and "stress-buffering" effects described in the previous chapter. Another extremely important issue is the fact that some of the most common neuroleptic side effects tend not to be recognised for what they are and are thus not responded to appropriately. Misunderstanding the true nature of common side effects such as neuroleptic-induced agitation (akathisia), for example, could result in affected individuals being given even more medication when a *reduction* in dosage is called for. There is no doubt that diagnosed people are sometimes condemned to suffering persistent side effects which, in more severe cases, may be sufficiently debilitating to compromise recovery. This statement by an authority on neuroleptic treatment of schizophrenia alludes to such a situation:

> Psychopharmaceuticals, especially when co-prescribed [two or more psychoactive drugs at one time], are often responsible for unfavourable mental and behavioural responses. It is not uncommon to observe psychiatric patients who are lethargic, disinterested, asocial, or behaving oddly. Frequently, these symptoms are attributed to illness and not to medication. Yet, when dosages are reduced or drugs discontinued, a favourable transformation occurs in these patients. They become alert, talkative, sociable, show a broadening of interests, have more drive, and much of their odd behaviour vanishes. Clearly, these patients were "drugged" and much of their strange behaviour was medication-induced.[37]

While the advent of atypical neuroleptics and the general trend toward the use of lower dosages of medication has resulted in a reduction in the incidence of some of the more severe side effects, it has not eliminated these problems entirely. Furthermore, many people are still being treated with the older drugs, some of which are notorious for their propensity to cause debilitating side effects (this includes most currently available long-acting depot medications). Worryingly, some common neuroleptic-induced side effects have proven to be highly resistant to effective treatment.

Neuroleptic Side Effects Are Common

All neuroleptic drugs work by selectively blocking receptors in specific parts of the brain. Since the brain's various neurotransmitter systems are connected by complex networks of delicately balanced synergistic relationships into a functionally integrated whole, blocking receptors in one brain area will inevitably cause some unintended effects in areas *other* than those specifically "targeted" by the medication. As well as acting directly on the brain and central nervous system, neuroleptics can affect the functioning of virtually every tissue and organ system in the body. These facts have extremely important implications, as Norman Cousins explains:

> No greater popular fallacy exists about medicine than that a drug is like an arrow that can be shot at a particularised target. Its actual effect is more like a shower of porcupine quills. Any drug – or food, for that matter – goes through a process in which the human system breaks it down for use by the whole. There is almost no drug, therefore, that does not have some side effects. And the more vaunted the prescription ... the greater the problem of adverse side effects.[38]

The various *unwanted* effects of medications take the form of a wide variety of possible symptoms, both physical and mental. These are the drug's adverse effects, commonly referred to simply as its "side effects". Neuroleptic side effects can occur in virtually any part of the human body, with the following being among the most common:

- Sedation (drowsiness, sleepiness, tiredness, lack of energy)
- Autonomic disturbances such as dry mouth, blurred vision, constipation
- Metabolic disturbances including weight gain, elevated cholesterol, diabetes
- Dermatological effects such as photosensitivity (skin burns easily in sunlight)
- Cardiovascular disturbances, including changes in blood pressure
- Blood disorders, including reduced white cell count (*agranulocytosis*)
- Endocrine disturbances, including breast engorgement, menstrual irregularities, and various kinds of sexual dysfunction (e.g. diminished libido, impotence)
- Neurological symptoms, known collectively as *extrapyramidal side effects*
- Cognitive symptoms (e.g. impaired concentration, learning difficulties, reduced capacity for abstract thinking, memory problems)
- Seizure disorders ("convulsions" or "fits")

Different neuroleptics tend to vary somewhat in terms of their most predominant side effects and experienced clinicians soon become familiar with what is referred to as the "side-effect profile" of various drugs. Indeed, when psychiatrists are trying to decide which particular neuroleptic to prescribe, its likely side effects are often one of their primary considerations. An oft-used clinical rule of thumb says: "The differences between the major tranquillisers are in the extent and severity of side effects, not in their anti-psychotic action."[39] "Much of the art of managing patients with schizophrenia", says one authority, "is in the diagnosis and management of side effects".[40]

Diagnosed people also vary considerably in regard to their individual susceptibility to side effects. A number of factors are known to influence this variability. For instance, it has been found that the amount of active neuroleptic medication in the bloodstream can vary by up to a hundred-fold between individuals who have been given identical doses of the same drug (e.g. if two people are given precisely the same amount of chlorpromazine one could eventually have up to a hundred times as much of this drug in their system as the other).[41] The treated person's age, gender, ethnic background, state of physical health, weight, dietary habits, and use of substances (including social drugs such as tobacco and alcohol) can also play a part. Research has indicated that genetic factors can strongly influence a person's tendency to experience medication side effects, with one recent report suggesting that up to 70% of the human population may carry a genetic variation that causes them to metabolise many pharmaceutical drugs particularly slowly.[42]

Fortunately, many neuroleptic side effects are relatively minor and amount to little more than a nuisance (e.g. dry mouth). Some may gradually disappear after a person has been taking the medication for a short while (e.g. a few weeks). Far more problematic side effects can and often do occur, however, as surveys of diagnosed people consistently reveal. For example, while 57% of the 516 people interviewed in one recent survey said they found the medication helpful, more than 60% reported experiencing severe or very severe side effects.[43] In another survey, carried out by the British mental health charity SANELINE in 1994, many respondents complained about severe side effects. Some said their medication made them feel like a "zombie" while others complained about feeling they were separated from the world by a glass screen, that their senses were numbed, their willpower drained, and their lives meaningless.[44]

Attitudes Toward Side Effects Are Highly Individual

Despite its importance, the *subjective* response of people to the side effects they experience is very often overlooked. In general, the unwanted or adverse effects of any medication are likely to be far more tolerable if they are outweighed by its perceived benefits. Thus, it may be relatively easy to put up with even quite severe side effects during the early stages of treatment if medication brings relief from overwhelming anxiety and distress. Later, when psychotic symptoms such as delusions and hallucinations have become less prominent or possibly disappeared altogether, the benefits of the medication may no longer be so obvious even though its side effects may still be very much in evidence. Diagnosed people often tend to become less enthusiastic about taking medication during what is referred to as the *maintenance* phase of treatment when its prophylactic effect (i.e. helping to reduce the risk of relapse) is often more evident than its therapeutic action (e.g. reducing the intensity or frequency of hallucinatory experiences and disturbing thoughts).

The personal significance of overtly similar side effects can also vary greatly from one individual to another, to the extent that what may be merely a nuisance to one person could be virtually intolerable to someone else. An intellectually inclined person, for instance, might not be particularly bothered about being a bit slowed down physically but may feel very distressed about medication-induced memory impairment or even a relatively minor reduction in their mental clarity or acuity. By contrast, someone who is usually a physically active "sporty" type may be extremely worried about gaining weight or having less energy or slower reflexes. Furthermore, people may attribute very different meanings to the side effects they experience.* Thus, while one individual may see them as clear proof that they are being poisoned by noxious chemicals, another may view them as evidence that their medication is actually working.

Clinicians' attitudes toward side effects also vary considerably. Thus, while some do their utmost to ensure prescribed treatments cause the least possible distress and discomfort, for various reasons others may be inclined to display a more casual, even dismissive, attitude. A clinician's stance on this issue can have important implications for

---

* Researchers have found that placebo treatment elicits a greater therapeutic response when the dummy pills contain substances that cause physical symptoms since subjects tend to assume these are side effects of the "medication" they believe they have taken. So great is the power of autosuggestion that some authorities argue that "active" placebos - rather than inactive ones which have no side effects - should always be used in experimental trials designed to determine the effectiveness of new therapeutic drugs. (See *Chapter Five* for more about the placebo effect).

treatment satisfaction and medication compliance. Those taking medication are far more likely to develop trust and confidence in clinical personnel who show an active interest and demonstrate real concern. On the other hand, psychiatric patients who have only ever been subjected to cursory inquiries about side effects may eventually conclude that those providing treatment are not really interested in hearing about their experiences and concerns.

"I Thought It Was Me"

Discussing neuroleptic side effects in detail invariably raises concerns that doing so could frighten people and even cause some to stop taking these drugs. There is no strong evidence to suggest that this is actually likely to occur. In fact, researchers have found that providing diagnosed people with accurate information about side effects can help reduce fear without compromising compliance.[45] Nevertheless, such concerns are partly responsible for a tendency to play down this issue in certain quarters. As a result, *many readily available sources of information about neuroleptic medications - including many of the pamphlets and booklets routinely given to patients and their families - often fail to even mention some of the most common and important side effects.* Even professional resources are sometimes remiss in this regard. For example, the section in *DSM-IV* (the diagnostic manual often referred to as the "psychiatrist's bible") that deals with neuroleptic side effects is entitled "Medication Induced Movement Disorders" (pp.735–749). Both the title and contents of this section strongly emphasise the occurrence of observable physical side effects (movement disorders) while the more subtle but no less important adverse effects of the drugs are ignored or played down. For instance, the section on Neuroleptic-Induced Parkinsonism makes no mention at all of the possibility that neuroleptics may cause slowing of mental functioning (bradyphrenia) in addition to physical slowing.

Failure to acknowledge the full range of possible side effects can have serious untoward consequences. For example, it sometimes happens that people who have been given a neuroleptic drug for the first time feel flat, lethargic, and lifeless (in extreme cases this is the "zombie" effect referred to earlier). If such feelings are only temporary they may be accepted as an unfortunate but necessary part of the price that must be paid for the benefits of treatment. However, if they were to persist for extended periods they may sooner or later start to undermine the treated person's morale. Indeed, anyone who continues feeling this way may fear that life is effectively over for them since they are unable to experience much joy or enthusiasm, and may no longer feel capable of doing anything meaningful or worthwhile. It is crucial for people in such circumstances to be told that, rather than being a permanent "part of their illness" – which is very often what they are told – such a state, if it occurs, may actually be due to medication. Knowing this allows room for hope since it leaves open the possibility that a relatively simple modification of the medication regime may be sufficient to eliminate the problem. Psychiatrist Peter Breggin has described the relief one of his own clients experienced when he explained to her that her inability to think and feel was due to the neuroleptic drugs she had recently been given:

"It's the medication", I said. "It does that to everybody in the doses you've been given." "The medicine?" A small smile flickered across her face. "It's not me?" "No", I said, "It's not you." "Oh, God", she said, "I thought I had finally lost my mind." "No, it's nothing like that", I reassured her. "It will wear off."[46]

Ignoring the true nature of medication-related problems risks condemning some people to a state of hopelessness and despair which, if unrelieved, may lead to medication refusal, hostile non-compliance, and in certain instances, possibly even suicide. Indeed, researchers have found that in the last few weeks prior to their eventual suicides, some diagnosed individuals have made frequent complaints about their medications and repeatedly requested that they be stopped.[47]

Invisible Neuroleptic Side Effects

Because they are well known to experienced mental health clinicians many of the more common neuroleptic side effects are readily identified as such. Examples of these include dry mouth, blurred vision, sedation, and weight gain. However, for a number of complex reasons, some side effects are less well known or less easily identified. In addition, side effects are systematically under-reported. Harvard Medical School research psychiatrist Dr Joseph Glenmullen has recently noted that the US Food and Drug Administration (FDA) allocates a mere 4% of its annual budget to monitoring side effects of new drugs once it has approved their use. Dr Glenmullen further noted that, "to monitor the safety of the more than 3,000 drugs already on the market and being prescribed to millions, the agency has a professional staff of just five doctors and one epidemiologist." In 1993 the then commissioner of the FDA estimated that only about 1% of serious medication side effects are ever reported to his agency.[48] Health professionals (and others) who have assumed that side effects are relatively uncommon tend not to be on the lookout for them and may not recognise them even if they do see them.

Certain side effects tend to be overlooked because of their particular nature. For example, researchers have estimated that between 30% and 60% of people on conventional neuroleptics will experience various kinds of sexual dysfunction (disturbances of erection and ejaculation, changes in libido, and priapism in men; decreased libido, orgasmic dysfunction, menstrual irregularities in women).[49] To avoid embarrassment many may never complain about such problems. Clinicians do not always inquire about such matters either for similar reasons. Ironically, people who are inclined to complain a great deal about medication side effects may end up in a situation in which treating professionals tend to become rather sceptical about the validity of their complaints. In such cases it may eventually become very difficult for *anyone* to be sure whether a person's medication is truly causing problems or if they are simply "blaming" the medication for other problems in their life (which might include the fact that they have to take medication). Nevertheless, studies have shown that the majority of diagnosed people are actually quite good at correctly ascertaining whether or not they are experiencing medication side effects.[50]

One of the main obstacles hindering recognition of neuroleptic side effects is undoubtedly the fact that some of the most significant of them closely resemble behaviours widely considered to be symptoms of schizophrenia. Common side effects such as lack of energy, reduced motivation, and emotional indifference, for example, are often assumed to be negative symptoms (*akinesia* and *Neuroleptic Induced Deficit Syndrome* are discussed below). Some people may experience severe restless agitation as a side effect. Rather than being identified as drug-induced (see *akathisia* below) this restlessness may be viewed as a psychiatric symptom such as anxiety, or it may be interpreted as a sign that the person concerned is becoming psychotic again ("getting sick"). In 1992 a group of senior psychiatrists, expert in the therapeutic use of neuroleptics, made the following comments regarding the difficulty of correctly identifying the presence of "invisible" medication side effects:

> An unwanted by-product of treatment with these medications ... is the blockage of brain dopaminergic receptors other than the ones most directly involved in the manifestation of psychosis. This incidental blockade produces some of the most tenacious and disturbing side effects of neuroleptics. Some of these side effects are easily recognised and clearly attributable to the use of medications. Tremor, muscular rigidity, and dystonia have been linked to acute dopaminergic blockade in the part of the brain that controls non-voluntary movements, the extrapyramidal system ... Other more subtle side effects of medications, however, are often misunderstood and mistaken for depression, anxiety, or manifestations of schizophrenia. These effects are potentially devastating. They are caused by the very medications that were meant to help bring these patients more easily

into contact with others …Two of the most disabling subtle adverse effects of neuroleptics are akinesia and akathisia, which can more easily be missed or misinterpreted …[51]

The erroneous assumption that such side effects are an inherent part of the person's psychiatric condition has undoubtedly resulted in some people being afflicted with these problems for years on end with little respite.

Extrapyramidal Side Effects

Among the most troublesome of the more common neuroleptic side effects are those which occur as a result of the fact that these drugs can reduce activity of dopamine and other neurotransmitters in parts of the brain other than those they are intended to affect. The resulting neurological effects frequently involve the brain systems responsible for controlling and coordinating movement. These are known collectively as *extrapyramidal side effects* (EPS). It is often forgotten that in addition to observable *physical* symptoms such as stiffness and tremor, these side effects can also manifest on a *mental* level in the form of various degrees of impairment of the affected person's memory, ability to concentrate, and capacity for abstract thought.[52] Some early researchers coined the term *behavioural toxicity* to refer to adverse overt and covert behavioural changes that can be caused by neuroleptic drugs.[53] The following comments regarding neurological side effects were made by noted psychopharmacologist Dr John Kane in the *British Journal of Psychiatry* in 1994:

Among the neurological (or extrapyramidal) side effects found in association with neuroleptic medication, perhaps the most troublesome represent the extremes of movement disturbance – from akinesia at one pole to akathisia and dyskinesia at the other. EPS occur in up to 90% of people taking conventional neuroleptics, and cause both physical and mental impairment, as well as tending to be associated with poor compliance.[54]

Fortunately, some people only experience minor extrapyramidal side effects or none at all. Furthermore, atypical neuroleptics are reputed to be less likely than the older drugs to cause these problems (see *Chapter Three*). However, certain drugs that may be administered along with neuroleptics, such as antidepressant medications belonging to the class known as *serotonin-specific re-uptake inhibitors* (SSRIs), can increase the likelihood of EPS as they are also known to cause these side effects.[55]

Since EPS are generally more likely to occur with high doses, they sometimes only become severe when people are taking large amounts of medication, as might happen when someone is hospitalised in a severe psychotic crisis. As unpleasant as these side effects may be at such times, they can usually be expected to diminish quite substantially as the treated person's medication dosage is reduced, which will usually occur as their mental state starts to become more stable. It should be noted, however, that a small subgroup of diagnosed people, estimated to be between 5% and 10%, seem to be especially susceptible to the dopamine blocking effect of neuroleptic drugs. Dr David Healy has pointed out that even on low dosages such people can develop severe neurological side effects, "so much so that the taking of these drugs may be quite distressing and in the long run possibly harmful to mental health."[56]

Of far greater concern are the possible physical, social, and psychological consequences of extrapyramidal and other side effects which persist over long periods of time. This may occur when people remain on long-term maintenance medication for years on end with little variation in the type or dosage of neuroleptic. There is little doubt that, for some diagnosed people, the cost of controlling symptoms with high doses of neuroleptics comes in the form of diminished quality of life, reduced ability to participate in psychosocial rehabilitation and other activities of ordinary life, and possibly compromised recovery.[57] Professor Manfred Bleuler was especially cautious about prolonged use of neuroleptic medications for these very reasons:

> Long-term dispensing of neuroleptic drugs is a measure I strive to avoid because it also often dampens the vitality and the initiative of a person. Patients under such long-term medication are sometimes more impersonal, more "adynamic", and less sharply defined in personality ... by no means always, but sometimes. So we see that long-term maintenance with neuroleptics is fraught with some of the same disadvantages that are ascribed to lobotomies.[58]

Among possible negative consequences of such invisible side effects, Professor Bleuler specifically noted "loss of the ability to establish or sustain friendships or love relationships while under medication" and a "loss of energy and happiness".[59]

Of the various extrapyramidal side effects discussed below the more dramatic kinds such as tremor or severe muscle spasms are generally quite easy for mental health workers and others to identify. It should be noted, however, that EPS are frequently *not* correctly diagnosed even by experienced clinicians. Indeed, a study published in the *American Journal of Psychiatry* in 1987 found that extra-pyramidal symptoms were under-diagnosed by clinical staff "at an alarmingly high rate".[60] A predictable consequence of this unfortunate state of affairs is that many affected persons may fail to receive appropriate assistance from prescribers and other helpers.

(a) Neuroleptic-Induced Acute Dystonia

Neuroleptic drugs can cause muscular spasms (*dystonia*) in various parts of the body. Spasms can involve the muscles of the neck and shoulders causing abnormal positioning of the head ("wry neck"); the jaw and tongue causing difficulty speaking or swallowing; or the entire trunk, resulting in abnormally twisted, bent, or extreme postures. Of the so-called acute dystonic reactions the most dramatic involves the muscles that control eye movement, causing the affected person's eyeballs to roll upwards (*oculogyric crisis*). Neuroleptic-induced muscle spasms tend to occur within a week of a person commencing medication, or increasing the dosage, or stopping a drug used to treat or prevent the occurrence of EPS. Although muscle spasms are rarely life threatening they can be very frightening and alarming, especially the first time they occur or if it is not realised that they are caused by medication. Neuroleptic-induced acute dystonia occurs most commonly among young males receiving high potency drugs.[61] Acute dystonic reactions can usually be alleviated rapidly by administering so-called anti-parkinsonian drugs such as benzhexol (Artane), biperiden (Akineton), orphenadrine (Norflex), or benztropine (Cogentin). In a crisis benztropine can be administered by intramuscular injection. (*These and other drugs, commonly referred to as "side-effect medications", are discussed in more detail in Appendix B*).

(b) Neuroleptic-Induced Parkinsonism *(also known as "pseudo-parkinsonism")*

This state closely resembles Parkinson's disease, a neurological disorder which also involves a lack of dopamine in certain areas of the brain. Characteristic features include: tremor; muscular rigidity; stooped, shuffling gait; bland, expressionless or mask-like face; "pill-rolling" movement of fingers and thumbs; *seborrhoea* (greasy skin); and drooling. The American Psychiatric Association states that at least 50% of people receiving long-term conventional neuroleptic treatment will experience parkinsonism at some time, with the symptoms usually developing within two and four weeks of commencing the medication, increasing the dose, or stopping a drug used to treat or prevent EPS. Symptoms may develop rapidly but can also develop insidiously over time.[62] Parkinsonian rigidity involves generalised muscular tenderness or stiffness, impaired coordination and muscle or joint pain.[63] Affected individuals may walk with a characteristic shuffling gait ("Modecate shuffle") and, in more severe cases, may have a distinctly "robot-like" appearance involving limited spontaneous movement, short steps, stooped posture, and absence of normal arm swing when walking. It should be noted that in some instances Neuroleptic-Induced Parkinsonism can occur in more subtle forms which, while being more difficult to diagnose correctly, are potentially no less disabling:

> Sometimes, patients manifest a subtle form of parkinsonian disease, which is seen as emotional blunting or zombie-like appearance rather than a clear parkinsonism. One should be alert to subtle parkinsonian-like symptoms because they can be confused with emotional withdrawal or retardation ... Indeed, one should not only watch for the conventional parkinsonian symptoms, such as mask-like facies and shuffling gait, but also be aware that patients who appear apathetic, lacking in spontaneity, relatively unable to participate in social activities, lifeless, zombie-like, or drowsy, may be demonstrating subtle extrapyramidal side effects.[64]

It is well known that parkinsonism often involves a general slowing down and reduction in physical movement (*bradykinesia*). Less well known is the fact that those affected may also experience a generalised slowing down of *mental* activity (*bradyphrenia*). The technical term for slowing of movement and thought is *psychomotor retardation*. While the *physical* (motor) aspects of Neuroleptic-Induced Parkinsonism are widely acknowledged, many authorities fail to even mention the *mental* (psycho) aspects of this syndrome (*DSM-IV* is remiss in this regard). However, as renowned neurologist Dr Oliver Sacks has pointed out:

> Arrest (akinesia) or profound slowing (bradykinesia) are equally evident in other spheres – they affect *every* aspect of life's stream, including the stream of consciousness. Thus, Parkinsonism is not 'purely' motor

– there is, for example, in many akinetic patients, a corresponding 'stickiness' of mind or bradyphrenia, the thought stream as slow and sluggish as the motor stream.[65]

Some researchers have pointed out that *cognitive and emotional parkinsonism* is indeed a common occurrence among those treated with conventional neuroleptics.[66] The consequences can sometimes be severe:

Affected individuals may appear slowed down, clumsy or stupid. They may not respond to things that are going on around them. There may be lengthy delays before they respond to questions. If severe the person may appear like a zombie, sitting immobile in a chair with a flat, vacant expression, not responding to things going on around him or her.[67]

The American Psychiatric Association has stated that symptoms of Neuroleptic-Induced Parkinsonism may persist for up to three months *after* a person stops taking oral neuroleptics and for up to a year if they have been receiving medication in the form of long-acting injections.[68]

(c) Akinesia and the Neuroleptic-Induced Deficit Syndrome

The physical and mental slowness characteristic of Neuroleptic-Induced Parkinsonism can occur in the *absence* of overt physical symptoms such as tremor and muscular rigidity. The term *akinesia* (literally, lack of movement) refers to a state of diminished spontaneity characterised by apathy, difficulty initiating everyday activities, and reduced verbal and physical communicativeness (e.g. noticeably restricted use of expressive gestures and body language).[69] Akinesia and similar side effects are not always correctly diagnosed due to the fact that these behaviours often tend to be interpreted as negative symptoms of schizophrenia.[70] However, in recent years belated attempts have been made to more clearly differentiate between negative symptoms and what has been termed the *Neuroleptic-Induced Deficit Syndrome* (NIDS).[71]

Because akinesia is predominantly an inner, subjective state it is very difficult for others to appreciate what an affected person is experiencing (it has been called an *invisible* extrapyramidal side-effect for this reason). People with severe akinesia are emotionally inexpressive ("blunted" or "flat" affect) and lack motivation. Some affected individuals have likened this "locked in" state to being confined in a chemical straitjacket:

> The patient can be left with a less emotionally expressive face, even a "bland", "stupid-looking", or "out-of-it" appearance. The voice may sound monotonous or indifferent ... Patients suffering this side effect behave as if their "starter motor is broken". As they sit in a chair and watch television, for example, they lack the spontaneity to turn it off and do something else, or even to change the channel when the show ends. Instead, they sit passively, witnessing whatever comes on next, no mater how uninteresting or unappealing. Although they will answer questions when asked or participate in activities when urged, patients with this side effect tend not to initiate conversations or activities themselves, even ones they might find pleasurable or interesting. This manifestation of akinesia easily

can be missed or misunderstood by all concerned as a deficit in motivation or drive or as an intrinsic deterioration in social skills and cognitive processes.[72]

People suffering a relatively mild degree of akinesia often become concerned about what is the matter with them. Zan Bockes has explained that she did not feel particularly concerned about taking neuroleptic medication, but said, "what bothered me most was my inability to get interested in anything, to be curious about anything, or to feel any emotion about anything ... I spent most of my free time lying on my bed."[73] Ironically, those who experience more *severe* akinesia may not complain about it. David Healy has suggested that such a situation is especially pernicious because people sometimes become "indifferent to being indifferent".[74] In some instances, a side effect such as akinesia, may actually be looked upon by treating personnel and others (possibly including the diagnosed person's relatives) as evidence that the individual concerned is improving:

> The patient may talk less of psychotic concerns but may also be less talkative altogether; he or she may seem to be less bothered by hallucinations but is less reactive to other stimuli as well. Many patients with akinesia experience a peculiar absence of emotions, appear emotionally flat, and often, when asked, reply that everything is all right. This is a type of "improvement" that may be acceptable when a patient is tormented by intractable psychotic experiences. In such cases, an akinetic dampening down of the entire mental life may indeed be necessary and "therapeutic" ...[75]

Akinesia frequently goes unrecognised as a neuroleptic side effect because apathy, lack of emotional expressiveness, and reduced spontaneity, are very often attributed to other causes, such as negative symptoms, depression, or demoralisation. Its prevalence is therefore uncertain, though some authorities have estimated that between 27% and 47% of people treated with conventional neuroleptics may be affected to some degree.[76] In one study of a group of 94 people diagnosed with schizophrenia, the researchers concluded that 30% had akinesia in the *absence* of any other parkinsonian symptoms (17% had akinesia combined with other EPS).[77] Experienced clinicians acknowledge that it can be extremely difficult to differentiate akinesia from negative symptoms, especially among those with "chronic" schizophrenia. Some authorities feel that the only truly reliable way of doing so involves reducing the affected person's medication dosage, switching them to a neuroleptic with fewer EPS, or commencing anti-parkinsonian treatment.[78]

One group of researchers has suggested that diagnosed individuals who are capable of responding spontaneously to other people or situations despite having some degree of negative symptoms are probably *not* suffering from akinesia.[79] Furthermore, people with akinesia tend to also experience some degree of daytime drowsiness as a result of the sedative side effects of their neuroleptic medications.[80]

(d) Akinetic Depression
Some diagnosed individuals who become depressed while taking neuroleptic medications may be suffering from an atypical form of akinesia characterised by a "wooden" appearance, profound emotional withdrawal, lack of

initiative, overwhelming fatigue, and disinclination to speak. One highly regarded researcher has estimated that between 10% and 15% of people on long-acting neuroleptic depot injections may develop a syndrome referred to as "akinetic depression".[81] It can be difficult to differentiate this type of *drug-induced* depression from depression related to psychological causes such as loss, sense of personal failure, or lack of meaning in life. However, researchers have noted that akinetic depression is often accompanied by some degree of drowsiness and that those affected often improve rapidly when they are given anti-parkinsonian medication:

> Not all patients with akinesia become depressed, but if they do they improve with treatment of akinesia ... Response to one test dose of antiparkinsonian medication was usually diagnostic. Not only did the subtle slowness improve, but so did the depression ... If the schizophrenia patient becomes depressed during the course of anti-psychotic drug therapy, the clinician should first consider the possibility that this is a "toxic" drug effect. The fact that the depression may be "understandable" or that the schizophrenic himself attributes it to his circumstances should not be accepted at face value. The response to a brief course of antiparkinsonian drugs should distinguish between akinetic depression and depression due to some other cause.[82]

(e) Neuroleptic-Induced Akathisia

Paradoxically, rather than inducing a state of apathy and reduced motivation, neuroleptic drugs can sometimes cause the opposite to occur. A drug-induced state of restless agitation called *akathisia* can develop soon after a person begins taking neuroleptic medication for the first time, or when the dosage is increased or a drug used to treat or prevent EPS is stopped. It is now known that this side effect sometimes first appears when the dosage of neuroleptic medication is being *reduced*, a phenomenon referred to as *withdrawal-emergent akathisia*. Affected individuals typically make constant fidgety movements or swing their legs while seated, rock from foot to foot or walk on the spot while standing, and pace about to relieve their inner restlessness. It may be impossible for a severely affected person to remain still for more than a few seconds at a time and they may experience considerable distress if requested not to move.[83] While akathisia is sometimes mild, in more severe cases it can manifest as an excruciating sense of torment involving "a strange fear inside", a state of "cruel restlessness" that has been likened to being "caffeinated". Severe akathisia has been described as like living with the sensation of someone scratching their fingernails down a blackboard twenty-four hours a day.[84] Peter Chadwick describes how akathisia makes it impossible to rest or experience stillness:

> With akathisia there is never *any* peace from this incessant urge to *move*, be it rock backwards and forwards in a chair, shuffle around the wards, kneel and huddle in a chair or go for a walk. It is like a tinnitus of the body, there is *never* a moment of inner silence. Indeed, going for walks, from the ward to the day hospital and back, from the ward to the chapel and back or out briefly along the Thames … were the nearest I could get to a state of physical equanimity when this side-effect was at its height.[85]

It is not difficult to understand why akathisia has been described as the most distressing extrapyramidal side effect.[86] Carol North has explained how she came to prefer her critical inner voices to incessant drug-induced restlessness and agitation:

> I couldn't sit still for five minutes. I could no longer pass the time by watching TV or knitting … I was being motorised … I felt as if I had an unstoppable motor running in my chest, twenty-four excruciatingly long hours a day, making me unable to sit or lie down or relax. The motor-chest made me walk. Hours on end, I paced from one end of the hospital to another, wearing trails down each of the hallways … I had never experienced restlessness like this before. It was so intense it was worse than pain. It felt like a live worm growing inside my chest, and as soon as it got big and strong enough it would burst right out my chest. In the meantime, it wiggled around inside me, giving me the wiggles too … I had to do *something*. So I quit taking the medication. Over the next few weeks the akathisia died away, but the voices grew more clamorous. Even so, I felt more comfortable without the medication.[87]

While it is not known precisely how many people will experience akathisia, the American Psychiatric Association recently estimated that 20% to 75% of people treated with conventional neuroleptics may be affected.[88] One study published in the *British Journal of Psychiatry* in 1994 found that 24% of a group of 120 long-term hospitalised patients were suffering from chronic akathisia. The researchers noted that those with akathisia also reported experiencing tension, panic, irritability, and impatience.[89] One reason the prevalence of akathisia is uncertain has to do with the little known fact that this side effect sometimes manifests as a primarily subjective *mental* state involving a minimal amount of overt restlessness such as pacing and fidgeting. This is described as a "subtle" form of akathisia which, while less obviously recognisable as a drug side effect, can nevertheless result in behaviours that are disturbing to both the affected person and others. Such behaviours may include intrusiveness, hostility, aggression, and a general tendency to "act out" in a socially inappropriate, disruptive manner:

> Gross akathisia has been well described. It makes patients pace, fidget, and feel restless. By and large, clinicians have been trained to recognise this uncomfortable state in patients. Subtle akathisia, on the other hand, can be difficult to recognise. As subclinical restlessness, it manifests as a predisposition to behaviour and action. It can be quite uncomfortable, making patients feel dysphoric [uneasy] and even desperate. In a way, it can be thought of as the opposite side of the coin from akinesia: these patients' "starter motors" refuse to turn off ... akathisia tends to get patients into trouble. They may say things better left unsaid, do or try things better left undone, or wander restlessly into someone else's "space", figuratively or even literally. Obviously these are not traits that will increase a person's popularity. Even worse, the unacceptability of these behaviours is compounded when all involved, including the patient, fail to recognise the source of the problem, attributing it instead to dynamic motivations,

weakness of self-control, innate lack of tact, or other developmental or psychological factors. [90]

Some neuroleptic drugs are reputed to be "energising" or "activating", a characteristic that endears them to clinicians who treat apathetic, unmotivated clients. It is possible that this effect is due in part to the fact that such drugs induce a degree of akathisia. Professor Nancy Andreasen has acknowledged that side effects such as akathisia "tend to be more severe with the more energising drugs".[91] People who take antidepressants belonging to the group known as *serotonin-specific re-uptake inhibitors* (SSRIs) in addition to neuroleptics may be especially likely to develop akathisia since SSRIs can also cause this side effect.[92]

Failure to correctly diagnose akathisia can have dire consequences. For example, akathisia symptoms such as irritability, restlessness, talkativeness, and aggression may be seen as signalling an impending psychotic relapse and lead a well-meaning clinician to increase a diagnosed person's medication dosage. Tragically, this may make the akathisia even *worse* and set in train a destructive vicious circle. Another possibility is that a person who develops akathisia may *incorrectly* interpret this to mean their illness is becoming more severe. A number of cases have been documented in which people who developed akathisia appear to have concluded that they were getting worse despite taking the medication prescribed for them and, believing that their situation was therefore truly hopeless, decided that their only way out was to commit suicide.[93]

Since restlessness and agitation can have a wide variety of possible causes – including the condition for which medication was prescribed in the first place – it can be difficult to determine whether or not someone is experiencing akathisia. However, the *abrupt* onset of restlessness soon after commencing or increasing the dosage of a neuroleptic drug tends to suggest the problem may be medication related. Often the only way to be sure is to see what happens when the dose of neuroleptic medication is reduced, or the affected person switches to a drug less likely to cause akathisia, or they take anti-parkinsonian medication. If someone has been taking neuroleptic drugs for a prolonged period it can take several months or even longer *after* the drugs are stopped before the akathisia finally disappears.[94] Some researchers believe that akathisia can become a relatively permanent condition (*tardive akathisia*), in which case reducing the neuroleptic dosage or stopping treatment entirely may *not* lead to a reduction in the severity of the symptoms.[95]

(f) Neuroleptic-Induced Dyskinesia

Neuroleptic drugs can cause a wide range of abnormal, involuntary movements known collectively as *dyskinesia*. The most common form of these movements is a tremor affecting the hands, arms, or legs often referred to simply as "the shakes". The tremor may be so mild it is barely noticeable, or so severe that the affected person has difficulty writing or holding a cup or glass without spilling its contents. A number of less common manifestations of dyskinesia can occur, including writhing movements of the arms, abnormal body posture, and unsteady gait. Dyskinesic movements usually begin very soon after someone starts taking neuroleptics and are generally alleviated by reducing the dose or concurrent administration of anti-parkinsonian medication. Unfortunately, movement disorders which develop as a result of *long-term* neuroleptic treatment, may be rather more difficult to treat (see below). A characteristic feature of this group of side effects is that they sometimes first appear when the dosage of neuroleptic medication is being *reduced* or when it has been completely stopped – a phenomenon referred to as "withdrawal emergent dyskinesia".[96]

Because extrapyramidal side effects can cause severe distress and have the potential to exacerbate physical and mental disability, it is worth emphasising that they are common accompaniments of neuroleptic treatment. In 2002 the *Australian and New Zealand Journal of Psychiatry* published a survey which noted that, among patients receiving the older neuroleptic medications in oral form (tablets), 48% complained of drowsiness and/or lethargy, while 60% experienced EPS and 48% had symptoms of akathisia.[97] (Unexpectedly high levels of EPS were also reported by people being treated with atypical neuroleptics – see *Chapter Three*)

Tardive Dyskinesia
People who have been taking neuroleptic medications for some time can develop a particular type of movement disorder known as *tardive dyskinesia* or TD ("tardive" means late onset). TD may affect the torso or extremities but most commonly involves the face and mouth. This causes involuntary rhythmical movements of the tongue, mouth, and jaw, such as chewing, lip-smacking, protrusion of the tongue, puffing of the cheeks, sucking, grimacing, and frowning. In addition to such disfiguring physical movements, clinical research has demonstrated a high incidence of cognitive impairment (marked impairment

of memory and learning) among those suffering from tardive dyskinesia.[98]

A person must have been taking neuroleptics for at least three months (one month if they are 60 years of age or older) for TD to be diagnosed. There has been considerable disagreement regarding the exact prevalence of this serious neurological side effect. (In fact, for a very long time the psychiatric profession demonstrated considerable collective resistance to even acknowledging its existence.[99]) In 1994 the American Psychiatric Association stated that between 20% and 30% of people receiving long-term conventional neuroleptic drug treatment may be affected (up to 50% of older persons).[100] Research conducted at Yale University in 1993 suggested that 32% of people will develop TD after five years on conventional neuroleptics, 57% after fifteen years, and 68% by twenty-five years.[101] An individual's total cumulative exposure to neuroleptic drugs is widely considered a key risk factor, i.e. the higher the dosages and longer the treatment period the greater the likelihood that TD will eventually occur. Some evidence suggests that people who have developed parkinsonian side effects (described earlier) may be more likely to eventually develop TD.[102] It appears that alcohol abuse may increase the risk of TD.[103]

Tardive dyskinesia is exacerbated by stimulants, stress, and emotional arousal and, unlike some other extrapyramidal side effects, may actually be made *worse* by anti-parkinsonian drugs ("side-effect medications"). Since it often first appears when a person's neuroleptic medication is being *reduced*, one way to control TD is to increase the dose again. This generally masks the movements but may increase the likelihood that the underlying disorder will continue to worsen. The American Psychiatric

Association has stated that in about a third of cases TD will remit within 3 months if affected individuals remain off neuroleptics, and that after 12-18 months without this medication approximately 50% of cases will remit.[104] Some research has suggested that lowering neuroleptic dosages *very gradually* may reduce the severity of TD. Sadly, TD may be irreversible (i.e. permanent) in up to 50% of affected individuals (even more in older age groups).

The appropriate management of tardive dyskinesia is widely regarded as one of the most challenging issues facing contemporary psychiatry. With the advent of atypical neuroleptics it is hoped that it will become possible to prevent TD occurring in the first place. In the meantime, it is now widely accepted that neuroleptic and anti-parkinsonian drugs should only be used when truly necessary, and then very judiciously, i.e. the smallest possible dose for the shortest possible time. It is also advised that everyone taking neuroleptics should be closely monitored and systematically examined at least once every six months for abnormal movements. At the first sign of TD it is now recommended that the dosage of neuroleptic medication should be reduced. If it is not feasible to stop these drugs altogether it is increasingly common for those who have developed early signs of TD to be switched to one of the newer neuroleptics (at the present time clozapine is reputed to be the least likely to cause TD) in the hope that doing so may reduce the risk of an already-established disorder becoming worse.

Effects on Learning and Memory

Since neuroleptics were introduced in the 1950s, the question of what effect these drugs might have on a treated person's memory and ability to learn and retain new information, has been studied with great interest. Researchers have reached few firm conclusions, however, and there are very wide differences of opinion on this complex issue. Some authorities have been quite vociferous in their claim that these drugs have the potential to cause significant *impairment* of intellectual functioning and memory. Psychiatrist Dr Peter Breggin, for example, considers neuroleptics (and a number of other commonly used psychotherapeutic drugs) to be "brain disabling" due to their ability to induce a "chemical lobotomy":

> Thus the mechanism of action of neuroleptics is no mystery: *clinically* the drugs produce a lobotomy and *neurologically* the drugs produce a lobotomy ... The brain-disabling principle applies to all of the most potent psychiatric treatments - neuroleptics, antidepressants, lithium ... the major psychiatric treatments exert their *primary or intended effect* by *disabling normal brain function*. Neuroleptic lobotomy ... reflects impairment of normal brain function.[105]

Extreme opinions such as this tend to be dismissed out of hand by mainstream psychiatry. In fact, the opposite view tends to hold sway these days, with drug advocates saying that neuroleptic treatment may help to *improve* cognitive functioning among people diagnosed with schizophrenia. In particular, it is claimed, these medications can have beneficial effects on attention so that a treated person is better able to focus on specific tasks and can more readily switch their attention from one task to another. Some researchers believe this beneficial effect may be a result of the fact that neuroleptics selectively reduce a treated individual's susceptibility to being distracted by extraneous, task-irrelevant stimuli.[106]

To the extent that neuroleptic treatment helps to reduce anxiety and ameliorate potentially distracting symptoms (e.g. "voices", intrusive thoughts), it might be expected to have a beneficial effect on concentration and learning ability. There is little doubt, however, that neuroleptics have variable effects in this regard and, in certain circumstances, can result in an impairment of learning ability. This is especially true of some of the older drugs.[107] As mentioned above, a marked impairment of memory and learning is known to occur in association with tardive dyskinesia. A large body of scientific research has indicated that a wide range of mental effects, both positive and negative, are possible.[108] It is not difficult to imagine, for instance, how certain of the neuroleptic side effects already discussed (e.g. psychic indifference, sedation, bradyphrenia) might markedly reduce a person's ability to focus attention on learning tasks, thus impairing their ability to learn and retain new information. Many diagnosed people have difficulty reading or watching television. In some cases this may be attributed to blurred vision, itself a common side-effect. However, since most people with this problem do not have any significant visual impairment, the real culprit in some cases may be a "subtle" form of neuroleptic-induced akathisia (restless agitation) that interferes with attention, comprehension, and recall.

The advent of a range of new atypical neuroleptics was accompanied by the expectation that these drugs might have specific beneficial effects on cognitive functioning. So far there is little clear evidence to support these hopes.[109] However, if atypical neuroleptics do prove to have fewer extrapyramidal and other neurological side effects, it might be reasonable to expect them to at least have fewer detrimental effects on learning and memory than the older drugs sometimes have.

It is important to remember that, as well as receiving neuroleptics, people being treated for schizophrenia are often given various other drugs which could affect their cognitive functioning. Anxiety-reducing drugs belonging to the benzodiazepine family (Valium-type drugs) can impair learning, academic performance, intellect, and memory.[110] *Anticholinergic drugs* (so called because they block the neurotransmitter, acetylcholine), often used to help prevent or alleviate neurological side effects of neuroleptics, can cause impairment of short-term memory.[111] (Both these groups of drugs are discussed in detail in *Appendix B*). It is often forgotten that *most* neuroleptics, including both the older and newer drugs, have anticholinergic properties of their own and could, therefore, have a detrimental effect on a treated person's memory:*

> The majority of neuroleptics in clinical use have an inbuilt anticholinergic effect in addition to dopamine receptor antagonism. This is particularly true, of course, for clozapine [Clozaril] and thioridazine [Melleril] ... subtle, sub-clinical memory deficits, which could go unrecognised by either the doctor or the patient, might occur with therapeutic doses of anticholinergic medication and, more particularly, with unnecessary

---

* The atypical neuroleptic, risperidone (Risperdal) is an exception to this general rule in that it is believed not to have any anti-cholinergic properties. Thioridazine (Melleril) and clozapine (Clozaril), on the other hand, both have a very *high* level of anti-cholinergic effects.

"as required" [PRN] doses ... It is important to bear in mind that the bulk of the serum anticholinergic activity may be due to the neuroleptics themselves rather than to additional anticholinergic drugs.[112]

Most authorities agree that neuroleptics have few predictable effects on cognitive function. In other words, while treatment with these drugs might prove beneficial in some cases, in others it is likely to have no obvious positive effects and may possibly even be detrimental. Since learning and memory play such an important role in rehabilitation, it is essential that every effort is made to prevent or minimise side effects which might compromise these and other key cognitive functions. To this end treatment must be individually tailored, i.e. the right drug (or combination of drugs) at the optimal dosage for the appropriate duration. Adopting a flexible attitude and being prepared to experiment may mean the difference between a treatment regime which will help recovery and one which may actually hinder it.

It should be stressed that while it is a fact that learning difficulties and memory problems can sometimes occur as a result of taking neuroleptics and other psychoactive drugs, it is also the case that some people may experience an even greater degree of impairment if they are *not* taking such medications. Indeed, disorganised thinking, hallucinations, and other symptoms can become so disruptive at times that it is virtually impossible for some diagnosed individuals to participate in conversations, work, or function adequately in social situations. As discussed earlier, use of potent psychiatric drugs always involves an effort to find an acceptable balance between their potential benefits and their possible negative effects.

Psychological and Social Side Effects

In addition to the various adverse effects already described, neuroleptic drugs can have a number of untoward consequences which might be thought of as their psychological and social side effects. These may sometimes be secondary to physical effects of the drugs, e.g. weight gain or EPS such as the "shakes", slowness, or tardive dyskinesia could cause shame, guilt, and embarrassment. Medication side effects may further stigmatise a treated person by functioning as the inescapable "badges of patient-hood" which make visible to others the fact that someone is a "psych patient" even though their behaviour may be normal or even exemplary in every other regard. Peter Chadwick summed up his own experience thus:"I looked like everybody's image of a mental patient – but it was entirely a medication effect."[113] As Susan Estroff's sociological research has shown, well-meaning helpers who constantly reiterate the need for medication may inadvertently reinforce a diagnosed person's sense of dependency and compound feelings of inadequacy, abnormality, and difference, all of which may serve to further entrench a "mental patient" identity:

> The embarrassment, the feelings of dependence, the despair, and the restriction of activity have consequences not only in terms of self-image but in terms of clients' ability to interact with persons to whom [medications] and side effects are strange or stigmatising … What I question is whether psychiatric personnel

are aware of the actual and potential social and inter-personal *costs* of [medication] ... although symptoms may be reduced, the dependency on medications and the visibility of side effects serve to magnify clients' deficiencies and differentness not only to themselves but to others. Clients who are told constantly in multiple ways that they need [medication], probably for the rest of their lives, are also being told that they will never "get well" ... they come to see themselves caught between a non-medicated world that is out of reach, and a medicated world that identifies them as crazy people with problems in their heads and in their lives.[114]

As well as contributing to a sense of hopelessness and demoralisation, medication-induced embarrassment and stigmatisation may cause some treated people to become increasingly isolated, e.g. limiting their social contacts to a relatively small circle, often fellow members of the "psych scene" who understand and share their predicament and medicated way of life. Side effects may thus contribute to an exacerbation of the social withdrawal and relative lack of supportive, intimate relationships that is the lot of many long-term psychiatric patients. Even when relatively mild, side effects such as akinesia may be sufficient to seriously compromise a diagnosed person's ability to relate with, and be accepted by, others. It is not difficult to imagine how even a relatively modest reduction in non-verbal expressiveness (manifesting as a monotonous voice, blank or immobile face, little spontaneous body language) could have potentially devastating personal and social consequences:

This side effect can be extremely damaging socially because so many subtle cues in social interactions – such as attention, interest, understanding, need for further information or elaboration, friendliness, and trust – are mediated through facial expression and tone of voice. Patients who, on the basis of a medication side effect, communicate poorly in this crucial non-verbal realm are at a distinct disadvantage. Who would want to hire such a person? Who would want to introduce such a person as a member of his or her family? Who would want to go out on a date with such a person? Even worse, people in daily contact with the patient usually fail to recognise the actual source of the problem: the friends don't know, the family doesn't know, the employer doesn't know. In fact, even the patient and the physician may fail to realise the true nature of the problem ... who would want such a person for a friend? And, again, who would wish to see such qualities (or lack of qualities) in himself or herself, especially without having a clear idea of how they came about or what to do about them?[115]

Akathisia can also interfere with a person's ability to develop and sustain relationships with others. The restless agitation associated with severe akathisia (inability to sit still, pacing, fidgeting) can be extremely distracting and off-putting in social situations and is likely to further exacerbate problems such as low self-esteem and lack of self-confidence. Even relatively mild akathisia can cause problems such as poor concentration and reduced ability to sustain attention. Difficulties like these make it hard for an affected person to participate in conversations and other types of ordinary social interaction. As well as contributing to reduced quality of life, such medication-related effects may compromise social and occupational adjustment, education, rehabilitation, and recovery.[116]

While there is no doubt that some psychological and social side effects are directly related to the effects of neuroleptic medication, others probably have more to do with the treated person's feelings about having to take these drugs and their attitude toward psychiatric treatment generally. Even if they experience no obvious medication side effects, the very fact that they are required to take "psych" drugs (as opposed to drugs for ordinary medical conditions) may cause some people considerable distress. Medication non-compliance or even outright refusal is sometimes at least partially motivated by a desire to reject the stigmatised identity which taking these drugs so often implies. As one person said, "I didn't take my medicine at times because I didn't want the disease, its problems, and its stigma. I wanted to be normal."[117] John Modrow has given a graphic illustration of the kind of troubled relationship some people have with neuroleptic drugs and other psychiatric medications:

> I had come to the psychiatric clinic with the conviction that I was a very unique person with a sacred mission, but I walked away from the clinic miserably clutching a bottle of Stelazine [trifluoperazine] with the vague and uneasy suspicion that I might not be anything more than an emotional cripple. This vague and uneasy suspicion grew more and more into a certainty each time I took one of my Stelazine tablets. More than words could ever have done, taking

those pills indoctrinated me with the notion that I was a defective person whose only claim to uniqueness consisted of a chemical defect, probably genetic in origin.[118]

Supersensitivity: A Possible Long-Term Effect of Neuroleptic Treatment

In treating people diagnosed with schizophrenia, psychiatrists face the challenging task of trying to determine which particular medication will be of most benefit to a given individual, the hope being that a treatment regime can be devised which is therapeutically effective while causing a minimum of problematic side effects. Quite often this will necessitate a process of trial-and-error which may extend over a considerable period. However, even if a satisfactory regime *is* eventually found, a significant problem may still exist. Put simply, nobody is presently able to say with any certainty what consequences could be associated with prolonged use of these potent psychoactive drugs. Among the various possible long-term effects of neuroleptics, those of greatest concern have to do with what might occur as a result of the sustained presence within the human brain of these foreign chemical substances.

A phenomenon referred to as *neuroleptic-induced dopamine-receptor supersensitivity*, which some researchers believe may be caused by long-term exposure to neuroleptics, has been a contentious subject in psychiatric circles since the 1970s. In order to appreciate how such supersensitivity might come about, it is helpful to review the dopamine hypothesis which has for several decades strongly influenced psychiatric thinking about schizophrenia. In simple terms, this theory proposes that the occurrence of psychotic symptoms is associated with receptors in certain parts of the brain (the limbic system in particular) being overly reactive to the neurotransmitter dopamine. In line with this view, the therapeutic efficacy of conventional neuroleptics is believed to rest on their ability to block some of these receptors, thus reducing the overall level of dopamine activity – an effect sometimes referred to as *dopamine blockade.* A simplistic way this is often put is to say that neuroleptics rectify the chemical imbalance (excessive dopamine activity) which some believe is responsible for causing schizophrenia symptoms.

Researchers who have studied the possible long-term consequences of dopamine blockade have become concerned that, in an attempt to overcome this unnatural situation, the brain may utilise its remarkable adaptive capacity (termed *neural plasticity*) and change in various ways which could have untoward consequences.[119] For example, long-standing blockade appears to lead to an increase in both the number and sensitivity of the very dopamine receptors the neuroleptic drugs have targeted. As a result, drugs originally given in order to *reduce* receptor sensitivity may eventually cause it to *increase.** It is now widely accepted that the neurological side-effect tardive dyskinesia (TD) is a result of neuroleptic-induced supersensitivity in the area of the brain responsible for controlling and co-ordinating movement (the striatum). Scientific evidence suggests that supersensitivity can also occur in the

---

* Animal research has established that dopamine receptor supersensitivity can develop after a *single dose* of a neuroleptic drug and that the affected neurons may take four to six weeks to return to normal (longer after repeated dosing). See: Baldessarini, R. and Tarsy, D. (1979) "Relationship of the Actions of Neuroleptic Drugs to the Pathophysiology of Tardive Dyskinesia". *International Review of Neurobiology,* Vol. 21

mesolimbic system – the very brain region proponents of the dopamine hypothesis believe is causally related to schizophrenia.[120] This could potentially have a number of extremely significant consequences:

The brain responds to neuroleptics – the blocking of dopamine transmission – as though it were a pathological insult. To compensate, dopaminergic brain cells sprout more D2 receptors. The density of such receptors may increase by more than 50 percent. At first, this compensatory mechanism may alleviate some of the physical and emotional deficits caused by neuroleptics. Parkinson's symptoms may diminish and extreme emotional lethargy may lift. But the brain is now "supersensitive" to dopamine, and this neurotransmitter is thought to be a mediator of psychosis. The person has become more biologically vulnerable to psychosis and is at particularly high risk of severe relapse should he or she abruptly quit taking the drugs.[121]

Careful study of this phenomenon has led psychiatrist Richard Warner to summarise the "neuroleptic dilemma" as follows:

An important potential hazard of the neuroleptic drugs should now be apparent ... The basic neurochemical defect in schizophrenia may well be [an over-reactivity] of dopamine receptors. The immediate action of the neuroleptic drugs is to minimise the effects of that defect; on this basis rests the great value of these drugs in psychiatry. The long-term effect of the neuroleptics, however, may be *a worsening of the basic*

neurochemical defect in schizophrenia. As in tardive dyskinesia the supersensitivity effect may be temporary,
gradually disappearing over the course of weeks or
months after drug withdrawal, or − if drug treatment
continues long enough − it may become permanent
… this formulation, if correct, has serious implications
for drug treatment in schizophrenia.[122]

The most important question for diagnosed people and
their helpers concerns the possible consequences of neuroleptic-induced supersensitivity, should it occur. One possibility is
that the effectiveness of neuroleptic medication could decrease
over time so that ever-increasing doses are needed to maintain
control of symptoms. Though it is often claimed that tolerance
does *not* occur with neuroleptics, there is good evidence to
suggest otherwise. It is well known that experimental animals
do develop a tolerance to the effects of neuroleptics.[123] The
fact that a considerable number of diagnosed people are liable
to experience relapse, even though they are receiving maintenance neuroleptic treatment, also points in this direction
(see *Table One* in *Chapter Six*). This fact cannot simply be due
to medication "non-compliance" as similar relapse rates have
been noted among groups of people who receive neuroleptics
in the form of long-acting injections. One study found that
44% of such persons required their dosages of neuroleptics to
be increased over a seven-month period in order to maintain
their stability.[124] Recent investigations have revealed that a
considerable proportion of schizophrenia patients do indeed
receive progressively higher dosages of neuroleptic medication
over the course of their treatment.[125]

Of even greater concern is the possibility that neuroleptic-induced supersensitivity might result in some diagnosed

people becoming *more* prone to relapse – and, if relapse does occur, for it to be *more* severe – than may have been the case if they had never received neuroleptics in the first place. Such an increased predisposition to relapse is most likely to become obvious if a person's neuroleptic dosage is being reduced or if they stop it completely. Noted psychopharmacologist Professor Leo Hollister has summarised the situation as follows:

> If tardive dyskinesia is due to pharmacologically-induced supersensitivity of dopamine receptors in the nigrostriatal system, does a similar supersensitivity exist in the mesolimbic system? Current evidence suggests that it does. If so, the spectre has been raised that in the long run, anti-psychotic drugs may aggravate the very disorder that they initially treat so well. Thus, schizophrenics treated over long periods with these drugs may have the underlying pathogenetic mechanism worsened, so that when the drugs are withdrawn they relapse, possibly even to a state worse than that which existed before drug treatment. Thus, we might inadvertently be producing patients who are dependent on these drugs lest their psychosis becomes even worse than it was before treatment.[126]

A group of senior psychiatric researchers at the US National Institute of Mental Health (NIMH) were among the first to draw attention to the possibility that neuroleptic treatment might result in an increased risk of relapse for some diagnosed people. In an article published in 1977 in the *American Journal of Psychiatry* these experts elaborated their concerns:

There is *no* question that, once these patients are placed on neuroleptics, they are less vulnerable to relapse if maintained on neuroleptics. But what if these patients had never been treated with drugs to begin with? ... we raise the possibility that anti-psychotic medication may make some schizophrenic patients more vulnerable to future relapse than would be the case in the natural course of their illness. Thus, as with tardive dyskinesia, we may have a situation where neuroleptics increase the risk for subsequent illness but must be maintained to prevent this risk from becoming manifest.[127]

Some authorities believe that dopamine receptor supersensitivity may result in an increased likelihood that affected individuals will develop psychotic symptoms if their medication dosage is reduced, a phenomenon that has been termed *Neuroleptic-Induced Supersensitivity Psychosis*.[128] Researchers note that those who have developed neuroleptic-induced supersensitivity sometimes make statements such as, "Before, I was not taking my medication regularly and I was readmitted once a year or every two years. Now since I take my medication regularly, I get sick as soon as I miss a single injection or stop taking my medication."[129]

If a diagnosed person's symptoms do reappear or become worse, the usual explanation is that their neuroleptic dosage is simply too low to control their underlying illness. Another possibility is that the newly emerging symptoms are actually manifestations of a "rebound psychosis" that is a direct result of medication-induced supersensitivity.[130] Researchers who have closely studied this phenomenon have concluded that a distinguishing feature of supersensitivity psychosis is that it occurs *very soon* after a reduction in neuroleptic dosage or complete cessation of treatment.[131] By contrast, if relapse is due to a person's medication being insufficient to control their symptoms effectively, there is often a substantial time lag between dosage reduction and symptom exacerbation. This can range from a number of weeks to many months.* Researchers have suggested that another distinguishing characteristic of supersensitivity psychosis is that it is likely to be accompanied by the emergence or exacerbation of symptoms of tardive dyskinesia (TD) since these abnormal involuntary movements are also related to dopamine receptor supersensitivity. Individuals who develop supersensitivity also often experience sexual dysfunction of various kinds such as reduced sex drive, erectile impotence, and inability to experience orgasm.

The phenomenon of neuroleptic-induced dopamine receptor supersensitivity is not widely acknowledged by mainstream mental health clinicians. Psychiatrist Philip Thomas believes that an important consequence of this neglect is that symptoms which may actually be a neuroleptic drug withdrawal syndrome, tend instead to be seen as signs of impending relapse which call for an immediate increase in medication dosage. In Dr Thomas's view, the rebound psychosis which can occur following a rapid

---

* Residual anti-psychotic effects of neuroleptics may be partly related to the persistence in the body of the active drug itself as well as various metabolic by-products. For example, metabolites of some neuroleptics can still be detected in the body several months after a person has stopped taking them. Some long-acting injectable neuroleptics can take 8 to 10 months or longer to be completely cleared from the body.

reduction of neuroleptic dosage is comparable to the familiar withdrawal syndromes known to accompany cessation of a wide range of potent psychoactive drugs:

> Most people are familiar with accounts of what happens when someone stops minor tranquillisers after taking them for any length of time. In such circumstances minor withdrawal symptoms such as anxiety, insomnia, and mild depression are very common. Similar, but more severe, disturbances occur after stopping alcohol or barbiturates, when hallucinations and delusions are not uncommon. Withdrawal states ... are usually rapid in onset, and start almost immediately on stopping the drug. Given the fact that most psychiatrists are familiar with this scenario – the appearance of a disordered mental state in response to the discontinuation of a drug that has powerful effects on the brain – it is perhaps surprising that this model has not been proposed as an explanation for the relationship between the reappearance of psychotic symptoms on stopping neuroleptics. To put it more directly, under some circumstances, could the "relapse" of schizophrenic symptoms on stopping neuroleptics in reality be a neuroleptic withdrawal syndrome rather than a true relapse of the illness? ... There is evidence that this indeed may be the case ... The difficulty here is that so far, no research study has seriously addressed the possibility that symptom recurrence in schizophrenia on stopping neuroleptics is effectively a drug withdrawal syndrome.[132]

One of the most important implications of these challenging ideas is that they raise the possibility that diagnosed individuals may become enmeshed in a vicious circle, in which some of the symptoms they experience might actually be a direct result of the treatment they have been given. For example, at some point a person who is "stable" may wish to try reducing their regular medication dosage. In some cases doing this may result in the development of a withdrawal syndrome (rebound psychosis), *especially if the dosage is reduced rapidly*. Since such withdrawal symptoms are rarely recognised for what they are, the person may be told that they are beginning to relapse and must promptly return to their original neuroleptic dosage – possibly to an even a *higher* dosage in order to ensure their stability. Some people receiving neuroleptics in the form of depot injections may develop withdrawal symptoms as the drug's effects gradually wear off. Since this often occurs as the time for the next injection approaches, the assumption may be made that the injection is overdue, or that the interval between injections needs to be shortened to prevent symptoms from re-emerging. Something similar may also occur with oral medication. For example, some people who take all their tablets at once (e.g. before going to bed at night) may experience an increase in the frequency or severity of symptoms in the late afternoon or early evening when the amount of drug in their body is at its lowest level. If the possibility that an apparent worsening of symptoms may sometimes be a withdrawal phenomenon is not taken into account, diagnosed persons in situations such as these have little hope of ever being able to stop taking neuroleptic drugs or even of managing a sustained reduction in dosage. An article pertaining to this issue was published in the *Canadian Journal of Psychiatry* in 1980. It ended with a sobering reflection:

One wonders how many patients are currently receiving maintenance medication as a consequence of a psychotic episode following attempted discontinuation of neuroleptics where the aetiology [i.e. cause] may have actually been a withdrawal phenomenon and not a "relapse" of an underlying chronic illness ... If so, it is possible that [the] further years of treatment with neuroleptic medication may not have been necessary.[133]

Most of the research on neuroleptic-induced supersensitivity was done well before second-generation neuroleptics began to be introduced in the 1990s. These newer drugs are often referred to as atypical neuroleptics and are reputed to cause fewer neurological side effects, especially tardive dyskinesia. Several of these drugs are described as *broad spectrum* since they act on a wide range of receptors, including those for dopamine. It is unclear at present whether prolonged treatment with atypical neuroleptics might also result in the development of supersensitivity. However, it is already well known that rebound psychosis can occur when clozapine is stopped abruptly. Indeed, some researchers believe this problem is even *more* likely to occur with clozapine than with the older neuroleptics, as they explained in a 1996 report in the *Schizophrenia Bulletin*:

> Several authors have described rebound psychoses in patients withdrawing abruptly from clozapine. Such cases of rapid-onset psychosis or rapid relapse are postulated to be due to specific properties of clozapine or to mesolimbic supersensitivity ... Supersensitivity of

mesolimbic dopamine receptor sites may also occur, perhaps to a greater extent with clozapine than with "typical" antipsychotics … greater inhibition of limbic dopamine receptors with clozapine than with other antipsychotics may make patients more prone to psychosis after clozapine treatment than after treatment with other antipsychotics.[134]

The supersensitivity phenomenon has a number of practical implications for those being treated with neuroleptics. One of the most important of these is that the risk of experiencing a rebound psychosis can be significantly reduced if neuroleptic dosages are lowered very gradually. Practical guidelines for doing this are outlined in detail in *Chapter Ten*.

Side Effects of Depot Neuroleptics

Many people diagnosed with schizophrenia receive psychiatric treatment in the form of long-acting intramuscular injections (*depot medication*) given at regular intervals – typically weekly or fortnightly, though in some cases they may be as infrequent as once every three months or more. This has a number of advantages. Firstly, because the medication is administered by injection it is far more likely to be adequately absorbed, whereas a large proportion of an orally administered drug may actually be excreted from the body before it has a chance to take effect. For this reason, some people who fail to respond to oral medication may respond better when treated by injection. This mode of treatment also makes it easier for clinical personnel and others (such as relatives) to know whether or not a given individual is actually receiving neuroleptic medication and, if so, precisely how much of which particular drug they are getting. Finally, there is no doubt that some diagnosed people prefer having injections as this arrangement frees them from the need to remember to take their tablets every day.

Depot neuroleptics have a number of potential disadvantages, the most significant being that most have numerous possible adverse effects. Extrapyramidal side effects are especially common with many of these preparations. A recent Australian survey found that of those treated with conventional depot medications, 58% experienced EPS, while 56% reported having problems with akathisia.[135] In addition to EPS, sedation occurs frequently (particularly with zuclopenthixol decanoate and fluphenazine decanoate) as do various anticholinergic side effects, e.g. memory impairment (especially with flupenthixol decanoate and zuclopenthixol decanoate). A potential complicating factor is that, if side effects are severe enough to warrant a dosage reduction, it can take a relatively long time for the concentration of drug in the body to diminish to a level at which the problem begins to be alleviated. (As noted earlier, it can take 8 to 10 months or longer for all traces of a depot neuroleptic to be eliminated from the body.)

One of the great ironies associated with contemporary treatment of schizophrenia is that people who refuse to take prescribed medications because of concerns about its side effects may find themselves being forced to accept treatment with depot drugs *more* likely to cause problematic neurological side effects than are many of the oral neuroleptics now available (see the next chapter). For reasons that are yet to be fully clarified, Australia is reputed to use depot medications more often than most other countries, with a 1999 report suggesting that up to 43% of diagnosed people receive medication in this form.[136] A rather more conservative estimate, published in *Schizophrenia Research* in 2002, suggested that around 38% of all neuroleptics prescribed for schizophrenia in Australia were given as depots.[137] A survey published in the *Australian and New Zealand Journal of Psychiatry* in 2003 estimated that over 18,500 Australians had received depot medication during the latter half of 2001, with fluphenazine decanoate (Modecate) the neuroleptic most often given (this estimate did *not* include drugs prescribed by public hospitals and community mental health clinics).[138]

Conclusion

The material discussed in this chapter demonstrates that neuroleptic side effects represent far more than a minor source of irritation or temporary inconvenience. Indeed, they are a complex, multi-faceted issue which has many important ramifications for diagnosed individuals and those who care for them. Medication compliance, the treated person's general quality of life, and their long-term physical and mental health are all influenced, to one degree or another, by the side effects they experience now and in the future. While not denying the potential benefits of these drugs, it is an unavoidable fact that they can have a variety of untoward effects, both physical and mental. For these reasons it is most important that this issue is dealt with in an open and honest way, an undertaking that begins with the acquisition of a sound knowledge of the wide range of side effects that neuroleptic treatment can entail. Armed with this knowledge, it may be possible to devise strategies which minimise potential problems without compromising therapeutic effectiveness unduly.

Interested readers will find a range of practical strategies for preventing, minimising, or managing neuroleptic side effects outlined in Appendix B.

Partly in response to increasing lay and professional concern about neuroleptic side effects – particularly tardive dyskinesia – attempts have been made to develop drugs with fewer adverse effects. While the ever-expanding range of drugs that have been gradually introduced over the past decade or so has had an unprecedented impact on many aspects of schizophrenia treatment, it has unfortunately not eliminated problems related to side effects. Rather, while certain once common adverse effects now tend to occur less frequently, others have become far more prevalent than used to be the case. The next chapter tells part of this unfolding story.

Chapter Three

ATYPICAL NEUROLEPTICS – LIGHT AT THE END OF THE TUNNEL?

Perhaps the newer medications for schizophrenia will make for a smoother journey of reintegration for younger people now diagnosed ... Perhaps their journeys will be very different from mine, a little easier. I hope so.

Simon Champ[139]

THE INTRODUCTION OF CLOZAPINE in 1990 has been vigorously promoted as marking the beginning of a new era in pharmacological therapy of schizophrenia, with this particular drug often described as representing the first major innovation in neuroleptic treatment since the advent of chlorpromazine in the early 1950s. During the past decade, a number of other drugs known as *atypical neuroleptics* have been introduced and all are now in widespread use. At the time of writing the most frequently prescribed members of this group include clozapine (Clozaril), risperidone (Risperdal), olanzapine (Zyprexa), quetiapine (Seroquel), amisulpride (Solian), and aripiprazole (Abilify). Many potential new medications are currently undergoing pre-clinical testing and a host of others await official approval for human clinical trials to begin. Why have these drugs generated so much interest? Do they really amount to a major step forward in schizophrenia treatment? This chapter attempts to answer these and other questions regarding the "second-generation" neuroleptics.

Clozapine's Resurrection

Clozapine is not actually a new drug. It was originally developed in the 1960s and had been in use for a number of years before growing concerns about certain of its side effects led to it being withdrawn from regular use in 1975. Interest in this drug was rekindled when a 1988 study claimed it had proven effective in treating a group of people with "chronic" schizophrenia who had not improved despite prolonged treatment with the older neuroleptic, chlorpromazine.[140] A major factor in clozapine's resurrection was the observation that it appeared to cause few of the extrapyramidal side effects (EPS) which have long detracted from the therapeutic usefulness of the neuroleptics. Furthermore, researchers eventually realised that, unlike the earlier drugs, clozapine's therapeutic effects are not solely determined by its ability to block dopamine receptors. Indeed, it is known to affect *many* neurotransmitter systems, including those involving dopamine and serotonin (for this reason clozapine and similar drugs are sometimes referred to as *broad-spectrum receptor antagonists*). This is highly significant because pharmaceutical research under the influence of the dopamine hypothesis had

previously confined itself to the study of dopamine blocking agents. The realisation that neuroleptics may work by
blocking receptors other than those for dopamine gave
impetus to the search for new drugs that are not simply dopamine antagonists. In clozapine's wake a veritable
tidal wave of psychoactive substances have been studied
to determine whether or not they might prove useful as
effective "anti-psychotic" agents.[141]

Advent of second-generation neuroleptics has had a
profound impact on many aspects of mainstream psychiatric practice. These medications, which are often referred
to as *atypical* to distinguish them from the *typical* original neuroleptics, are reputed to have a number of unique
features which justify the assertion that they constitute a
significant breakthrough in the pharmacological therapy of
schizophrenia. In particular, the following claims are often
made about atypical neuroleptics:

- They provide effective therapy for treatment-
  resistant schizophrenia
- They cause relatively few extrapyramidal side effects
  (including TD)
- They are an effective treatment for negative
  schizophrenia symptoms
- They have fewer problematic side effects than the
  older neuroleptics

Because of the rapidly growing popularity of this group
of drugs, a closer examination of these claims is warranted.
Before proceeding with this discussion it should be pointed
out that, as with the original neuroleptics, reliable and
unbiased information about the effects and side effects of

the newer drugs can be difficult to obtain. (Some reasons for this are outlined in *Chapter Eleven*.) Readers should bear this fact in mind when considering the material that follows.

Are Atypical Neuroleptics More Effective Than The Older Drugs?

A considerable number of people diagnosed with schizophrenia are relatively unresponsive to the anti-psychotic action of conventional neuroleptics. In other words, they will continue to experience positive symptoms such as hallucinations, delusions, and thought disorder, despite being given these drugs, even if they receive large or very large dosages. It has been estimated that around 30% of diagnosed people experience limited benefit from conventional neuroleptic treatment and that a further 20% experience no beneficial effects whatsoever.[142] Many people also experience what are termed *negative symptoms* such as restricted emotional expressiveness (blunted or flat affect), poverty of thought, lack of motivation, and social withdrawal, all of which have proven largely unresponsive to conventional neuroleptic treatment. People with persistent positive and negative symptoms are sometimes said to be *treatment resistant* or to suffer from *refractory schizophrenia*.

Until relatively recently, psychiatrists faced with the problem of treatment resistance had little choice but to give their patients ever-increasing dosages of medication (which, in some cases, became *very* large) or to try one neuroleptic after another in the hope of eventually finding one that would work satisfactorily. Combinations of various drugs were often tried as well. Since response to neuroleptic treatment is known to be highly idiosyncratic, simply changing to a different drug *may* in itself some-times be sufficient to elicit a more favourable therapeutic response. (As explained in *Chapter Four*, the phenomenon known as the placebo effect undoubtedly plays a significant although rarely acknowledged role as well.) The discovery in the 1980s that some people who had not previously benefited from such measures sometimes improved when given clozapine, raised the hope that an effective therapy for treatment-resistant schizophrenia had finally been found. Subsequent experience has tempered these early expecta-tions and it is now accepted that only around 30% or so of people with long-standing refractory schizophrenia may benefit from treatment with clozapine. Some researchers claim this percentage may increase with treatment that is sustained over a long period.[143]

Despite its relatively limited effectiveness, the advent of clozapine nevertheless ushered in an era which has seen a significant increase in the range of available neuroleptics. However, as a group, the newer drugs have *not* proven more effective in terms of their anti-psychotic action than the older ones, nor are they generally effective against treat-ment resistance – clozapine stands alone in this regard thus far. Significantly, a growing body of evidence has begun to show some of the earlier glowing claims about the atypicals in a rather more modest light. For example, in 1999 the journal *Schizophrenia Research* published a review of evidence regarding the effectiveness of three of these drugs (olanzapine, quetiapine, and risperidone) which concluded that they are "more effective than placebo, but the magnitude of the effect is only moderate".[144] A report compiled by researchers for the National Schizophrenia Guideline Development Group in the UK represents one of the most thorough investigations yet carried out on this matter. Published in the *British Medical Journal* in 2000, this review examined the results of 52 randomised trials in which the responses of 12,649 diagnosed individuals to either atypical or conventional neuroleptic treatment were compared. On the whole, these researchers found no evidence to suggest that the then available atypical drugs differ substantially from one another in regard to their effectiveness in treating either positive or negative symptoms, i.e. they are essentially therapeutically equivalent in this regard. Most importantly – and contrary to widely held opinion – they found little scientific support for the frequently made claim that the new drugs are vastly superior to the older ones. "There is no clear evidence," they concluded, "that atypical antipsychotics are more effective or are better tolerated than conventional antipsychotics."[145] In line with this finding these experts do *not* recommend the preferential use of atypical neuroleptics to treat those experiencing psychosis for the first time: "Conventional antipsychotics should usually be used in the initial treatment of an episode of schizophrenia unless the patient has previously not responded to these drugs or has unacceptable extrapyramidal side effects."[146*]

A recent review of the US Food and Drug Administration (FDA) database on clinical trials of medications used to treat schizophrenia, concluded that the average level of

---

* For various reasons some other advisory groups take a different view. Recent Australian and New Zealand Guidelines recommend that, in first-episode psychosis, atypical neuroleptics *should* be used in preference to conventional neuroleptics. Exceptions to this general rule arise when depot medication is unavoidable or atypical drugs are poorly tolerated. See: McGorry, P., et al. (2003) 'Summary Australian and New Zealand Clinical Practice Guideline for the Treatment of Schizophrenia', *Australasian Psychiatry*, Vol. 11, No. 2.

symptom reduction was 17.3% for the older neuroleptics and 16.6% for the newer ones.[147] These findings echo the views of a growing number of experienced clinicians who have begun to question whether the new drugs are actually as effective as the older ones. For instance, researchers have described cases in which a good initial response to olanzapine has been followed by unexpected early relapse, despite the absence of any obvious causative factors, such as excessive stress.[148] Similar observations have been made in regard to risperidone, with some individuals experiencing a recurrence of psychotic symptoms after 3 to 6 months despite good initial response and strict compliance with treatment.[149] A clinical review published in the *Schizophrenia Bulletin* in 1997, which summarised research done on risperidone up until that time, included these comments:

> It is possible, based on the available studies, that risperidone is not as effective as standard neuroleptics for typical positive schizophrenia symptoms (e.g. delusions, hallucinations, thought disorder) in schizophrenia patients ... There are other suggestions in the recent literature supporting the idea that risperidone may not be as effective as standard neuroleptics.[150]

Some commentators have challenged these views and argued that drugs such as risperidone are at least as effective as older neuroleptics.[151] It would appear, however, that diagnosed people whose positive symptoms respond to neuroleptics (i.e. who are *not* treatment resistant), are generally no more likely to benefit from the newer drugs than they are from the older ones. It is certainly true, nevertheless, that some people who have not done well on the older neuroleptics may improve substantially when changed to one of the newer ones. While this might appear to indicate that the new drug is more effective, in some cases factors *other* than its therapeutic efficacy may be responsible for the observed improvement. As psychopharmacologist David Healy has pointed out, the fact that drugs such as clozapine generally have a lower incidence of debilitating neurological side effects, may be especially important in this regard:

> On clozapine, it appears that around 30% of individuals who are unresponsive to other neuroleptics improve. The reason for improvement in such cases is a matter of some conjecture. One possibility stems from the fact that clozapine acts more potently on the serotonergic (5HT) system, in addition to its action on dopamine receptors, than do other neuroleptics. As there appears to be a cooperative action between the dopamine and serotonin systems, this might explain its efficacy. Another possibility stems from the fact that clozapine binds less effectively to dopamine receptors than do other neuroleptics. Accordingly it is much less likely ... to bring about a worsening of mental state as a result of distressing side effects. If the poor response of some individuals put on conventional neuroleptics results from the development of side effects such as akathisia, then one might expect some such individuals to improve once their "poisoning" ceases. Whatever the reason, there is a clear benefit for some people ...[152]

This view would appear to be consistent with the observation that the treatment resistant patients who can be predicted to improve most on clozapine are those who have had the highest level of EPS while being treated with the older drugs and who subsequently experience the greatest reduction in these side effects during the course of treatment with a newer one.[153]

What really distinguishes atypical neuroleptics from the earlier drugs is that they have a different side-effect profile, presumably due to the fact that they act on different combinations of neuroreceptors.* Most importantly, they tend to have fewer extrapyramidal side effects (EPS) such as akathisia, parkinsonism, and TD which, as well as encouraging medication non-compliance, may contribute to disability and reduced quality of life even if they are relatively mild. One expert commentator recently summarised the present situation thus:

> We all agree there is no scientific evidence that newer antipsychotics are superior to classical neuroleptics, at least regarding positive symptoms. Antipsychotics, whether typical or atypical, may differ in tolerability rather than efficacy.[154]

The relatively greater tolerability of neuroleptics with an atypical side-effect profile means they may prove acceptable to hitherto "treatment intolerant" individuals who have previously been unable to benefit from medical treatment as a result of their heightened tendency to develop

---

* The advent of atypical neuroleptics has led to a significant shift in thinking regarding the neurochemical basis of schizophrenia. After several decades during which dopamine was considered the most likely "culprit", many now question the validity of the dopamine hypothesis. Though the hypothesised chemical imbalance has long been thought of as involving excessive dopamine activity, many now believe that serotonin and other neurotransmitters are also implicated.

severe adverse reactions such as akathisia, dysphoria, and other debilitating side effects.

Do Atypical Neuroleptics Cause Extrapyramidal Side Effects?

Although researchers are not yet able to say precisely how atypical neuroleptics work, it is known that they act on a wide range of neuroreceptors in various parts of the brain. It has been suggested that the "anti-psychotic" efficacy of these drugs is related to the fact that they block serotonin and other receptors, as well as those for dopamine (though these ideas are purely speculative at present). Particularly important is the fact that these drugs appear to interfere relatively less with dopamine transmission in the *nigrostriatum* — the brain region responsible for the control and coordination of movement. An important consequence of this characteristic is that, on the whole, these drugs tend to have fewer acute (short-term) extra-pyramidal side effects (EPS).

Many exaggerated claims have been made regarding the newer drugs, to the extent that it has sometimes been suggested that they do not cause *any* EPS. Such statements are misleading. Indeed, evidence has accumulated over the past few years which raises the suspicion that some of the original claims may have been deliberately exaggerated. *It is now clear that these drugs are not as free of neurological side effects as some people appear to believe.* The British researchers who compiled the National Schizophrenia Guidelines concluded that, while the atypical neuroleptics do tend to cause fewer extrapyramidal side effects than the older drugs, they only offer "a modest advantage" in this regard.[155] The authors of a survey published in the *Australian and New*

Zealand Journal of Psychiatry in 2002, expressed surprise at the relatively high incidence of extrapyramidal side effects among those receiving atypical neuroleptics. Commenting on the finding that 49% of the survey respondents experienced neurological side effects associated with atypical treatment (as compared to 60% of those receiving the older drugs), the researchers said:

> We draw attention to aspects of the patient-reported profile of side effects that are somewhat at odds with data from clinical trials. Some form of extrapyramidal side effects was described by the majority of respondents, for both typical and atypical antipsychotics, although their frequency was slightly lower in those on risperidone/olanzapine ... the high rates of reported EPSE in patients on clozapine are unexpected ... Similarly, akathisia – one of the most distressing side effects of antipsychotic medication – was predictably reported most commonly by patients on typical depot agents, but, unpredictably also by nearly half of those on any of the atypical agents.[156]

It has been found that even clozapine, the atypical reputed to have the *lowest* tendency to cause EPS, is not free of such side effects. In a recent study, signs of parkinsonism were observed among 33% of a group receiving clozapine (as compared to 61% of those receiving conventional neuroleptic treatment).[157] Some researchers have suggested that akathisia (restless agitation) may occur just as often with clozapine as it does with conventional neuroleptics, leading the authors of a 1991 report published in *Biological Psychiatry* to comment:

Contrary to expectation, akathisia was present as frequently in patients receiving either medication ... Our
raters could not tell akathisia in the patients receiving standard neuroleptics from akathisia in patients
receiving clozapine ... The results suggest that the
production of akathisia may be a common property
of all anti-psychotic drugs, including not only standard neuroleptics but atypical anti-psychotics, such as
clozapine, as well ... although akathisia may not be
as severe in patients receiving clozapine as in patients
receiving standard neuroleptics, it seems appropriate to
suggest that patients receiving clozapine be specifically
monitored for akathisia.[158]

There have recently been reports of *severe* akathisia
associated with olanzapine[159], *severe* withdrawal-emergent
dyskinesias and dystonias with clozapine[160], and tardive dyskinesia occurring with both olanzapine and risperidone.[161]A
report published in the journal *Schizophrenia Research* in
2000, challenged the claim that clozapine does not cause
any EPS, and tardive dyskinesia (TD) in particular. After
studying 200 diagnosed individuals who had been treated
for several years with one of the older neuroleptics or with
clozapine, the researchers stated:

On the whole, long-term relatively extensive use of
clozapine has not markedly reduced the prevalence of
extrapyramidal syndromes in our psychiatric in-patient
population. In particular, we failed to demonstrate a
beneficial effect of clozapine on prevalence of TD
... This finding does not preclude the possibility that
there might be TD patients who profit from clozapine

treatment; however, it is ... possible that TD amelioration in the proportion of patients suffering from this
condition and switched from typical neuroleptics to
clozapine is not due to the clozapine therapy as such
but is due to spontaneous remission ... in some patients,
TD manifests in the course of clozapine treatment for
the first time.[162]

In general, it seems fair to say that extrapyramidal side
effects tend to be less problematic with atypical neuroleptics han they are with the older drugs, *especially if the
dosages are kept low*. On the other hand, it has been found
that some of these drugs are just as likely to cause EPS as
the older ones, if dosages exceed a minimum level. For
example, it is known that the incidence of EPS with risperidone (Risperdal) is dose dependent, and that dosages
above 6 mg per day can result in levels of EPS comparable to haloperidol, an older neuroleptic notorious for its
propensity to cause neurological side effects.[163] A recent
study found that people who had not previously been
treated with any neuroleptics (*neuroleptic naïve* individuals)
developed EPS identical to those caused by haloperidol,
even on very low dosages of risperidone (around 3 mg
per day).[164]

While it is certainly true that promotion of the newer
drugs has tended to foster unrealistic expectations, there
is no doubt that the belated advent of medications which
do not generally cause severe extrapyramidal side effects
is a significant development.[165] Having a lower propensity to cause EPS is arguably one of the major advantages
of atypical neuroleptics, especially since these side effects
often contribute to the behaviours referred to as *negative*

symptoms (see below). It is interesting to note that a number of highly regarded psychiatric authorities have commented that this relative advantage of the newer drugs – fewer EPS – would be significantly reduced if the older drugs were to be used in low doses.[166] It is now widely recognised that, in general, treatment with low doses of conventional neuroleptics is just as therapeutically beneficial as treatment with high doses, though the latter approach is still common in everyday clinical practice. Richard Bentall, a professor of clinical psychology and noted schizophrenia authority, recently observed that despite clear advice to the contrary from their professional bodies, "psychiatrists continue to treat many of their patients with bizarrely high doses of neuroleptic drugs".[167] His conclusions were based on the findings of a survey carried out in the UK between 1995 and 1998 on 212 hospitalised psychiatric patients. To his surprise, Professor Bentall discovered the median dosage of neuroleptic medication was equivalent to 600 milligrams of chlorpromazine per day, while approximately a quarter of the patients were given the equivalent of 1000 milligrams or more per day.

Do Atypical Neuroleptics Treat Negative Symptoms?

In the long-term, negative symptoms such as reduced emotional expressiveness and diminished motivation, often represent a far greater problem for diagnosed individuals and their helpers than do positive symptoms, though the latter often tend to be the main focus of medical treatment. Since negative symptoms generally respond poorly to conventional neuroleptics, they have come to be seen as one of the major components of treatment resistance (the other being persistent delusions and hallucinations). The advent of atypical neuroleptics has been hailed as a breakthrough in regard to negative symptoms, with the claim frequently being made that it is now possible to treat these problems with medication. Graphic reports have appeared in professional literature and popular lay media of the dramatic changes – sometimes described as near-miraculous "awakenings" – that have occurred when people have been put on one of the new drugs, usually after having received prolonged treatment with one or more of the older ones.[168] In other instances the changes, though somewhat less dramatic, have sometimes resulted in a substantial and sustained improvement in the diagnosed person's motivation, attitude, energy, and general outlook on their life and the future.

Some people *do* become noticeably more animated and energetic – as though some kind of invisible veil had been lifted – when one of the older drugs is replaced by a new one. In some instances, switching drugs may even set the scene for a series of changes which mark the beginning of a definite turning point toward recovery. In such cases it certainly *appears* as though the new drug is indeed treating negative symptoms, especially if amelioration of such problems has coincided with its introduction. A closer examination of the awakening phenomenon suggests a rather different interpretation, however. In particular, there is reason to believe that this effect is often largely a result of the relatively reduced incidence of extra-pyramidal side effects with the newer drugs (as described above). Although most discussions of EPS tend to focus on *physical* symptoms such as stiffness and tremor, in many cases the mental and emotional manifestations are more significant and potentially far more problematic. As noted in *Chapter Two*, side effects such as parkinsonism, bradyphrenia, akinesia, and the Neuroleptic-Induced Deficit Syndrome (NIDS), tend to occur far more often with the older drugs than many people realise. The following anecdote graphically illustrates the profoundly negative impact these side effects can have on mental and emotional functioning. The neuroleptic in question, Moditen (fluphenazine enanthate), was once a widely used as a depot injection:

> Four years ago I began having fortnightly injections of Moditen, and since then my periods of psychosis have stopped (and you can see why I must keep on with the injections). Unfortunately, my personality has been so stifled that sometimes I think that the richness of my pre-injection days − even with brief outbursts of madness − is preferable to the numbed cabbage that I have become … in losing my periods of madness I have to pay with my soul, and the price of health seems twice as high as Everest. I have become a neuroleptic with a skylark's shattered wing, and can no longer write a poem … whereas once I lived in a fascinating ocean of imagination, I now exist in a mere puddle of it. I used to write poetry and prose because it released and satisfied something deep inside myself; now I find reading and writing an effort and my world inside is a desert.[169]

This description refers to a rather extreme situation, such as might generally be expected to only occur on relatively high doses of medication. It is interesting to note, therefore, that the most dramatic awakenings are sometimes observed in people who, before starting the new medication, had received prolonged treatment with large dosages of high potency neuroleptics, often as a result of determined attempts to overcome their treatment resistance. It should also be remembered that some people are extremely sensitive to the effects of dopamine-blocking drugs and can experience severe adverse reactions even on very small doses.

Whether debilitating mental and emotional side effects are a result of small or large doses of EPS-inducing neuroleptic drugs, anything which helps to reduce them is invariably a significant, possibly even life-altering, experience for the individuals concerned and for their helpers. In some cases it may involve a deep sense of release accompanied by a dramatic resurgence of feelings and energies that have long been buried. An experience described by Simon Champ indicates just how profound such changes can sometimes be:

> Recently, talking to my friend Helen, who also started feeling so much better on the same medication I switched to six months ago, she said of the medication, "It gives you back your mind". The drug company would love that as a testimony, I'm sure.[170]

At first glance, statements such as this do indeed seem to provide a glowing testimony to the new drug's powerful efficacy against negative symptoms such as "poverty of thought" (*alogia*). However, elsewhere in this same report, Champ described some of his own experiences with older neuroleptics, in which their profoundly debilitating impact on his mental and emotional state are vividly described:

The medications had changed how my very being felt to myself. The medications I was taking dulled my thoughts and robbed me of familiar emotions and feelings I had always known. The post-psychotic world seemed colourless in comparison with the world I had known before becoming ill. Trying to decide what was normal or sane was like negotiating a foreign city without a map. I felt like a stranger to myself ... At the early stages of my illness the nurses were the oppressors of my mind ... enforcers of mediocrity and the status quo. I called the nurses "soul fuckers" for the medication seemed to eat at my very soul. They were the ones that administered the injections, the "mind death".[171]

It seems clear from this first-hand account that the neuroleptics Champ was given had a profoundly deleterious effect of his mental clarity and sense of self-identity, thus raising the suspicion that the seemingly miraculous ability of a new drug to "give you back your mind" may actually be related to its relative *lack* of such mental and emotional side effects. Is it possible that Champ's experiences were simply a highly subjective idiosyncratic response to the drugs? Many competent authorities believe not. Indeed, effects like these have been described as a kind of neuroleptic-induced "chemical lobotomy" with the suggestion that they are not at all uncommon.[172] Some researchers have specifically investigated the relationship between the mental and emotional side effects of the older drugs and the extraordinary awakenings sometimes reported to occur on the newer ones and reached similar conclusions to those proposed here. For example, the following statement was made by a highly regarded expert in a report published in the prestigious psychiatric journal, *Acta Psychiatrica Scandinavica*, in 1994:

A side-effect that has escaped close attention is akinesia, or the "zombie effect" induced by classical [typical] neuroleptics; this is probably one major reason for low compliance … not only muscular but also cognitive and emotional rigidity are induced by classical neuroleptics, and the terms cognitive and emotional parkinsonism seems appropriate … One of the clinical impressions, among many others, is a dramatic awakening in many patients when changing the treatment from a classical neuroleptic to an atypical one such as clozapine. They may report a clearing of the mind, an ability to think and to feel. *Our interpretation of that awakening is the disappearance of cognitive and emotional parkinsonism.*[173]

Claims that the newer drugs provide the first effective treatment for negative symptoms have obvious appeal and for this reason have been strongly emphasised in promotional campaigns. Nevertheless, even researchers who were initially inspired by these claims have tended to become rather more circumspect with the accumulation of further evidence. This gradual change in focus is especially evident in regard to some of the original claims made about clozapine, widely regarded as the prototype of atypical neuroleptics. Two recent reviews concluded that clozapine does *not*, in fact, have specific ameliorative effects on primary negative symptoms associated with schizophrenia.[174] The following summary statement appeared in a recent

review of current knowledge regarding the pharmacotherapy (neuroleptic treatment) of schizophrenia:

> A third hallmark of the new pharmacotherapy of
> schizophrenia is the emphasis on better treatments
> for negative symptoms (i.e. alogia, apathy, anhedo-
> nia, blunted affect) [because these] often represent
> the real stumbling blocks for patients trying to lead
> more fruitful and satisfying lives. Several studies have
> suggested that long-term outcome for patients with
> schizophrenia is associated with negative symptomatol-
> ogy. Although early reports suggested that clozapine
> has superior efficacy for negative symptoms, more
> recent studies suggest that this finding many actually
> be related to clozapine's lack of EPS.[175]

Similar conclusions have been reached about other
atypical neuroleptics. For example, in a review published
in the *Schizophrenia Bulletin* in 1997, the author opined
that, "Regarding negative symptoms, the reported superiority of risperidone, compared with haloperidol, may result
primarily from the relative lack of EPS from risperidone
at the doses used."[176] Since the two other commonly prescribed atypical neuroleptics, olanzapine and quetiapine,
are also reputed to cause relatively few extrapyramidal side
effects compared to the older drugs, it can be presumed
that similar comments would also apply to them.

Given their disabling nature, any reduction in negative
symptoms is obviously welcome, however it is achieved.
Nevertheless, it is potentially misleading to claim that
atypical neuroleptics are an effective "treatment" for these
problems when it now appears more likely that what

these drugs actually do is to cause fewer neurological side effects such as parkinsonism and akinesia, the very side effects which often represent a major component of negative symptoms such as loss of drive and lack of emotional responsiveness.

A final comment: it is important to understand that negative symptoms are not simply a biological phenomenon. Although they are often spoken about as though they were *entirely* a result of brain malfunction ("broken brain"), it has long been clear that a wide range of psychological and social factors can contribute to their development and persistence.[177] For example, at some point many diagnosed people lose hope, purpose, and a sense of direction and some eventually succumb to depression and demoralisation. When tackling the problem of negative symptoms, therapeutic approaches which fail to take into account basic human concerns such as the search for identity, meaning, and purpose in life, are certain to be only partially effective. While it is very important to attend to medication issues, especially in terms of finding a drug regime which causes a minimum of potentially debilitating side effects, it will never be possible to invent a pill that will provide an instant "cure" for complex and multi-faceted human problems. For this, only a truly holistic approach is likely to be successful in the long run.

Do Atypical Neuroleptics Have Fewer Side Effects Than The Older Drugs?

The promotional zeal surrounding the newer neuroleptics has sometimes tended to encourage the impression that these drugs, as a group, have few side effects. This perception is erroneous. While EPS generally tend to be less of a problem – as long as the proviso regarding the importance of keeping dosages low is adhered to – it is now clear that a wide variety of other side effects occur frequently.[178] Although some of these are relatively minor, others can be far more troublesome, and some are potentially life threatening.[179] At the time of writing, the most worrisome side effects are those which result in adverse changes to various metabolic systems and processes (see below).

Many side effects that regularly occur with these drugs are similar to those associated with the older ones, the most common of these being sedation, drowsiness, dry mouth, blurred vision, constipation, urinary retention, and low blood pressure (*hypotension*). A tolerance effect may occur with some of these side effects so that they tend to become less troublesome or even disappear after the first few weeks of treatment. Atypical neuroleptics can have various other side effects, among the most important of which are the following:

(a) Agranulocytosis
The side effect that has caused the greatest concern since atypicals were introduced is undoubtedly agranulocytosis. This condition, which has only been noted with clozapine, involves a significant reduction in the number of white blood cells which could leave the person concerned vulnerable to infections of various kinds. Although reversible (i.e. the white cell count begins returning to normal when the offending drug is stopped) it can be life threatening if not detected early. Concern about this side effect has led to the requirement that people receiving clozapine have regular blood tests, usually weekly for at least the first 4-6 months of treatment.

Research and clinical experience have shown that the risk of clozapine-induced agranulocytosis is low, with the cumulative incidence said to be less than 1%. The likelihood of developing this condition is somewhat greater for females and increases with age. The risk of developing agranulocytosis appears to decrease substantially after the first six months of treatment.[180]

(b) Sedation

Sedation is a side effect of many neuroleptics including the newer drugs. Its various manifestations include somnolence (sleepiness, drowsiness) and a general feeling of tiredness and lack of energy. Sedation is one of the most common side effects of clozapine treatment with up to 40% of people being affected. Other atypical neuroleptics also often cause sedation. While this side effect tends to be less severe with lower dosages and may gradually diminish after the first few weeks, tiredness and a lower level of energy can become a more persistent problem for some people.

(c) Seizures

All neuroleptic drugs increase the likelihood of seizures. At low doses, the incidence of seizures associated with clozapine appears not to be any greater than with the older drugs, but approximately 6-8% of persons on doses over 600mg per day have experienced seizures. The incidence may be further increased at higher doses.[181] There has been no suggestion that any of the other atypical neuroleptics cause an increase in the incidence of seizures any greater than is known to occur with the older drugs.

(d) Elevated Prolactin

Prolactin, a hormone produced by the pituitary gland, has the function of regulating production of milk by the mammary glands. All of the older neuroleptics cause a marked increase in the level of prolactin in the bloodstream.[182] While this sometimes has no obvious physical consequences it may result in various symptoms including *galactorrhoea* (production of breast milk by men or women who are not breast-feeding), *gynaecomastia* (breast enlargement in males), *amenorrhoea* (absence of menstrual periods), *menorrhagia* (menstrual periods too long and too heavy), and reduced libido (diminished sex drive). Studies have shown that olanzapine, risperidone, and amisulpride can cause an elevation in prolactin.[183] With risperidone this effect is dose related (higher doses cause greater elevation than smaller ones). It should be borne in mind that the intimate nature of the side effects associated with elevated prolactin may cause them to be under-reported. Consequently, it is quite possible that they occur more frequently than is generally realised.

(e) Sexual Dysfunction

A wide range of disturbances of sexual functioning, presumably related to altered hormonal activity, are known to occur in association with neuroleptic treatment. David Healy has estimated that up to 50% of people taking these drugs may experience these side effects.[184] In males these can include the loss of libido, delayed ejaculation, ejaculatory failure (orgasm without ejaculation), and erectile impotence (inability to sustain an erection). Females may experience loss of libido, reduced sexual arousal, and anorgasmia (inability to experience orgasm). Though it is claimed that such sexual problems are relatively uncommon with atypical neuroleptics, it should be born in mind that these side effects are especially likely to be under-reported or attributed to the affected individual's mental condition. Drugs which cause an increase in prolactin levels (see above) have the potential to cause sexual side effects. Various kinds of sexual dysfunction have been reported by people on risperidone and olanzapine, while cases of *priapism* (persistent involuntary erection) have occurred in association with clozapine treatment.[185]

(f) Weight Gain

Many people put on weight while taking neuroleptics, a side effect which is very common with the newer drugs, especially clozapine and olanzapine. Studies have shown that significant weight gain is a problem for up to 80% of people on clozapine, with gains of 10 kilos or more not unusual and the extra weight tending to persist for longer than with other neuroleptic drugs.[186] Weight gain with risperidone may be less severe than with clozapine and olanzapine and seems to be dose-dependent (i.e. increases tend to be greater at higher dosages). The weight increase that occurs with clozapine appears to be independent of medication dosage.[187] It is important to appreciate that this side effect is not trivial or inconsequential even if it is sometimes implied that it is merely "cosmetic". While not as obviously disabling as EPS, the potential negative impact of significant weight gain should not be underestimated. As well as discouraging medication compliance, this side effect can have a devastating effect on a diagnosed person's self-esteem and self-confidence which could, in turn, undermine their psychological recovery (see the earlier discussion regarding the psychological and social side effects of neuroleptic medications). Excessive and persistent weight gain can have many detrimental effects on physical health and general wellbeing, some of which may eventually result in serious medical consequences (see below).

(g) Metabolic Disorders

Atypical treatment can contribute to increased risk of a wide range of potentially serious metabolic disorders. Among those presently causing greatest concern are:

- Obesity, i.e. body weight 20% or more above statistical average for height
- Abnormally elevated levels of fats in the blood, including cholesterol and triglycerides (*hyperlipidaemia*)
- Alterations in glucose metabolism (insulin resistance, impaired glucose tolerance) and abnormally elevated blood sugar (*hyperglycaemia*)
- Adult onset (type 2) diabetes

Research has demonstrated that the risk of developing these metabolic disorders is substantially greater for people being treated with atypical neuroleptics than it is for those taking conventional neuroleptics or no medication. Presently available medications may vary in regard to their potential to cause these side effects. Current evidence indicates that the greatest level of risk is associated with clozapine and olanzapine.

A study published in the *Archives of General Psychiatry* in 2002, reported that people who received olanzapine were three times more likely to develop *hyperlipidaemia* (elevated blood fats) than those on conventional neuroleptics, and five times more likely than diagnosed individuals not taking neuroleptic medications.[188] In 2004, an expert panel reported that clozapine and olanzapine tend to cause the greatest increases in total cholesterol and are associated with raised levels of LDL ("bad") cholesterol and reduced levels of HDL ("good") cholesterol. Risperidone and quetiapine were said to have an intermediate effect on lipid levels.[189] Medical authorities agree that people being treated with neuroleptic drugs should have their blood lipid levels measured on a regular basis in view of their increased risk of hyperlipidaemia.[190]

It is now clear that atypical neuroleptics can increase the likelihood of treated individuals developing diabetes.[191] A study published in the *American Journal of Psychiatry* in 2002, noted that diabetes was significantly more common among patients who received clozapine, olanzapine, and quetiapine, but not risperidone. However, for patients below 40 years of age, *all* of these atypical neuroleptics were associated with a significantly increased risk of diabetes.[192] At present, the level of risk remains uncertain. One recent study reported that, among a group of 82 patients who switched from conventional neuroleptics to clozapine, 30 individuals (36.6%) developed new-onset diabetes during a five-year follow-up period.[193] It is noteworthy that this was *not* necessarily accompanied by substantial weight gain, i.e. some people who did not gain weight while taking clozapine still developed diabetes. The researchers noted that weight gain was characteristic of individuals who developed insulin-requiring diabetes.

In February 2004, four prominent US medical

organizations took the unprecedented step of issuing a joint statement regarding the potentially serious health risks that may be associated with use of atypical neuroleptics. In their statement, The American Diabetes Association, American Psychiatric Association, American Association of Clinical Endocrinologists, and North American Association For The Study of Obesity, noted that there was a lack of long-term data due to the fact that, with the exception of clozapine, the drugs in question have only been available for a relatively short time. Nevertheless, on the basis of information now available, an expert panel representing these groups stated that, if atypical neuroleptics are generally found to increase the risk of obesity, high cholesterol and diabetes, "this should be of major clinical concern".[194] It was noted that certain medications often given in combination with atypicals (e.g. valproate, lithium) may further increase the likelihood of health problems. Given the potential risks involved the panel recommended that all candidates for atypical treatment be thoroughly assessed, before commencing the drugs, and that they be closely monitored throughout the course of treatment. The panel further advised that anyone whose weight increases by 5% or more, at any time during treatment, should immediately have their medication regime reviewed and that an effort should be made to change them to a drug with fewer adverse health effects.

In addition to being a concern in their own right, the adverse health effects noted above can contribute to other problems. Obesity, elevated cholesterol levels (especially "bad" cholesterol), and diabetes are all associated with a significantly increased risk of heart disease, stroke and a wide variety of other medical conditions. Physical inactivity (sedentary lifestyle), cigarette smoking, and poor dietary habits compound the dangers. Clearly, many diagnosed individuals are now exposed to multiple, potentially life-threatening, risk factors.

(h) Supersensitivity

As discussed in *Chapter Two*, long-term exposure to neuroleptics might lead to the development of receptor *supersensitivity*, one result of which could be that abruptly decreasing the dosage elicits a withdrawal syndrome involving a dramatic exacerbation of psychotic symptoms. Because some atypical neuroleptics have only been in use a relatively short time it is hard to say with certainty whether similar problems will eventually occur with these drugs (if they do they will presumably entail supersensitivity of serotonin, dopamine, and possibly other receptors). Nevertheless, recent research has shown that atypical neuroleptics can cause an abnormal increase in brain D2 dopamine receptors.[195] Furthermore, there is now clear evidence of a supersensitivity effect and an associated severe withdrawal syndrome (*rebound psychosis*) characterised by hallucinations, delusions, hostility, and paranoia following abrupt reduction in clozapine dosage.[196] Recent reports suggest that a similar phenomenon can occur with olanzapine.[197]

(i) Obsessive-Compulsive Symptoms

A number of cases have been reported in which people on clozapine have developed symptoms of obsessive-compulsive disorder (OCD) such as repetitive checking or ritualistic hand washing.[198] In at least some instances these behaviours appear to have been transient, with the symptoms having subsided after a few weeks.[199] Similar problems have also been reported with olanzapine.[200]

Note: see Appendix B for practical advice regarding the management of neuroleptic side effects.

A Neuroleptic Dilemma

As the catalogue of problematic side effects grows, it becomes increasingly clear that, whatever their advantages, the atypical neuroleptics are far from being the harmless "wonder drugs" they are sometimes made out to be. Indeed, some authorities have recently suggested that the metabolic and other physical side effects of the atypical neuroleptics are potentially as serious a cause for concern as were the extrapyramidal side effects (EPS) of the older drugs:

> Atypical antipsychotics can compound a patient's risk for developing metabolic, endocrine, and cardiac complications that may be comparable, if not worse, than risks associated with extrapyramidal side effects and tardive dyskinesia ... This reminder becomes especially pertinent today as we stand only one decade after the introduction of atypicals and begin to realise that these medications carry their own adverse effects, the long-term consequences of which are only just emerging. The key question to be considered is whether atypicals are in fact safer and better or whether they are merely different in their side-effect profiles, compared with the older, typical neuroleptics.[201]

It has been suggested that the generally lower incidence of EPS with the newer drugs may sometimes be counteracted by their greater propensity to cause various other side effects. A recent report in the *Schizophrenia Bulletin* lends credence to this idea. In this study 423 people diagnosed with treatment-resistant schizophrenia were given either haloperidol or clozapine over a twelve-month period. When researchers analysed the results, they were surprised to discover that, while treatment personnel rated the newer medication (clozapine) as more effective than the older one (haloperidol), patients' subjective evaluations told a different story. As it turned out, those treated with clozapine did *not* have a more positive opinion of their medication than those treated with haloperidol. And, while the treating clinicians considered the clozapine patients to be more likely to have shown dramatic improvement by the end of the twelve month study period, when given a quality of life assessment, these patients did not rate themselves any higher than those who had been given haloperidol. In fact, while they were less likely to complain of EPS or akathisia, the clozapine-treated patients were more likely to report other side effects and a greater overall number of severe side effects. These rather unexpected findings led the researchers to comment:

> It is notable that the side effects that have received the greatest emphasis in evaluations of atypical anti-psychotics have been EPS, on which atypical [drugs] are clearly preferable to conventional agents. However, consideration of a wider range of side effects and patient-rated assessment of both their relationship to the current medication and their severity suggests that the side-effect profile of clozapine may be less acceptable than that of conventional medications,

on the whole, at least from the patient perspective ... Further, the study suggested that even when standard instruments and clinical judgement indicate that newer treatments are more effective than standard [neuroleptic] treatments, subjective patient responses may show no effect or even a negative effect.[202]

These thought-provoking findings are especially noteworthy in view of the fact that this study compared patient's feelings about clozapine, reputedly one of the most "user friendly" of the atypical neuroleptics, with haloperidol, an older drug renowned for its numerous side effects!

Conclusion

The advent of atypical neuroleptics arguably represents an important forward step in psychiatry's on-going effort to develop more satisfactory pharmaceutical treatments for schizophrenia and other psychotic disorders. However, as the preceding discussion makes clear, rather than being the major innovation that is sometimes claimed, it would probably be more appropriate to say that the newer drugs simply allow a degree of fine-tuning of previous treatments. Indeed, it may even be the case that the new generation of anti-psychotic drugs "do not at present appear to be a radical departure from what has already been available", as David Healy recently observed.[203] Given the variable and highly individualised nature of treatment responsiveness, the most that can be said at present is that *some* people – though certainly not all – who have done poorly on older medications, may do better on atypical neuroleptics. On the other hand, it is possible that some people may feel *worse* on the newer drugs, despite their reputation as being "more tolerable". Very recent research has shown that, contrary to popular expectation, introduction of the newer drugs has *not* resulted in any substantial improvement in medication compliance.[204]

Even if they do not prove substantially more effective than the older drugs in terms of their ability to alleviate positive symptoms, the fact that atypical neuroleptics are generally less likely to cause debilitating neurological side effects provides grounds for cautious optimism. Whether or not they actually prove to be a genuine boon to diagnosed people, their relatives, and clinicians, will depend on a number of factors. In particular, any potential advantage of these drugs could be lost if they are used without great skill and sensitivity, something which might easily occur if they are prescribed in excessively high dosages or for unnecessarily prolonged periods, or they are given to people who really do not need them. If these (or any other drugs) are looked upon as the only truly important component of treatment, the temptation will always exist to keep increasing the dose (or add other kinds of drugs) if diagnosed people do not quickly respond in ways that are considered adequate – exactly as occurred with the original neuroleptics. Furthermore, anyone who is seduced into thinking that all they need to do is take the "right" medication, may find themselves developing a complacent attitude which will eventually become a barrier to recovery.

The development of second-generation neuroleptics has catalysed a frenzied search for more substances with "anti-psychotic" properties. One of the most significant legacies of the newer drugs is the tremendous impetus they have given to biomedical conceptualisations of schizophrenia and other mental disorders. While there are many who view this as a promising development and a mark of real scientific progress, others – including a growing number from within the ranks of the mental health professions – question whether there is not now too much emphasis on trying to "fix" complex human problems by manipulating brain chemistry. In an article published in the *American Journal of Psychiatry* in 1992, Professor Glen Gabbard cautioned his psychiatric colleagues about the consequences of losing "the complexity and richness of human functioning in the quicksand of neurotransmitters and molecular genetics".[205] Others have expressed grave concern about the extent to which the pharmaceutical industry increasingly controls both the nature and direction of medical research. Professor Ross Baldessarini, one of the world's leading authorities on psychiatric drugs, has recently lamented the fact that "psychiatry is now strongly influenced by aggressive marketing of newer antipsychotics". Baldessarini added that, "much more independent research is required to assess their long-term cost-benefit relationships."[206]

In order to safeguard against excessive or inappropriate use of neuroleptics and the related tendency to dehumanise those receiving such treatment, it is vital to understand that the potential benefits of these drugs can only be realised if they are used in a holistic context. Such an approach moves beyond a narrow focus on symptoms and biology to consider the diagnosed person's total social, psychological, and spiritual needs and circumstances.

Chapter Four

TREATING SCHIZOPHRENIA HOLISTICALLY

As the central concept of disease is dis-ease, the central concept of therapy is ease: everything which promotes the ease of the patient reduces his pathological potentials, and assists the fullest coming to terms which is possible.

Oliver Sacks[207]

MEDICINE'S EARLY SUCCESSES IN developing effective drug treatments for a wide variety of infectious diseases fostered a way of thinking that has exerted a powerful influence upon psychiatry. Thus, just as medical science created "magic bullets" (antibiotics) capable of destroying disease-causing micro-organisms, the advent of chlorpromazine in the early 1950s led to the confident expectation that psychiatry, too, would soon acquire its own arsenal of powerful drugs to use as "weapons" in the "war" on schizophrenia. Wholesale application of this paradigm to psychiatric disorders has resulted in a heavily medication-centred approach, which tends to pay scant attention to vital social, psychological, and spiritual aspects of mental health and emotional well-being. It has also seriously overshadowed clinical interest in therapeutic modalities other than drugs. The contemporary trend toward seeking purely biochemical solutions to mental distress stands in stark contrast to the ethos of earlier times. Previously, mental health professionals still believed that the real value of neuroleptics lay in their potential to help highly disturbed people feel calmer and less distracted, thus enabling them to benefit from "talking" therapies and other psychologically-oriented treatments.[208]

Given the explosive growth of popular interest in holistic healing and natural therapies that has occurred over the past couple of decades, it is curious that mainstream psychiatric treatment of psychotic disorders like schizophrenia has tended to become ever more narrowly focused during this period. While development of new medications has brought certain benefits, excessive concern with controlling or eliminating symptoms has sometimes led to situations in which people have had to pay a heavy price in terms of the side effects of prescribed treatment. As one person said about the medication he was given, "It fixed my problem but ruined my life". Situations such as this serve to highlight the importance of looking beyond symptomatic effects of treatment to consider how it is affecting a person's life as a whole. The study discussed at the end of the previous chapter, in which the effects of clozapine and haloperidol were compared, illustrated this point well. It also highlighted the fact that those receiving treatment are generally in the best position to assess how medication is affecting their overall quality of life.

Anton Boisen's Legacy

In order to gain a better understanding of what a more holistic approach to treatment might entail, it is instructive to consider the views of Anton Boisen, founder of the pastoral psychology movement in the USA and a true pioneer in this area. As a minister of religion and clinical psychologist, who himself experienced several severe psychotic episodes, Boisen was uniquely qualified to comment on these matters. While working as a mental hospital chaplain in the early 1920s, Boisen set out to discover why some people who experience acute psychosis manage to recover fully and go on to lead meaningful and productive lives, while others seem to become stuck or even go downhill, with some eventually lingering in a shadowy netherworld of severe and prolonged mental and social disability. Years of sensitive observation led him to conclude that social and psychological factors play a key role in these developments. Among these, Boisen believed, the following are especially important:[209]

- The amount and quality of social support diagnosed people receive
- The honesty and sincerity with which they face their difficulties
- The balance of assets and liabilities in their character and life situation

Although Boisen made his observations well before the advent of modern psychiatric medications (the book in which he first set out his ideas, *The Exploration of the Inner World*, was originally published in 1936), there is no reason the factors he identified should be any less important in our present medication-centred era. Indeed, it could be said that a truly holistic approach would involve paying careful attention to basic human issues such as those Boisen identified, and combining these efforts with judicious use of medication if it proves helpful. As the ensuing discussion shows, it is not possible to determine what role medication can or ought to play without taking account of the treated person's total social, psychological, and spiritual circumstances.

People Do As Well As Their *Total* Circumstances Allow

Pharmacologists have long understood that human beings do not exist in a social or psychological vacuum and that medical treatment *always* involves a complex interaction of numerous factors, both physical and non-physical. The drugs a person takes are but one of the many components in what is invariably a dynamic and multi-dimensional process. Given this, the notion that a particular class or type of medication always has a specific and predictable effect on a certain type of patient, is an extreme over-simplification of what actually happens in reality. Professor Steven Rose explains:

> The effect of a drug varies enormously with the time, place, and circumstances of taking ... [which makes] evaluation of the effects of a particular drug on behaviour an almost impossible task; the nearest one can get to such an evaluation is to be able to describe the properties of a *system*, which includes the drug, the doctor prescribing it, the individual taking it, and his or her environment. Chemicals do have effects on the

brain, but so do all the other factors in the environment, and the interactions may be more interesting than the supposed "monolithic" effects of the agent. Such a view tends to be unpopular among doctors. For them, it is easier to regard the patient as a relatively passive recipient of treatment, *to* whom drugs are given and *on* whom they act ... The successes claimed for drug therapy and the effects which the drugs are claimed to have, must all be seen in the light of these remarks.[210]

The vast amounts of time, energy, and money now devoted to pharmaceutical research and the development of new psychiatric drugs far outweighs that allocated to investigating other types of therapy for people diagnosed with schizophrenia. Despite this narrow focus, scientific research carried out during the past few decades has clearly demonstrated that a wide range of psychosocial factors can significantly influence therapeutic outcomes for better or worse. In some instances, these factors appear to operate relatively independently of medication, while in others they work with it in a complementary or synergistic manner.[211] It is now understood that the most effective kinds of treatment involve a combination of therapeutically beneficial influences:

> Time has taught us to be more modest in our claims for the benefits of any type of chemotherapy [drug treatment] when used alone. Considerable research evidence has shown the additional benefits of combination treatment utilising social therapy, rehabilitation, and psychotherapy along with regular medication.[212]

Contemporary approaches to effective management of hypertension (high blood pressure) illustrate the benefits of applying holistic principles, such as paying careful attention to the specific needs and circumstances of the individual concerned, and utilising the combined effects of a variety of different therapeutic modalities. It is now understood that, even with a physiological condition such as this, the use of drugs is not always necessary or desirable and that a range of treatment options are feasible, the most appropriate being determined by the affected person's specific circumstances. A substantial proportion of people with hypertension are able to reduce their blood pressure using relatively simple lifestyle measures, such as losing weight, reducing consumption of alcohol and salt, giving up smoking, getting adequate exercise, and learning to use effective stress-management techniques. Some people may require anti-hypertensive drugs either temporarily (until the lifestyle measures begin taking effect) or for longer periods. The latter group would include those who, for various reasons, are unable or unwilling to reduce their blood pressure without medications. Similar considerations apply to diabetes, a medical condition with which schizophrenia is often compared. Thus, while some people with this condition (around 10%) require regular insulin injections and others manage with the help of tablets, many manage their diabetes without drugs, by adopting a lifestyle involving careful attention to diet, weight, exercise, and stress management. Interestingly, it has recently been found that for some people, stress-reduction techniques such as progressive muscular relaxation, breathing exercises and relaxation, can be just as effective as drugs in helping to control symptoms of diabetes.[213]

A substantial body of evidence has shown that many people diagnosed with schizophrenia can reduce their need for long-term neuroleptic medication, and increase its effectiveness, by adopting a holistic approach, which integrates judicious use of medication with careful attention to lifestyle measures, stress management, and various other psychosocial factors. Pioneer community psychiatrist Professor John Wing, has summarised the relationship between a diagnosed person's social circumstances and their need for medication as follows:

> Drug treatment and social treatments are not alternatives but must be used to compliment each other. The better the environmental conditions, the less the need for medication; the poorer the social milieu, the greater the need (or at least the use) of drugs.[214]

Unfortunately, there is still a tendency to rely almost exclusively on medications in many instances. In fact, as psychiatrist Richard Warner has noted, very often "antipsychotics have been used not as an *adjunct* to psychosocial treatment, as John Wing recommends, but as an *alternative* to such care."[215] Some of the psychosocial factors that are now known to influence the need for and effectiveness of neuroleptic medications are discussed below.

The Therapeutic Alliance

The treatment of people diagnosed with schizophrenia does not occur in a social vacuum but in the context of relationships of various kinds. Even if medications are the central focus of treatment, an interpersonal dimension is *always* involved since a person (more likely, a number of people) has to prescribe, supply, and supervise the drugs. While it is often assumed that the relationship a person has with those providing treatment is largely irrelevant to a drug's effects, there is good reason to question this belief. For example, research has shown that an individual's need for and response to medications given for ordinary physical illnesses can vary significantly, according to the nature of their relationship with treatment personnel. It has even been found that the insulin requirements of people with diabetes can fluctuate in response to changes in the nature of their relationship with the treating physician.[216] Similar effects are bound to occur in the context of psychiatric treatment where issues like trust, confidence, and expectation play such a vital role. As Professor Philip May points out, both the therapeutic effects and the side effects of psychotropic drugs can be strongly influenced by social factors, including those associated with the clinician/client relationship:

> It is frequently assumed that drug treatment requires no particular skill and no particular attention to the transactions of the therapeutic relationship. This is a serious error. The effectiveness of any kind of treatment depends on a good relationship with the patient and his family, and the vicissitudes of these relationships have a profound impact on the course of pharmacotherapy [drug treatment]. Establishing a continuing positive relationship must therefore occupy a central position in the overall strategy for treating the schizophrenic patient, whatever the form of treatment employed.[217]

The clinician's behaviour and the nature of the therapeutic alliance can exert a powerful influence for better or worse in a number of ways. On a psychological level the diagnosed person's willingness to comply with prescribed medication is often strongly influenced by the relationship he or she has with the prescriber and others (such as case managers) responsible for monitoring the drug's effects. The confidence, skill, and understanding of those who provide treatment can help to instil hope and positive expectations. These may themselves have a number of beneficial effects (as well as contributing to the placebo-effect, discussed in detail later in this chapter). Researchers have found that, among people with psychotic disorders like schizophrenia, establishment of a positive therapeutic alliance is associated with improved clinical outcomes and significantly reduced neuroleptic dosages.[218]

Stress Management

Most mental health clinicians now accept the *stress/vulnerability concept*, which sees people diagnosed with schizophrenia as having a specific predisposition ("vulnerability") to developing psychotic symptoms when exposed to excessive stress.[219] While stress does not actually *cause* schizophrenia, research has demonstrated that people with this diagnosis are often highly sensitive to stressful stimuli. Some may be prone to experiencing an exacerbation of their existing symptoms, or possibly even another acute psychotic episode (relapse), if exposed to stress that exceeds their coping abilities. It is important to appreciate that the kinds of stressors which seem to "trigger" the onset of a psychotic episode are often highly idiosyncratic, i.e. the individual concerned may react adversely to situations or experiences that most people might not find excessively stressful. The kinds of situations most likely to cause overwhelming stress often seem to be ones that the person concerned experiences as hurtful or injurious because they touch on his or her exquisite sensitivity or threaten an already precarious self-image.

As explained earlier, the fact that neuroleptic drugs induce a state of psychic indifference allows them to function as effective buffers against the potentially destructive impact of stress. In line with this observation Professor Luc Ciompi has noted that neuroleptics are especially indicated when there is a danger of emotional over-taxation. One of the most important implications of the schizophrenia/stress connection is that diagnosed people who can find ways of reducing the overall amount of stress they experience, or who learn to handle unavoidable stress more effectively, will often have less need for the protection medication can provide (the "neuroleptic shield"). In short, use of effective stress management techniques increases the possibility that a diagnosed individual will be able to do well on smaller amounts of medication or, in some cases, possibly no medication at all.[220] Professor Wing offered the following summation of the view that creating an environment in which social stress is minimised can lead to a substantial reduction in the need for neuroleptic drugs, especially for those with a high level of vulnerability:

> The schizophrenic patient with a fairly severe degree of … vulnerability is balanced, at the optimum, on a knife-edge. On one side is the tendency toward overdoing the protective social withdrawal. On the other side, particularly if the patient is forced into social interaction with no possibility of controlling the degree of stimulation, there is the danger of acute

relapse ... The optimal social environment therefore is structured, with neutral (i.e. not highly emotionally involved) stimulation to perform up to achievable standards, with little necessity for complex decision making, but with some degree of control over the amount of social stimulation left in the patient's own hands. It is in these circumstances that a relationship of trust and confidence is most likely to develop with professional staff or family members and the need for [neuroleptic] medication is likely to be minimal.[221]

As explained below, the therapeutic value of stress reduction within families has been incontestably demonstrated.

Family Education and Support

It has been known since the early 1970s that a diagnosed person's family can significantly effect his or her long-term wellbeing for better or worse.[222] In particular, it has been found that people are much more likely to experience relapse if the family in which they live is fraught with stress and tension, while relapse is much less likely in families whose "emotional climate" is characterised by warmth, acceptance, and supportive attitudes. Various methods have been devised to help families become more supportive, e.g. family therapy that helps resolve specific conflicts, and educational programmes (referred to as "psychoeducation") which foster greater tolerance and increased support as a result of helping family members acquire a better understanding of schizophrenia. A great deal of research has shown that in supportive families a diagnosed person's medication can often be safely reduced to a much lower level than would be possible in a more stressful environment.

Just how important the emotional climate of the family can be was demonstrated in a series of highly regarded studies conducted in London, under the auspices of the Social Psychiatry Unit of the Medical Research Council (MRC). One study of a group of 128 diagnosed individuals found that 51% of those from high-stress families had experienced a relapse by the end of the nine-month research period, whereas only 13% from low-stress families had relapsed during the same time.[223] Of particular significance was the fact that while neuroleptic medication helped to substantially reduce the risk of relapse in high-stress families (individuals in this situation appear to need the protective, stress-buffering effect of the "neuroleptic shield"), it made little difference to relapse rates among those from low-stress families.

Attitudes and Expectations
It is increasingly clear that a diagnosed person's attitudes, beliefs, and expectations – together with those of others closely involved with him or her – can strongly influence both their current state and their future prospects. For example, research has shown that the less negative a person's attitudes are toward their psychotic experiences and the future, the better their prospects are generally likely to be.[224] Absence of negative attitudes appears to be especially important in this regard. Professor Ciompi's research on the numerous factors which together determine a person's prognosis, led him to conclude that expectations often act as "self-fulfilling prophecies". He summarised this view in an article published in the *British Journal of Psychiatry* in 1989:

A favourable or unfavourable outcome seems to depend less on genetic and biological than on psychosocial and situational factors, such as available therapeutic and rehabilitative facilities, family atmosphere and "affective style", economic and cultural conditions, etc. – all of which are in continuous interaction with the pre-existing vulnerability. Among the most important determining factors are the expectations of the family, the professionals, and the patients themselves; at least in part, these seem to act as self-fulfilling prophecies.[225]

Just how powerful an influence a diagnosed person's attitude can be was clearly illustrated in research conducted by Professor John Strauss, in which he interviewed people whose condition had improved significantly after ten years or more of severe mental disorder. Professor Strauss was struck by the way a change of attitude – particularly the development of a more hopeful outlook – seemed to provide an impetus to general improvement and in some cases marked a turning point toward recovery. An especially noteworthy observation was that some people said that their long-standing symptoms became less severe when they began developing a more hopeful attitude:

Somehow, after an extended period, they found themselves wanting not just to live with their illness but to have a life along with it or in spite of it. Some stated that they came to accept their disorders. But this was not the kind of giving–up resignation that often seems generated by the attempts some professionals make at helpful teaching (e.g. "You have an illness like diabetes and will have it all your life. You'll need to stay on medication and there are certain things you'll never be able to do.") The acceptance described by these subjects was one that involved hope for a better life and the resolve to work for it. In several instances, subjects noted that symptoms — even delusions and hallucinations — then started to become less dominating and often faded considerably.[226]

The fact that the development of a more hopeful, accepting attitude can sometimes lead to a reduction in the severity of schizophrenia symptoms *in the absence of any changes to medication regimes* raises important questions about the nature and origin of these symptoms. In particular, it suggests that the severity of a given individual's symptoms (both positive and negative) is more closely intertwined with their psychological and emotional state than is usually realised. At the very least, it calls into question the wisdom of attributing symptoms to a chemical imbalance that is independent of the affected person's subjective state.

Medication itself can have a range of different effects on a diagnosed person's attitude and expectations. Especially if it is forced upon someone, it can be an ever-present bone of contention and an on-going cause of anger and frustration. Such a situation may seriously compromise an individual's sense of autonomy, hopefulness, and expectations for the future. Certain side effects can seriously erode a person's emotional vitality and life energy. On the other hand, medications that are effective in reducing the intensity of debilitating symptoms and which provide a degree of protection against the impact of stress, can foster a greater sense of confidence and control. These feelings may in turn contribute to the development of a more hopeful outlook, both in those receiving treatment and in others, such as relatives, friends and mental health workers responsible for providing care and support.

Self-Help

Medication does not work in isolation from all the other influences that together shape a person's life. Of the many things that can help bring about an improvement in a diagnosed person's mental health and general wellbeing, their own efforts may be among the most important. In a recent Australian survey in which people were asked to identify factors that had helped their recovery, the vast majority of respondents nominated various kinds of self-help as being extremely important.[227] The factors nominated by the greatest number of respondents were these:

- Determination to get better (74%)
- Finding their own way to manage their illness (64%)
- Recognising the need to help themselves (54%)

Esso Leete is just one of many people who have discovered that their recovery did not begin until they were willing to take responsibility for doing everything they could to help themselves:

> Over the years I have reluctantly become an expert in the area of my illness ... I have learned coping mechanisms to deal with my mental illness ... Sadly, for years I had expected someone else to "fix" me. However, I finally realised, after many clinical disappointments,

that this task fell to me alone and that no one else could really make me better. I approached this task very seriously, conscientiously working to get my life back together. For the first time, I then felt ready to take responsibility for myself, including management of my illness, and I feel it was at this point that my recovery really began ... We did not choose to be ill, but we can choose to deal with it and learn to live with it. By learning to modulate stress, we will manage our illness more effectively thus endowing ourselves with an ongoing sense of mastery and control. I find that my vulnerability to stress, anxiety, and accompanying symptoms decreases as I gain more control of my own life.[228]

Nobody truly recovers by relying on medication alone. Indeed, it is increasingly clear that the potential benefits of medication can only be gained when it is used in the context of a holistic approach in which self-responsibility is strongly emphasised. In recent years psychiatric researchers have discovered that there are many things people diagnosed with schizophrenia can do, apart from taking prescribed medication, to help improve their mental health and wellbeing.[229] The following are some of the many ways people can learn to play an active role in their own recovery:

(a) Self-understanding and self-education
Learning as much as possible about schizophrenia, and the medications used to treat it, can lead to a greater sense of control, as well as providing a sound basis for understanding one's own experiences and behaviour.

(b) Cultivating a realistically hopeful attitude

As explained earlier, positive attitudes and expectations can act as self-fulfilling prophecies which exert a beneficial influence on recovery. Minimising negative attitudes and pessimistic expectations is especially important in this regard.

(c) Learning to manage stress

Many people discover through experience that excessive stress can cause their symptoms to worsen and might even trigger the onset of psychotic episodes (relapse). Consequently, effective stress management ought to be a central component in every diagnosed person's repertoire of coping and survival skills.

(d) Adopting a healthy lifestyle

As well as being necessary to sustain physical and mental health and wellbeing, a nutritious diet, regular exercise, and adequate sleep and rest, can all help to strengthen the natural healing powers of body and mind which play a vital role in recovery.

(e) Avoiding substance abuse

Since abuse of illicit and social drugs can exacerbate pre-existing symptoms as well as having a wide range of detrimental effects on physical and mental health, use of these substances should be avoided altogether or their consumption severely restricted.

(f) Monitoring prodromal symptoms

Learning to recognise the characteristic warning signals that may indicate an imminent psychotic episode increases the likelihood that a diagnosed person will be able to take appropriate steps to reduce stress and restore their mental equilibrium before they reach a point of no return. Prodromal symptom monitoring is an essential skill for people whose treatment involves using medication on an intermittent "as needed" basis (see *Chapter Nine*).

(g) Using counselling or psychotherapy

As explained below, "talking therapy" provides an opportunity to identify and address important emotional, social, and psychological issues, such as loss of self-confidence, low self-esteem, and lack of trust. The on-going support of a trusted therapist or counsellor provides an ideal setting in which to work on issues concerning self-identity, interpersonal relationships, and personal goals.

(h) Cultivating self-esteem

The stigma and general negativity associated with mental illness can have a very damaging effect on a diagnosed person's self-image and self-esteem. Making a conscious effort to counteract these destructive influences, and working to develop and maintain a personally acceptable identity and sense of self-worth, are crucial tasks for those intent on recovery.

(i) Respecting and nurturing spirituality

Although it is not always acknowledged as such, spirituality is a profoundly important dimension in the life of every human being. Deeply spiritual issues and concerns sometimes arise in the context of psychosis but are rarely dealt with in an appropriate or helpful manner. Many people have found that grounded spirituality provides them with an invaluable source of strength, comfort, guidance and meaning.

(j) Learning practical strategies for managing symptoms

Research conducted in recent years has demonstrated unequivocally that a wide range of non-drug strategies and techniques can be useful in dealing with both positive and negative schizophrenia symptoms.[230] For example, many diagnosed individuals have found that it is possible to reduce, or sometimes even stop disturbing voices, simply by listening to music through stereo headphones. Simple techniques such as this can often be used in conjunction with neuroleptic treatment and may, in some instances, allow lower dosages to be used. Non-drug techniques are sometimes sufficiently effective to be used instead of medication.

(k) Seeking and accepting help

Living with schizophrenia is a difficult and challenging task, even if effective medical treatment is available. While some diagnosed individuals are understandably reluctant to accept that they need the support and assistance of others, many eventually discover the truth of this GROW aphorism: "You alone can do it, but you can't do it alone".

In the following anecdotes, Richard Weingarten describes some of the many things he has done to actively nurture his mental health and emotional wellbeing:

> My health really began to improve in 1986 when I saw that my therapists were limited in what they could do for me, and I began to do things for myself, like

get involved in the Consumer Movement. Another danger is that I tended to blame everything on my "illness". As it turned out, I had many problems that were caused or made problematic by the lack of meaningful activities and a strong social network, or just being out of tune with my environment. Perhaps the biggest danger was seeing myself as a "sick person". It *had been* an important step for me to accept the fact that I had an illness, and I needed to make a strong commitment to work on my problems. But I began to make real progress when I took control of my life and began doing things that utilised my strengths and abilities and received some recognition ... when I began to take on real challenges and saw that I could meet them successfully, I felt more hopeful about myself and my future. It was about this time also that I began to see myself as a therapist and devised coping mechanisms to deal with my problems and situations that were causing me difficulty.[231]

It is worth noting that, while he acknowledges the personal value of medication, Richard nevertheless emphasises the many *other* things that have helped him recover his mental health and contributed to improving his overall quality of life:

I try hard to keep the amount of stress I encounter to a minimum. I get the exercise I need, eat the right foods, get the right amount of sleep and rest – very important – and generate the amount and kinds of activities I need that allow me to keep my life interesting and moving forward ... I regard my susceptibility to depression as a problem that I deal with preventively. I regard getting in touch with my anger and rage, improving my self-image and self-esteem, finding and sustaining a sense of inner wholeness and integration, keeping busy, etc., as essential elements to my daily living free of depression ... Paranoia has also been a persistent and long-term problem, though I feel I've reduced it considerably. The medication I take – Prolixin [fluphenazine] – wonderfully eliminates much of it. Because I am practically off of Prolixin, I feel that other measures I've taken have also made a difference. For example, getting in touch with my anger and learning how to express it have stopped me from projecting my anger onto other people. Testing my perceptions of situations and relationships with my therapist and friends has also been helpful ... As with depression, raising my self-esteem has also made feeling fearful of others less of a problem.[232]

Accounts such as these highlight the essential contribution constructive self-help makes to recovery. While many diagnosed people learn this through their own experience, the importance of such activities is not always acknowledged and affirmed by others. It is not uncommon for any positive changes that occur in a diagnosed person's life to be immediately attributed to the effects of medication rather than to their own efforts. The real danger of such responses is that they can inadvertently disempower people and encourage them to see themselves as mere passive recipients of treatment, rather than as active agents whose own efforts, creativity, and resourcefulness are of inestimable value.

Psychotherapy and Counselling

The growing emphasis on biological aspects of schizophrenia in recent decades has resulted in a gradual loss of interest in the "talking therapies" which once clearly distinguished psychiatry from other branches of medicine. Indeed, many practicing mental health professionals now take it for granted that psychotherapy is ineffective at best, and possibly even harmful, for people diagnosed with schizophrenia. The relatively rapid and occasionally quite dramatic results achieved by drug treatment have undoubtedly added considerable impetus to this attitude. Despite these trends, there has recently been a belated resurgence of interest in psychotherapy among some sections of the mental health professions.[233] Indeed, some psychiatrists have come to believe that their profession's collective rejection of psychotherapy as a valid treatment modality is based on faulty assumptions and inappropriate research methodology. Critics have pointed out, for instance, that some of the most influential studies purportedly demonstrating the lack of efficacy of psychotherapy utilised poorly trained and inexperienced therapists and only continued for six months, a period generally regarded as far too short to allow valid conclusions to be drawn.[234]

Some psychiatrists now acknowledge that, even if schizophrenia is viewed as an essentially biological illness, psychotherapy can still play an invaluable role in helping to address the human issues involved, including such important matters as the diagnosed person's feelings about having a mental illness and their struggle to adjust to profoundly altered personal circumstances.[235] Most importantly, despite considerable professional scepticism, many diagnosed people testify to having experienced significant personal benefit as a result of participating in psychotherapy of various kinds.[236] The results of a recent survey of a large group of diagnosed people who had received individual psychotherapy for an average of about twelve months, strongly underscored its potential value. Most (72%) reported that therapy had produced positive changes in their life, whereas only a small minority (14%) reported negative changes or said that therapy had no effect (14%).[237] When asked in what specific ways therapy had helped them, the following were reported as being among the most useful aspects:

- Receiving practical advice from the therapist
- Getting in touch with feelings
- Learning how they affect other people and how others affect them
- Reflecting on how they usually feel or act and understanding why
- Understanding the impact of the past on current feelings and behaviour

Mary McGrath is not alone in pointing out that symptoms are not all there is to schizophrenia, and that talking therapy can help people deal with personal issues and concerns that are very often neglected in conventional psychiatric treatment:

In the most recently published book I've read, a doctor writes that psychotherapy is useless with schizophrenics. How could he even suggest that without knowing me, the one over here in this corner, who finds a lot of support, understanding, and acceptance with my therapists? Marianne is not afraid to travel with me in my fearful times. She listens when I need to release some of the "poisons" in my mind. She offers advice when I'm having difficulty with just daily living. She sees me as a human being and not only a body to shovel pills into or a cerebral mass in some laboratory. Psychotherapy is important to me, and it does help.[238]

It has become increasingly clear that certain kinds of psychotherapy may be extremely beneficial for people diagnosed with schizophrenia, especially those which concentrate on practical problem solving and which focus on the here and now rather than on the past. Far from being ineffective or even destructive, it has been found that skilfully conducted psychotherapy can help ameliorate problems that have proven largely unresponsive to drug treatment, including negative symptoms such as retardation, apathy, and denial.[239] Therapists who are experienced and skilled in working with diagnosed individuals understand that it is important to attend to positive aspects of a person's life as well as to problem areas. Indeed, Professor Manfred Bleuler felt that the essence of the therapist's task involves relating constantly and actively to a client's "healthy" aspects.[240] Thus, as well as assisting people with problems, truly effective therapists also endeavour to help them recognise and affirm their strengths, abilities, achievements, positive attributes and characteristics, and the validity of their personal aspirations and goals (this endeavour is sometimes referred to as "supportive psychotherapy").[241] At times, supportive therapists may also need to function as carriers of hope for their clients, many of whom have attested to the importance of having had someone who continued to believe in them when they were unable to believe in themselves. The following testimony to the value of on-going therapy was provided by a person with a diagnosis of paranoid schizophrenia:

> I have heard it said that psychotherapy is not very effective for schizophrenia, and as I strongly disagree with this, I would like to list a few of the benefits I have received from it: The human connection I have developed with the therapist has helped me to reject the idea that I will never be able to relate to people or fit into society like a "normal" person. I got a lot of much needed encouragement which has allowed me to have some hope for the future rather than to feel my life is over. The therapist encouraged me to believe that my emotions, behaviour, and symptoms would improve and that I could try to add people and things to my life that would improve the quality of my life. I am reasonably certain that if it had not been for this effective encouragement, I would have given in to my disturbances much more and felt helpless to have anything but a low level of functioning with no hope for the future. The therapy was a great help to me in identifying which situations were particularly tension-producing and also in developing strategies to deal with symptoms when they appear, to try and prevent them from intensifying. I have gotten a lot of insight into how my background shaped my personality, and I can see where I got some "raw material" for developing my particular brand of delusions, paranoia, and other symptoms.[242]

In reflecting on the possible value of counselling or therapy, it is important to remember that different people have different needs which may change considerably over time. For example, some people may be reluctant to talk about what they are going through when first diagnosed, but their reluctance may decrease in time as they gradually adjust to their new circumstances. On the other hand, those with a strong natural desire to speak about their feelings and experiences, may feel extremely frustrated with treatment that does not provide them with an adequate opportunity to do so. Being denied a chance to discuss their experiences freely is not just frustrating – it may even constitute a significant hindrance to recovery for some people. Jungian psychiatrist Dr John Perry tells of an invaluable lesson he was fortunate to learn very early in his career:

> Psychiatry has developed a new habit in this era of "sane-making" drugs: that of non-hearing, of an interdiction against listening to the "patient's" non-rational concerns. My own start in the field got off on a different footing. When I was first entering upon medicine on the way toward psychiatry, my cousin's wife told me about a psychosis she had had and about the ideas, feelings, and delusional beliefs that had filled her mind. She wound up her account with one emphatic admonition: "What makes the crucial difference to a patient is to be able to talk to someone who will really listen." She clearly pointed to this as the one thing that allowed her to get over her psychosis. I have never forgotten that tip, and have always put it into practice; many others since have

told me of their recovering from psychosis when they found an understanding listener.[243]

The opportunity to be oneself in relationship with another person, together with the feeling of being accepted for who one is, can itself be a powerful healing experience. Indeed, Carl Jung once said that "a schizophrenic ceases to be a schizophrenic when he meets someone by whom he feels understood"[244] One of the truly invaluable aspects of effective therapy is that it provides a safe space in which people are permitted and encouraged to express themselves freely and openly. Those who have gotten into the habit of bottling up their feelings and thoughts often experience great relief when they discover a counsellor or therapist with whom they can at last let down their guard and just be themselves. This is often a significant issue for people who have been diagnosed with schizophrenia since they have often learnt to conceal certain thoughts and feelings, for fear of being judged or rejected by others. Sadly, bottled-up feelings or hidden thoughts and wishes can become a source of considerable stress, all the more difficult to deal with because they cannot even be spoken about.

Diagnosed people who may wish to discuss their psychotic experiences very often find few avenues available too them, due to the widespread fear that talking about such things will somehow reinforce them. This questionable belief has led to the creation of a virtual taboo that effectively prevents open discussion of matters which may be of great personal significance. There is no doubt that some people gain considerable therapeutic benefit when given the opportunity to speak freely about their dream-like psychotic experiences, as Simon Champ attests:

If a person has a powerful dream, particularly if it is a frightening dream, he/she tends to share it at breakfast with family, lover, or friends. It is an acceptable practice and sometimes provides psychological insights and diminishes some of the fear the dream holds for the dreamer. However, symptoms of mental illness frighten our colleagues and family, so the contents of delusions are still rarely shared or explored. The domination of biochemical theories of illnesses like schizophrenia have further stifled discussions about the often frightening contents of psychotic episodes. We are so often encouraged to repress the fears we feel from our symptoms or have the whole experience lost to the mental fog of higher doses of medication. I found that I needed to talk about the contents of delusions to dissipate the fear they held for me. The best staff allowed me to go over my psychotic experiences thus gradually diffusing the power they held over me, and they helped me to integrate the delusions as best I could, into some sense of being whole and earthed again. I desperately needed to understand what psychosis was and extract some kind of meaning from the experience. I could only do that by telling it over many times.[245]

It is important to understand that, whereas it used to be believed that talking therapies and use of psychotropic medications were mutually exclusive, it is now widely accepted that they are not only compatible but may, in some cases, actually complement one another.[246] Many diagnosed people who have participated in therapy agree with this view. Thus, while 16% of the respondents in a recent survey said that medication was the most useful aspect of their treatment, 25% said they found talking most useful, and 60% believed a combination of talking and medication was best.[247] Scientific support for the potential benefits of combining these two distinctly different forms of treatment was provided by a recent study which found that diagnosed individuals who received psychotherapy in addition to drugs experienced a substantial reduction in the amount of time they spent in hospital over a period of 20 months (from 112 days to 43 days).[248] To the extent that they help to enhance coping, boost self-confidence, bolster self-esteem, and alleviate subjective distress (e.g. bottled-up feelings), talking therapies may actually reduce the need for the "stress-buffering" effect of neuroleptic medications. It should be noted that for some diagnosed people at least, participation in psychotherapy may not be possible without the calming and stabilising effects of medication. On the other hand, even quite subtle medication side effects can sometimes impair a person's ability to participate in and benefit from counselling and other kinds of talking therapy.[249] A recent survey found this to be a common experience: "Many stated that in this time of deep turmoil, they wanted to talk about their problems but the side effects did not allow this".[250]

Beginning therapy often requires a considerable leap of faith. Sensitised as they are by past painful experiences, it takes great courage for those diagnosed with schizophrenia to even consider what might occur should they venture to delve into their own personal can of worms in therapy. Indeed, people with fragile egos are often advised to avoid intensive psychotherapy. While this is undoubtedly sound advice for some, a person with considerable experience in therapy has pointed out that "a fragile ego left alone remains fragile".[251] As Patricia Ruocchio explains, many people feel certain that psychotherapy can contribute significantly to recovery:

Things that psychotherapy can do make it a necessary complement to medication. Psychotherapy helps with emotional problems that would have been there despite the illness as well as problems that may have developed because of the illness ... Therapy can help the schizophrenic develop feelings that are realistic and correct mistaken feelings ... Psychotherapy cannot relieve all the symptoms, but it can improve coping mechanisms and help the schizophrenic avoid some symptoms by discovering what triggers them. By talking to a therapist after a symptom occurs or after a psychotic episode, the schizophrenic can understand the psychological and emotional components of the illness and become less afraid and perhaps less prone to have the symptom ... For the schizophrenic who is lucky enough to be able to participate in psychotherapy, even in a minimal way, the process can often enhance a life that was once only dark and painful. In many cases, it can alleviate some of the worst manifestations of the illness, such as fear and loneliness. It provides a relationship that teaches one how to interact with others ... To learn how to relate to another person can be a major breakthrough in beginning the socialisation process ... In reality, a therapist who cares is not an intrusion but a godsend who can help to enrich a life that once seemed lost. Psychotherapy can probably help almost every schizophrenic to some degree.[252]

It is often assumed that psychotherapy has its principal effects on the psychological and emotional level. Interestingly, recent developments in neuroscience have drawn attention to some possible effects of psychotherapy that have previously gone unrecognised. In particular, a growing body of scientific research has indicated that the human brain is a uniquely malleable organ which undergoes structural and functional change in response to a wide range of psychosocial influences – a phenomenon known as *neural plasticity*.[253] There is now abundant evidence that, in certain circumstances, psychotherapy may have a favourable effect on biochemical processes occurring in the brain. For example, Professor Glen Gabbard noted, in a report published in the *British Journal of Psychiatry* in 2000, that recent research in Finland showed that psychodynamic psychotherapy may exert a beneficial effect on cerebral serotonin metabolism. Before commencing a year of such therapy, the brain of a man with borderline personality disorder and depression was imaged with single photon emission computed tomography (SPECT). Another man with similar problems who acted as the experimental control also underwent brain imaging but did not receive psychotherapy or any other form of treatment. Professor Gabbard believes this research shows that psychotherapy is sometimes just as effective as pharmacological treatment in helping to rectify a pre-existing chemical imbalance in the brain:

Initial SPECT imaging showed that both men had markedly reduced serotonin uptake in the medial prefrontal area and the thalamus, when compared with ten healthy control subjects. Repeat SPECT imaging showed that the man who had received one year of psychodynamic therapy had normal serotonin uptake, while the control patient who did not receive psychotherapy continued to have markedly reduced serotonin uptake. Since the patient who received psychotherapy did not take medication in conjunction with the therapy, the finding suggests that the dynamic therapy itself may have normalised the serotonin metabolism.[254]

When combined with what has already been said about the various psychological, social, and emotional benefits of psychotherapy, thought-provoking findings such as these suggest that its therapeutic benefits can extend beyond the non-physical level to include a positive influence on the physiological activity – and possibly even the structure – of the treated person's brain.[255] In light of this new, scientifically validated understanding of the beneficial effects of talking therapies on the brain as well as on the mind and emotions, it seems rather incongruous that psychiatrists who view schizophrenia as a "brain disease" still tend to rule out psychotherapy as a potentially valuable form of treatment.

The Placebo Effect: Nothing Works!

The fact that a person's beliefs and expectations can exert a powerful influence on their health and wellbeing is now firmly established. Because medication plays such a central role in the treatment of schizophrenia, it is worth taking time to consider a phenomenon that is frequently overlooked in contemporary psychiatry's determined effort to become more scientific, namely the extent to which the effects of drugs are influenced, for better or worse, by a person's beliefs and expectations about them. As professors Timothy Lambert and Harry Minas explain, it is well known that the effects of medications are not determined solely by their pharmacological properties, but rather by a complex interaction between these and a host of psychological and social variables:

> The prescribing and taking of medications is a complex social act which cannot be divorced from the "scientific" appraisal of a drug's actions and outcomes. The effects (and effectiveness) of medications are profoundly influenced by the symbolic significance of the interaction between the clinician and patient, the meanings attributed to the taking of medications, and the characteristics and qualities attributed to the drugs themselves. *The pharmacological properties of the drug are only one group (and not always the most important) of factors that will influence drug response and side-effect profile.* These factors should be considered together with a knowledge of the pharmacological actions of the drug.[256]

The power of these interactions is exemplified in a phenomenon referred to as the *placebo effect*. Physicians have long known that when people are given an inert substance – sometimes referred to as a "dummy" or "sugar" pill – in the belief that they are receiving an active therapeutic drug, many will respond as if they had indeed ingested a real medicine. The specific responses that a placebo "medication" elicits will be largely determined by the *expectations* of the person taking it. Thus, if people suffering from anxiety believe that the pills they are given will help reduce their anxiety, that is often precisely what occurs, even if the pills are actually only sugar or some other inert substance. The powerful influence of expectation on an individual's response to drugs of any kind is graphically illustrated in the following vignette:

In an experiment described by the psychopharmacologist C.R.B. Joyce, two groups, each of ten individuals, are placed in separate rooms. In one room nine are given a "sedating dose" of [sleep-inducing] barbiturates, one an "elevating dose" of amphetamine ["speed"]; in the second room nine receive amphetamine and the tenth barbiturates. In each room the odd individual out, rather than behaving in a way appropriate to the drug taken, behaves like the majority, either sedated on the amphetamine or high on the barbiturates. Not merely the extent but also the direction in which intake of a drug may change a person's mood, behaviour, and so forth depends materially upon the social context. Indeed, merely telling a person that he or she has been given a drug that will alter mood, ease pain or depression, or whatever, is enough in a large number of cases to result in the individual reporting improvement.[257]

The effect of expectation is so significant that it is now standard practice when a new drug is being tested, for half the research subjects to be given the active drug, while the remainder receive a placebo. This is usually done in such a way that nobody concerned knows who has had the real drug and who has received the dummy pills, until the testing is complete (this procedure is known as a double-blind placebo-controlled trial). The reason tests are carried out in this way is that a new drug is not considered worthwhile unless it has been proven to be significantly more effective than placebo in bringing about desired changes in the "target" symptoms for which it is to be prescribed, e.g. controlling delusions and hallucinations, reducing anxiety or depression.

The strength of the placebo effect can vary considerably from one person and situation to another. It is influenced by factors such as personality characteristics of the individual concerned, their beliefs and expectations about the drug, and the general attitudes that exist in the environment in which the drug is taken. This general environment includes the beliefs, attitudes and expectations of the prescribing doctor and other professionals involved in providing the treatment, together with those of relatives, friends, and the broader community. Even physical variables such as a placebo pill's size, shape, colour, and the route by which a placebo is administered can markedly influence its effects. Researchers Robert Ornstein and David Sobel summarised their findings thus: placebo injections are more potent than placebo capsules which are, in turn, more effective than placebo pills; small yellow pills seem to work well for depression while large blue pills have a better effect as sedatives; overall, a large brown or purple pill or a very small bright red or yellow pill seems to produce better effects than other size and colour combinations; the more bitter tasting the medicine, and the more difficult and unpleasant the treatment, the more likely it is to result in a pronounced placebo effect.[258] Nobody has yet been able to satisfactorily explain the placebo effect, even though it sometimes elicits responses comparable to those produced by active drugs:

> In certain predisposed persons, a placebo may produce extremely strong reactions with far-reaching consequences … placebos have been shown to evoke patterns of altered behaviour that are similar to and as long-lasting as those observed when a pharmacologically active drug is ingested. Thus, in analysing the pharmacology of a psychoactive agent, particular attention must be paid to the mental expectations, social setting, and the predisposition of the subjects taking the placebo if the pharmacological effects of a drug are to be described accurately. Certainly the placebo effect is a powerful element in drug-induced responses.[259]

The placebo effect is a mystery which has been largely ignored by mainstream medical science, despite the fact that it has been variously estimated to contribute between 30% and 70% of the total response to any given treatment.[260] Indeed, research has shown that up to 25% of people diagnosed with schizophrenia may experience a substantial improvement in their symptoms when they take placebo pills which they believe to be active medication.[261] Rather than dealing with the profound implications of these challenging facts, they are often treated rather dismissively ("Oh, that's just the placebo effect"). A far more creative response would be to try to understand what is going on and, more specifically, to investigate how so-called placebo responders are able to reduce the intensity and frequency of their psychotic symptoms, simply by *thinking* they have ingested an effective anti-psychotic medication.

It has been suggested that in a psychiatric context the placebo effect might be mediated via "self-liberation of endogenous neurotransmitters" including endorphins and catecholamines such as dopamine.[262] In other words, a person's beliefs and expectations are somehow capable of inducing tangible changes in the biochemical activity of their brain. Others view the placebo phenomenon from a more holistic perspective, regarding it as a specific manifestation of the ability possessed by all human beings to foster positive change by drawing upon innate healing powers that exist deep within. Some of the most innovative research on this subject, undertaken by Norman Cousins, is detailed in his seminal book, *Anatomy of an Illness*, in which he concluded that "the placebo is the doctor who resides within".[263] Cousins explains how:

> The placebo is not so much a pill as a process, beginning with the patient's confidence in the doctor and extending through the full functioning of his own immunological system. The process works not because of any magic in the tablets but because the human body is its own best apothecary and because the most successful prescriptions are those that are filled by the body itself.[264]

Herbert Benson, Associate Professor of Medicine at Harvard Medical School, has recently suggested that the placebo effect is best understood as a manifestation of "remembered wellness", a phenomenon that occurs as a result of the way human beings project their desire for wellness onto the medicines they take. Professor Benson believes that hope and positive expectations stimulate the body's innate healing mechanisms, which in turn allow the release of a range of natural healing chemicals from the "inner pharmacy".[265]

If it does nothing else, the placebo effect proves that a given drug's effects are not solely determined by its pharmacological properties, and that various psychological influences associated with its use are also extremely important. Indeed, the effects of hope and positive expectations sometimes prove to be even *more* therapeutically important than a drug's pharmacological effects. This fact is well illustrated in the following anecdote concerning an experiment which took place in the 1950s when tests were being conducted into the effects of chlorpromazine, the first neuroleptic to be used in psychiatry. As part of these trials, George, a long-term patient labelled a "chronic schizophrenic" was given an experimental dose of chlorpromazine (Thorazine) every day:

> No one had paid George any attention for years. Now doctors, attendants and nurses all talked to him and watched eagerly to see what effect the drug would have. His condition improved rapidly. After only two weeks of the drug treatment he was moved to a ward for less disturbed patients where he took part in a number of activities. Soon he was doing so well that he was promoted again. By this time he had lively relationships with the other patients and many members of the hospital staff. He began to spend several hours a day with paints and clay, using them to express the rich fantasy life that had previously interested no one. His doctors marvelled. Attendants praised his skill. George was released from the hospital thirty-eight days after his first dose of thorazine. While he was signing out he

remembered that he had left something behind, went back to his room, and returned with an old sock. The puzzled attendant who asked to see it found thirty-eight thorazine pills carefully stashed inside the sock. Why, then, had George suddenly come to life?[266]

George's unexpected recovery is reminiscent of the remarkable awakenings which have been reported in some people receiving treatment with clozapine or other atypical neuroleptics. It is interesting to think about what it is that sometimes allows such people to come back to life after a prolonged period of deterioration, isolation, and neglect. As explained earlier, switching to drugs with fewer disabling side effects is bound to substantially increase a diagnosed person's chances of recovery. Beyond this, the aura of hopefulness that surrounds the new drugs undoubtedly makes a significant contribution to their therapeutic efficacy. Many mental health professionals, carers, and diagnosed people have come to believe that the second-generation neuroleptics offer grounds for a greater sense of hopefulness than was previously possible. Such hope, together with a general increase in positive expectations, undoubtedly helps to awaken "the doctor who resides within". Holistic physician, Dr Larry Dossey, has noted that the tendency of patients to react favourably to new treatments about which their doctors feel confident and hopeful, is a familiar phenomenon in medicine: "For centuries physicians have recognised that new drugs can seem highly effective when first introduced, but stop working after a while. This phenomenon led the famous nineteenth-century French physician Armand Trousseau to observe, 'One should use a new drug as often as possible, while it still has the power to heal.'"[267]

A kind of mirror-image of the placebo effect, a phenomenon termed the "nocebo effect", has also been observed. Thus, *negative* attitudes and expectations can increase the likelihood of eliciting adverse reactions to drugs and other kinds of treatment. It is well known, for instance, that placebo pills can have side effects that may be just as severe as those produced by real drugs, as psychopharmacology researcher Dr Gordon Claridge explains:

> The potency of the placebo is seen even more dramatically in its side effects, which can be as frequent and as unpleasant as in the case of pharmacologically active drugs. After taking a sugar-pill the individual may complain of drowsiness, staggering gait, blurred vision, urinary frequency, ringing in the ears, and a host of other symptoms including, in one case, a severe itching rash which cleared up only when the "treatment" was discontinued. As with active drugs, the frequency and severity of these effects will increase roughly in proportion with the dose given – though the lethal dosage of placebo is unknown.[268]

As well as contributing to the development of side effects, under certain circumstances the nocebo effect might significantly reduce the effectiveness of a given treatment.[269] It is also likely to play a part in the development of various untoward reactions to neuroleptic medication. Thus, it is hardly surprising to learn that people who are strongly opposed to being given psychiatric drugs sometimes experience more adverse effects than do those who readily accept them, even if they both take the same drugs in the same dosages. (It would be a mistake, however, to suggest that a diagnosed person's negative attitude to neuroleptic treatment is ultimately to blame for *every* side effect they happen to experience. These powerful drugs have a wide range of physiological effects on the brain and other parts of the body that are largely independent of the taker's attitude. Consequently they are just as likely to occur in those who willingly comply with prescribed treatment as they are in those who resist it.)

Appreciating the extent to which beliefs and attitudes can influence a person's therapeutic responses to medication highlights the potent healing power of factors such as hope, confidence, and positive expectations. It is also serves as a reminder that, far from being mere passive recipients of treatment, diagnosed people are always more actively involved than even they may realise.

The World Is The Hospital Where Healing Takes Place

True healing requires that a range of positive influences, operating in concert, exert their beneficial effects on every aspect of a person's life and being. For those diagnosed with schizophrenia, the healing process can be facilitated by maintaining a realistically hopeful attitude, learning to manage stress, adopting a healthy lifestyle, and nurturing spirituality. While not denying the invaluable contribution medical treatment can sometimes make, the focus of a holistic approach goes beyond purely clinical concerns to attend to the diagnosed person's entire being and uniquely individual identity. At a time when mental health clinicians are often inclined to focus narrowly on the use of drugs to suppress symptoms, it is heartening to find that calls occasionally come from within the ranks of mainstream psychiatry urging the adoption of a broader, more holistic approach. Such a call was made by The Group for the Advancement of Psychiatry (GAP), a consensus committee of psychiatrists widely regarded as world authorities on schizophrenia and its treatment. In a report entitled *Beyond Symptom Suppression,* these experts said:

> The introduction in the 1950s of chlorpromazine ... created a turning point in the field of psychiatry. Suddenly, pharmacological agents known as neuroleptics or antipsychotics were available to counteract the most flagrant aspects of psychosis: hallucinations, delusions, fragmented thinking ... Enthusiasm for the capacity of neuroleptic drugs to tame this symptomatology was initially so great that the very definition of schizophrenia came to rely heavily on the observation of flagrant but potentially drug-responsive psychotic symptoms ... For almost three decades the circular logic created by this situation kept a focus on the acute psychotic manifestations of schizophrenia. Many clinicians became convinced that they were successfully treating this illness when those manifestations were suppressed. *Over time it has become clear, however, that containing psychosis is only the first step in treating schizophrenia. This step must be followed by a process that aims at broader healing of the patient as a person.* Thus, clinicians must now address how best to promote the recovery process.[270]

A holistic philosophy emphasises the fact that individual healing cannot occur in isolation from the rest of life. As neurologist Oliver Sacks has suggested, "the world is the hospital where healing takes place".[271] It is vital, for example, that recovering people be willing to seek and accept the help and support of others. As well as helping to reduce distress and instil hope and positive expectations, effective social support can actually enhance the beneficial effects of neuroleptic medications. Professors Ian Falloon and Robert Liberman reached precisely this conclusion as a result of their research into the possible interactions between drug treatment and psychosocial therapies for people diagnosed with schizophrenia: "The provision of a more supportive social milieu with effective problem-solving strategies may substantially improve the efficacy achieved by neuroleptic drugs."[272] Clinicians such as Oliver Sacks have also realised that a drug's therapeutic effects, and even its side effects, can be strongly influenced by various non-drug factors, such as the treated person's overall state of health and their general sense of wellbeing.

Of all the factors which help to promote healing and recovery, the quality of the diagnosed individual's relationships with other people are undoubtedly among the most important, as pioneer psychiatrist Dr Karl Menninger has testified: "Drugs cannot inspire or encourage or comfort. Only a person can heal a person."[273] Others believe that true healing ultimately requires the presence of love in a person's life. Psychiatrist Dr Peter Breggin has expressed this notion as follows:

> In the rich experience of life, there are so many ways to heal and be healed, and they are inseparable from the overall process of learning to overcome fear and helplessness and to love life. Indeed, to *love* is to be healed: to take joy in life, to be reverent towards life, to be immersed in life, to cherish oneself and

others, animals and plants, nature and existence itself.
The paths along this way are infinite ... all of them
exploring the delicate harmonies between helplessness
and independence, scepticism and faith, reason and
emotion, self and other, human beings and nature, and,
in religious terms, between all life forms and God.[274]

The personal experiences of many diagnosed people
and their helpers have borne frequent witness to the truth
of these sentiments.

Chapter Five

TREATING ACUTE SCHIZOPHRENIA
WITHOUT DRUGS

*The "patient" needs "asylum" in the sense of sanctuary, a safe
and congenial space to be … It must be in a community of
persons who are sufficiently familiar with this inner world not to
be afraid or condemning of it.*

John Perry[275]

THE PRACTICE OF ROUTINELY administering neuroleptic drugs
to people experiencing acute psychosis has become so deeply
ingrained in contemporary psychiatry that its appropriateness is now rarely questioned. In fact, many mental health
clinicians would probably consider it heretical to even pose
the question:"Should *every* person in an acute psychotic state
automatically receive neuroleptics as the first line of treatment?" Indeed, a growing number of professionals believe
it is justified to give medication to those they consider to

be at high risk of schizophrenia even *before* such individuals have become overtly psychotic.[276] Nevertheless, if the goal of psychiatric treatment is not simply to suppress symptoms but to promote healing of the whole person, it is legitimate to examine the role of medication and to ask if it is always necessary or helpful in this endeavour.

How one answers this question will be strongly influenced by what one believes psychosis to be. Mainstream biological psychiatry has wholeheartedly embraced the view that psychosis is a severe mental "illness" caused by some kind of malfunction in the diagnosed person's brain. In line with this conceptualisation, neuroleptic drugs are usually seen as the most helpful and appropriate therapeutic intervention. In fact, many proponents of what is referred to as the "medical model" would now consider it unethical to withhold such treatment (some have recently called for a ban on research in which psychotic individuals are given a placebo rather than an active drug). So ubiquitous are these attitudes that it is now almost impossible to find people diagnosed with schizophrenia who have never had any neuroleptic medication. This is increasingly the case in non-industrialised nations as well, despite the fact that research conducted by the World Health Organisation (WHO) has shown that before such medications were widely available, psychotic individuals in developing countries often had a significantly *better* prognosis than their counterparts in Western societies.[277]

Although most mental health clinicians now take the use of these medications for granted, scientific evidence occasionally emerges which raises questions about their role and effectiveness. A study published in the *Journal of Psychopharmacology* in 1999 did precisely this. The authors, a group consisting of some of the most highly regarded authorities in the field, wanted to know what the consequences would be of a four-week delay in commencing neuroleptic treatment. In an effort to answer this question they examined what occurred to people diagnosed with schizophrenia over a period of two and a half years. Some were initially given a placebo ("sugar pill") rather than neuroleptic drugs (subjects included individuals experiencing their first psychotic episode as well as some with one or more previous episodes). The researchers surmised that, if withholding medication did have a deleterious effect, during the subsequent two and a half years those initially given placebo would spend more time in psychiatric care, receive more medication, experience a greater decline in psychological and occupational functioning, have a higher level of substance use, more contact with police, and more symptoms. None of this occurred. In fact, the research failed to demonstrate that initial placebo treatment had *any* long-term negative effects:

> Examination of the many variables in this study suggests that there is no deleterious effect of delaying treatment for a month. On follow-up, patients who had initial placebo … required no more medication during the follow-up period, had no more decline in occupation, had no more symptoms at follow-up, had no more police contacts, and indeed had as good an outcome in returning to work. *There is no evidence from this extensive analysis that a month's delay in instituting active anti-psychotic medication results in any lasting harm.*[278]

In recent years many mental health clinicians have come to accept the idea that the longer a person has been psychotic without treatment, the worse their prognosis is likely to be. Uncritical acceptance of this notion has galvanised efforts to commence neuroleptic therapy at the earliest possible opportunity. However, when researchers recently examined the relationship between the duration of untreated psychosis (defined as the interval between the first appearance of psychotic symptoms and first psychiatric hospitalisation) and clinical outcomes after two years in a group of first-admission patients, they failed to find any evidence that prolonged periods without neuroleptic treatment had the severe negative consequences many have come to expect.[279] Another study, published in the *American Journal of Psychiatry* in 2000, found no support for the notion that a period of untreated psychosis is somehow toxic to brain structure and function in first-episode schizophrenia patients.[280] For various reasons findings such as these tend to have little impact on everyday clinical practice. Similar conclusions have been reached by others over the past few decades, but they have always tended to meet a similar fate.

Lessons From The Past

It is thought provoking to contrast contemporary approaches which strongly emphasise the use of neuroleptic medication with those of earlier times. For instance, in a 1977 report published in the *American Journal of Psychiatry*, a team of research psychiatrists affiliated with the US National Institute of Health (NIH), discussed the feasibility of treating people experiencing acute psychosis with minimal use of neuroleptic medications.[281] Combining their own clinical observations with a review of then current clinical research, psychiatrists William Carpenter, Thomas McGlashan, and John Strauss were led to question some of their profession's commonest assumptions regarding the treatment of people diagnosed with acute schizophrenia. They concluded that the following widely held beliefs are both *erroneous* and *unwarranted*:

1. Such individuals must be treated with drugs and failure to do so is unethical
2. Such individuals must be maintained on drugs after symptomatic recovery
3. Relapse must be prevented because the psychotic state is somehow "toxic"
4. No major treatment emphasis beside drugs is essential for such individuals
5. Relatively few hazards are associated with the use of neuroleptic drugs

So greatly do the views of these researchers differ from current orthodoxy that is worth stressing that they were put forward, not by rabid "anti-psychiatrists" or disgruntled ex-psychiatric patients, but by doyens of mainstream psychiatry. At the time this research was conducted, Dr Carpenter and Dr McGlashan were senior psychiatrists with the US National Institute of Mental Health (NIMH), and Dr Strauss was Director of Clinical Psychiatry Research at the University of Rochester School of Medicine. Upon what grounds were their now seemingly radical claims made?

The principle conclusions were based on impressions arising from a study conducted by the authors in which 49 people with a diagnosis of schizophrenia were admitted to an experimental ward which emphasised psychosocial treatment. On admission these individuals all had a similar pattern and severity of symptoms and similar prognoses. Despite having experienced psychosis on previous occasions, most had attained a reasonable level of social and work functioning prior to the onset of their present episode. During the study, 22 patients received neuroleptic medication while 27 remained drug-free. All participated in individual psychotherapy two or three times per week, and most also had group and family therapy once a week. Interestingly, the researchers found there were *no significant differences* in the overall severity of symptoms experienced by the two groups during their hospital stay. Furthermore, the drug-treated patients spent *longer* in hospital before they were considered ready for discharge (an average of 126 days compared to 108 days for the drug-free patients). A number of significant differences between the two groups were noted in the year following discharge: the drug-free patients were *less* likely to have been re-hospitalised than drug-treated patients (35% compared to 45%) and were also *less* likely to have been given any medication in the community (44% compared to 67%). The patients who had received neuroleptic medication were also noted to be more depressed at discharge than the non-drug patients and were significantly more likely to have experienced post-psychotic depression. Reviewing their somewhat unexpected findings, these researchers said: "we have demonstrated that failing to use neuroleptics during an acute psychotic episode does not necessarily result in a disadvantageous course and outcome, and it may have some advantages."[282]

A research project carried out in a specially created ward at the Agnews State Hospital in California between 1969 and 1971 produced findings comparable to those described above. This study involved young males experiencing an acute schizophrenic episode being randomly assigned to either placebo or neuroleptic medication (chlorpromazine). While those given active medication experienced a more rapid reduction in the intensity of their psychotic symptoms, significant differences were noted in favour of the placebo-treated patients during the post-discharge follow-up period. Of the 80 individuals studied, 73% of those who had received neuroleptic medication had been re-admitted to hospital by the end of the three-year study, compared to just 8% of those originally given placebo. Furthermore, those who had only received placebo in hospital, and who had remained medication-free over the next three years, were reported to have shown the greatest clinical improvement and the lowest levels of functional disability during this time. In summarising the findings of their National Institute of Mental Health funded research, Dr Rappaport and his colleagues commented in their 1978 report that, in their experience, "Anti-psychotic medication is not the treatment of choice, at least for certain patients, if one is interested in long-term clinical improvement."[283]

The Soteria Project

A number of other carefully conducted research studies have reached similar conclusions to those summarised above.[284] One of the most interesting and important of these was referred to as the *Soteria Project*. Its director, psychiatrist Loren Mosher, was Chief of the Centre for Studies of Schizophrenia at NIMH and editor-in-chief of the *Schizophrenia Bulletin*, a highly regarded international psychiatric journal. This research ran from 1971 to 1983 and involved the establishment of a small (6 bed) community-based residence which provided a home-like sanctuary for young people recently diagnosed with schizophrenia. A central tenet of the Soteria philosophy was that acute psychosis was considered a "crisis in development" rather than the outbreak of a serious and inevitably deteriorative mental disease. In keeping with this philosophy, Soteria residents received support and guidance from a team of specially selected staff, none of whom were mental health professionals.[285] Regarding the characteristics of Soteria's support staff, Dr Mosher commented:

> Another somewhat unusual group, the non-professional staff, also lived there to provide a simple, home-like, safe, warm, supportive, unhurried, tolerant, and non-intrusive social environment. Soteria staff believed sincere human involvement and understanding were critical to healing interactions with clients. The project's purpose was to find out whether this type of milieu was as effective in promoting recovery from madness as that provided in a nearby general hospital's psychiatric ward, which was oriented toward using anti-psychotic drugs.[286]

Ordinarily, Soteria residents did not receive medication during their first six weeks in the programme. If they did not appear to be improving after this time they were given a trial period of neuroleptic treatment on a case-by-case basis. During the initial five-year study period, there were fewer than a dozen occasions on which it was deemed necessary to administer medication to a resident during their first six weeks. Overall, only 8% of all Soteria residents received a therapeutic course of neuroleptics (defined as two or more weeks of chlorpromazine or an equivalent drug). For the purposes of research, a comparison was made between those who participated in the Soteria programme, and a comparable group of young people who received standard medical treatment in a conventional psychiatric facility. As Dr Mosher reported, one of the most important – and rather unexpected – findings was that, in the first six weeks, both groups experienced a similar degree of improvement in their acute psychotic symptoms:

> To our surprise, six weeks after admission our patients and control patients [those receiving standard psychiatric treatment] are basically indistinguishable in terms of symptoms, even though one hundred percent of the control patients have had therapeutic courses of neuroleptics and no Soteria subjects had. We did not expect symptoms to be alleviated by six weeks of interpersonal intervention. We thought it would take more like six months.[287]

The Soteria residents spent an average of five months in the programme, while those receiving conventional treatment were in hospital for about one month. Two years after being discharged from their respective programmes, the two groups were compared on various criteria.[288] This analysis highlighted a number of variations which reflected the difference in effectiveness of the two forms of treatment. In brief, it was found that during the two years following discharge:

- 53% of Soteria residents had been readmitted compared to 67% of those who had received hospital treatment

- 34% of the Soteria residents had taken neuroleptic drugs continuously or intermittently compared to 95% of the hospital-treated group
- 59% of the Soteria group had received some form of psychiatric treatment compared to 100% of those treated in hospital
- Soteria residents tended to be working at a significantly higher occupational level and were more often living independently or with peers than those treated in hospital

It has been suggested that the Soteria Project and other similar endeavours are historical anomalies whose success in minimising the use of neuroleptic drugs is somehow attributable to the influence of a more benign social era, now long-gone, such as existed between the early 1960s and late 70s. However, this view is contradicted by more recent studies conducted in Switzerland by Professor Luc Ciompi and his colleagues which achieved very similar results to those of the Soteria Project. This research, reported in the *British Journal of Psychiatry* in 1992, was conducted over a period of six years and involved providing milieu therapy, psychotherapy, and sociotherapy, rather than standard drug treatment, to sixty individuals with a diagnosis of acute schizophrenia.* A key feature of this innovative project was the provision of a small, home-like environment (6-8 beds) in which residents were

---

* "Milieu therapy" involves the use of influences in a person's immediate environment – particularly the social surroundings – to foster desired therapeutic change. Environmental qualities such orderliness, structure, and predictability are known to induce feelings of calmness and tranquillity, for example, while social interactions characterised by warmth, sensitivity, and acceptance facilitate the development of trust and security.

helped to grow through the "severe developmental crisis" of acute psychosis.[289] The majority of people remained in this programme for between one and four months. During this time neuroleptics were used only if a situation arose that involved serious danger to the resident or other people, or if no improvement had occurred during the first 3 to 4 weeks after admission, or if a resident appeared to be on the verge of impending relapse which could not be prevented by any other means.

Data from 51 residents was analysed on completion of the study. Among this group, 20 had received no neuroleptic drugs whatsoever during their time in the programme, while the remaining 31 received neuroleptic treatment for approximately 2/3 of this time. Average daily medication dosage for the drug-treated residents was equivalent to 172.5 mg of chlorpromazine, which the researchers estimated to be approximately 1/3 of the usual European dosage and between 1/5-1/10 of the usual American dosage. "Surprisingly," they commented, "patients who received no or very low-dosage medication demonstrated significantly better results." Summarising their findings, Professor Ciompi's team stated that, under emotionally favourable conditions, low-dose or even drug-free treatment, in combination with psychotherapy and sociotherapy, constitutes a feasible alternative to conventional neuroleptic treatment for many people diagnosed with acute schizophrenia:

> More than six years experience with a significantly sized group of schizophrenic patients show that the innovative therapeutic approach ... is applicable to clinical practice, and in terms of immediate outcome, has been successful in about two-thirds of cases. It

is particularly interesting that for certain patients, a remission of symptoms can occur without neuroleptic medication, and that drug-free or low-dose medication strategies have been correlated with better outcomes in several respects … in a special therapeutic setting which offers adequate and continual emotional support, comparable outcome in the long-term can be achieved despite a substantial reduction in the cumulative use of medication, while some drug-free patients are found to have positive outcomes after two years of study.[290]

Gentle Bridges

The approaches described above contrast sharply with contemporary trends which insist that people experiencing acute psychosis should be given neuroleptics as early as possible, in doses sufficient to eliminate their symptoms, lest they suffer serious adverse consequences as a result of the "toxic" effects of uncontrolled psychosis. It is rather startling to realise that a substantial body of carefully conducted research appears to contravene one of the most widely accepted tenets of conventional psychiatric practice! This research is so challenging that a careful analysis of its nuances and full implications is not only warranted but necessary. It would be both unwise and premature to conclude that medication is *never* necessary or that *every* person who experiences psychosis would be better off if they simply threw away their tablets and went to a quiet place to await spontaneous healing. (Many have opted for this course only to experience unpleasant or possibly even harmful consequences.) Nevertheless, a careful and dispassionate consideration of the available evidence suggests that somewhere between these extremes – over-emphasising the importance of medication, on one hand, and failing to recognise its potential usefulness, on the other – there lies a viable middle ground.

It is especially important to appreciate that a number of factors are crucial to the success of programmes which, like Soteria, restrict the use of neuroleptic medication. In particular, this type of approach appears to be primarily suited to people who are experiencing their first or second psychotic episode, and whose prior social and occupational adjustment has been reasonably good. By contrast, people with relatively lengthy psychiatric histories characterised by extended periods of institutionalisation, isolation, and poor interpersonal functioning are, in general, more likely to benefit from involvement in highly structured, reha-bilitation-focused programmes. Professor Ciompi and his colleagues commented that Soteria–style treatment was mainly suitable for those "who did not have the chance to learn the typical roles and behavioural patterns character-istic of psychiatric in-patients".[291] Experience demonstrates, furthermore, that people who are prone to experiencing persecutory feelings and beliefs (*paranoia*) often have great difficulty making constructive use of the opportunities a therapeutic community provides due to their limited ability to accept, trust, and co-operate with their fellow residents and support staff.

The success of medication-restricted therapeutic households is critically dependent on their ability to pro-vide an environment in which healing and recovery are truly supported. In order to do this they must address the entire spectrum of resident's physical, social, psycho-logical, and spiritual needs. As stated above, various styles and combinations of individual, group, and family therapy have been utilised to this end. It is interesting to note that there were no formal therapy sessions at Soteria. Rather, as Loren Mosher has explained, staff focused on developing "non-intrusive, non-controlling, but actively empathetic relationship with the psychotic person without having to do anything explicitly therapeutic".[292] Soteria was designed to function as a community in which the environment as a whole instilled positive expectations, as well as providing residents with an opportunity to develop greater self-understanding:

> Soteria's atmosphere was imbued with the expectation that recovery from psychosis was to be expected ... Perhaps the most important therapeutic ingredient in Soteria emerged from the quality of relationships that formed, in part, because of the additional treatment time allowed. Within staff-resident relationships, an integrative context was created to promote understanding and the discovery of meaning within the subjective experience of psychosis. Residents were encouraged to acknowledge precipitating events and emotions and to discuss and eventually place them into perspective within the continuity of their life and social network.[293]

Professor Ciompi's research programme endeavoured to provide "a special therapeutic setting which offers adequate and continual emotional support". The attitudes and personal characteristics of support staff are crucially important in this regard. Staff on the Agnews State Hospital research ward were individually selected and trained: "Of primary concern was their willingness to work closely and continually with even very [disturbed] patients and to accept as much as possible (rather than avoid) their own fears and fantasies about madness." The specific aim of this research was to investigate the therapeutic effect of providing a "space" in which the residents "were given room to express their energies in relative safety", the hope being that this would help them to eventually find ways to "re-balance" themselves. In keeping with this aim, Dr Rappaport and his colleagues believed it was most important that staff members demonstrated an "awareness of their own feelings and openness to the feelings of others". Such attributes, they felt, differed from those found in many conventional hospital settings.

Jungian psychiatrist John Perry believes staff in a therapeutic household must be keenly aware that individuals experiencing acute psychosis are extremely sensitive and highly vulnerable to suggestion. As a consequence, the attitudes and emotional responses of staff members can have a decisive impact, for better or worse:

> Everyday experiences teaches all of us who work in therapy with people in the schizophrenic state ... that what is absolutely crucial to the individual who is beginning to "space out" is the emotional response of the persons in his surroundings. If they are appalled, bewildered, and afraid, and have the feeling they are separated by a yawning chasm from this individual who has drifted into another world that is no longer recognisable as part of human experience, then the individual in the plight feels himself isolated and alone. Panic seizes him when he realises he has dropped out

of the world of human communication. When his sense of identity has dissolved inevitably in his turmoil, he is completely prey to whatever image of himself happens to come onto the mental stage. If he is looked upon by those around him as insane and crazy, that is exactly what he "becomes"; that is, it is the image he adopts of himself, and his behaviour will give expression to that. The other way, if he has friends who are not at all appalled at what he is undergoing ... and they regard it instead as an impressive and fascinating experience even if uncomfortable, then the individual does not feel crazy and does not act so.[294]

Dr Perry emphasised the need for support staff to "be trained in relating to the individual's altered state of consciousness and all his inner preoccupations as much as possible without anxiety and without pressure to make him conform to any expectation." It is essential, he adds, that their repertoire of skills should include the ability to know "how to let the individual alone when he needs to be."[295]

Psychosis: Mental Illness or Psychological Crisis?

A key feature of the Soteria philosophy was the adoption of a non-medical concept of psychosis. As well as helping to reduce some of the fear, stigma, and hopelessness that is so often associated with a psychiatric diagnosis, it was hoped that encouraging residents to view their experience as the manifestation of a profound "life crisis" would galvanise their desire to see this difficult period as an opportunity for change, growth, and personal development.

Few people today are aware that there is a long and rich tradition in psychiatry in which acute psychosis has been viewed, not as a mental illness *per se*, but as a profound psychological or psychospiritual crisis containing the possibility for positive as well as negative consequences. In this view, psychosis is considered to be a state of extreme "dis-ease" rather than a medical disease. (It is thought provoking to reflect on the fact that the medical term *psychosis* is derived from an ancient Greek word meaning "give soul or life to".) Psychiatrists of the stature of Carl Jung, Harry Stack Sullivan, Karl Menninger, Frieda Fromm-Reichman, and Silvano Arieti, together with many others whose professional stature is recognised internationally, founded this approach and based their treatment methods upon it. In recent years, this tradition has been carried on and developed by reputable psychiatrists and clinical psychologists such as Professor Manfred Bleuler, Professor David Lukoff, Dr John Perry, Dr Stanislav Grof, Dr Edward Podvoll, and Dr John Nelson. While the views of these pioneers have received scant attention from their more orthodox colleagues, it is heartening to note that, in recent years, the importance of attending to spiritual aspects of healing have occasionally been acknowledged in mainstream psychiatric literature.[296]

After experiencing a number of severe psychotic episodes for which she was treated with neuroleptic medication, Maryanne Handel formed a view remarkably consistent with those held by the highly regarded authorities mentioned above. Despite the very painful and at times emotionally overwhelming nature of her ordeals, she nevertheless considered her psychosis to be a "meaningful disturbance" from which she learnt a great deal:

Maybe there is a disturbance in your brain. But if that is so, then it must mean something about your brain, that it's indicating something about your emotional state. What is it indicating? What does it mean? My feeling was that the psychosis was there to teach me something. And it did teach me something! It did show me things and I did change through it and because of it I understood many things. Things I suppose that had always been wrong which perhaps I never would have come to understand if the psychosis had not happened to me, if I had not been through that absolute process. Maybe I would have gone on without ever really changing that much. I think, yes, it's a disturbance of course, but its a *meaningful* disturbance, and something that has to be understood before you can change and before it will go away.[297]

Treating psychosis as an opportunity for learning, growth, and healing, takes great courage and a willingness to face problems honestly. Therapeutic households which aim to foster personal growth strongly emphasise the need for residents to take responsibility for themselves and make a sincere commitment to doing the work of recovery. While it would generally be counter-productive to attempt to *force* people to confront personal issues raised by their psychotic experiences, a stable and emotionally supportive environment provides those who wish to "work on themselves" with a safe place to do so. Although most contemporary treatment approaches tend to actively discourage diagnosed people from exploring their psychotic experiences, there is reason to believe that, for some people at least, doing so may be beneficial. In a report published in the *American Journal of Psychiatry*, the researchers from the National Institute of Health (NIH), whose work was referred to earlier, explained that, while those who had participated in drug-free treatment often found it emotionally demanding, many also said that it was personally rewarding:

> These data suggest that patients found the NIH therapeutic program significantly different from programs they had participated in in other hospitals. Generally, [they] reported experiencing more anguish with our treatment approach, whereas they felt a greater sense of frustration and of being "frozen in the psychosis" in settings emphasising drug treatment. Many ... found their social experiences in the NIH ward both gratifying and informative, and they reported that their lives had been enhanced as a result of their therapeutic experience. A few patients made negative assessments; they felt their psychosis was destructive and their attempts to understand it were of no value.[298]

Individual Recovery Styles

The fact that some people feel they benefited from drug-free treatment, while others said they did not find it helpful, highlights the importance of providing a *range* of therapeutic options to people in acute psychosis. In particular, it is crucial to respect the fact that human beings vary considerably in terms of how they respond to and cope with disturbing experiences. Researchers have identified two distinct recovery styles in recently psychotic individuals which they have termed "integrating" and "sealing-over" respectively.[299] It has been noted that some people actively avoid talking about their psychosis and endeavour to put it all behind them as quickly as possible, i.e. the sealing-over recovery style. Others feel curious about their experiences and seek to understand and learn from them, i.e. the integrating recovery style. Therapeutic communities such as Soteria aimed to accommodate *both* recovery styles. Dr Mosher has pointed out that, while only around 60% of the Soteria residents chose to "face" their psychotic experiences, the community philosophy respected resident's personal choices in this matter:

> Some people who come to Soteria want nothing to do with their madness; they spend all their time running as fast as they can away from it, and that is all right. But if they feel that they in some way want to go through that process without anybody trying to abort it or force it into some pigeon hole or divert it, then we allow them to try to do this.[300]

By contrast, conventional psychiatric treatment settings tend to support the sealing-over recovery style. As a result, those who may wish to explore their experiences are often discouraged (either actively or passively) from doing so. This discrimination is often rationalised on therapeutic grounds – diagnosed individuals may be told it is potentially dangerous to their mental health to delve into such things. However, some commentators believe that many clinicians consciously or unconsciously encourage their clients to seal-over because this recovery style is less personally and professionally challenging.[301]

Containment Versus Suppression

It is important to emphasise that holistically oriented treatment does *not* necessarily totally prohibit the use of neuroleptic or other psychotropic medications. In both the Soteria Project and Professor Luc Ciompi's programme, neuroleptics were used in certain circumstances. When necessary, such drugs can provide a rapid and often highly effective means of controlling agitation, violent "acting out", self-injury, and other kinds of dangerous or threatening behaviour, whether directed at self or others. In some cases, on-going use of medication may be needed to ameliorate debilitating anxiety or to provide hypersensitive individuals with necessary protection against the impact of stress (the stress-buffering effect of neuroleptics).

While it is acknowledged that they may be very useful in certain circumstances, drugs are nevertheless assigned a different role in the context of holistic treatment than they are given in most contemporary clinical settings. The difference is largely a matter of emphasis. Thus, rather than giving medication simply to suppress unwanted behaviours, the real value of neuroleptics may lie in using them judiciously as one means of helping people contain rampant emotions and other distressing experiences by rendering them more manageable:

> One should also note … how medication was needed to help settle the patient's state of mind. Anti-psychotic medication viewed at a psychological level helps to provide a calming-down effect, so that emotions can be contained rather than continue to be violently projected. Medication does not have to be seen as just

producing a mental straight-jacket or as an alternative to dialogue, but can be recognised as facilitative within the rehabilitative process. In other words, medication should be considered for its helpful effects, rather than as a short cut to avoid meaningful emotional involvement with the patient.[302]

When combined with appropriate psychological support and guidance, this way of using medication allows people an opportunity to develop a better understanding of themselves and their experiences. This, in turn, is bound to provide them with a significantly enhanced ability to deal with their problems in a more balanced and constructive manner.

Considerable clinical and anecdotal evidence indicates that *some* acute psychotic episodes are self-limiting.[303] In other words, they only continue for a certain length of time before beginning to gradually "wind down" by themselves. People whose first contact with a mental health service happens to occur when they are at the *peak* of a self-limiting psychotic episode would be expected to improve spontaneously without any specific treatment, simply by spending a little time in a safe, protected, low-stimulus environment. As with colds and 'flu, providing the individual concerned with rest and appropriate support may be all that is required. The conventional psychiatric policy of administering psychotropic medication immediately upon admission, may inadvertently remove the chance to discover if natural self-healing processes would have been sufficient to resolve such a psychotic crisis, without the need for neuroleptic drugs.

Towards A Neuroleptic Nation

A considerable body of reputable psychiatric research has demonstrated that, in optimal therapeutic and social circumstances, people diagnosed with schizophrenia are often able to manage well with less medication.[304] Psychiatrist Richard Warner has summarised this research and commented on some of its major implications as follows:

> William Carpenter's study at the National Institute of Health and Loren Mosher's Soteria House ... demonstrated that the same observation holds true for young acute schizophrenics. Active, individualised, psychosocial treatment programs render anti-psychotic drug therapy unnecessary for a substantial number of patients ... psychosocial treatment programs [on] William Carpenter's research ward or at Soteria House were comprehensive attempts to shape a total therapeutic residential environment in such a way as to maximise the psychotic patients' chances of recovery ... We may conclude that when schizophrenics are in an environment which is protective but not regressive, stimulating but not stressful, and warm but not intrusive (whether it be their own family home or a residential treatment unit) many of these patients will not need anti-psychotic treatment. On the other hand, schizophrenics who are exposed to significant stress ... will have a high relapse rate and will require substantial doses of neuroleptic drugs to achieve minimal functioning levels. In Western society in recent decades, too few ... have been placed in the more therapeutic settings identified here.[305]

Sadly, rather than providing the kind of therapeutic environments that have been *proven* to be beneficial to people in the throes of acute psychosis, many modern treatment settings tend to do exactly the opposite. As Dr Mosher notes, "Psychiatric hospitals [are] not usually very good places in which to be insane".[306] Thus, people immersed in the emotional turmoil of a psychotic episode often find themselves cast (or dragged) into a hospital ward, in which their fears and confusion may be greatly exacerbated. Research has shown that the experience of involuntary hospitalisation and enforced treatment can be so stressful for some newly diagnosed people that it may even cause them to develop a post-traumatic stress disorder (PTSD).[307] Despite the best intentions of hospital staff and other helpers (such as police, ambulance crews, and relatives), newly admitted people are often assailed by a multitude of stimuli at the very time they are most in need of calmness and simplicity. In these circumstances, an escalating cycle of anxiety and emotional chaos can quickly develop and become self-perpetuating. Rather than providing people who are distressed and often highly agitated with the soothing and tranquil environments they so desperately need, most contemporary treatment settings have come to rely almost exclusively on pharmaceutical means to restore order and impose a degree of calm, i.e. chemical tranquillisation. Professor Ciompi's account of the kind of scenario that is typical of modern psychiatric care would be sadly familiar to many:

> In the acute [psychotic] phase patients are, as a rule, exposed to an appalling lack of continuity as far as environment and human contacts are concerned. In

the course of a few weeks they may pass through three or four hospital departments, each with its own staff, and in addition be exposed to the incessant coming and going of equally bewildered fellow patients. In other words, the already confused psychotic patient is overwhelmed by new impressions which would be difficult to handle even for a healthy person. Obviously, all this adds to fear, tension, and confusion which then have to be controlled by massive doses of neuroleptics and measures of restraint. The result is a vicious circle which increasingly affects the remaining healthy coping abilities. When the patient leaves the hospital the lack of continuity is even more pronounced.[308]

Many factors have contributed to shaping the way in which contemporary psychiatry views and responds to people experiencing acute psychosis. Some of the most influential of these deserve special comment. Over the past several decades a concerted effort has been made by a vast number of dedicated researchers to strengthen psychiatry's scientific foundations. As enlightening as this endeavour has been in certain ways, there are many who now feel that in its desire to be (and to be seen as) more scientific, psychiatry has become increasingly depersonalised. Indeed, in the highly technical language in which psychosis and schizophrenia are now discussed it is rare to find any reference to the *subjective* aspects of these quintessentially human experiences. Thus, vital matters such as the diagnosed person's feelings, his or her beliefs about the meaning of it all – to say nothing of the possible spiritual issues involved – tend to be completely ignored.

Psychiatrist Edward Podvoll believes a serious consequence of the growing "industrialisation of mental health" is the way modern treatment settings now inadvertently "promote a fear of the intimate relationships that are so precious and vital to the recovery from madness."[309] Adding further to this trend toward a more impersonal approach is a range of powerful social, economic, and political forces. These include the desire of health bureaucrats to minimise the cost of providing services and the ever-growing influence of the pharmaceutical industry.

One of the most decisive factors of all is the firmly entrenched hegemony of biological psychiatry which champions the view that *all* mental disorders – especially the more extreme kinds such as psychosis – are a purely physiological phenomenon, the end result of a malfunctioning or "broken" brain.[310] This narrow focus has had a range of negative consequences. Psychiatrist Colin Ross has said:

> Globally in psychiatry, I think, we have become sloppy clinicians in our study of schizophrenia because of the biological model of the illness. The tendency now is away from spending any amount of time talking with the schizophrenic patient in an attempt to understand his or her *mind*. Once we check off a few symptoms, make the diagnosis, and start medication, detailed study of the psychosis becomes clinically irrelevant, in much of daily practice. One monitors the patient only carefully enough to track treatment response, which is usually not very carefully. There is no reason to try to understand the patient's mind in detail, as there is in a long-term psychotherapy case, because the

symptoms are just biologically driven craziness that needs to be suppressed with medication.[311]

Clinicians working in contemporary psychiatric treatment settings often find themselves overwhelmed by time-constraints, burdened with unrealistically large caseloads, and subjected to frequent administrative demands to maximise their therapeutic "efficiency" in order to meet service goals. Constant exposure to these stressful and dehumanising influences, among a multitude of others, can eventually drive even the most sensitive, thoughtful, and caring practitioners to resort to "band-aid" solutions, despite their most heart-felt beliefs and intentions.

Psychiatry's Sacred Cow

In the early 1970s, pioneer psychiatrist Dr John Perry founded an innovative residential community called "Diabasis", where an attempt was made to provide a therapeutic milieu based on a Jungian understanding of psychosis.[312] Originally funded by Mental Health Services of San Francisco, the community eventually closed due to lack of adequate financial support. Some years later, Dr Perry described Diabasis as having been "one of the most beautiful experiences of community in my life" and "a natural expression of the kindly and humane atmosphere of the culture of that era"; an era he felt stood in stark contrast to the hard-nosed economic, political, and professional realities that had come to prevail by the end of the millennium:

> It is a matter of great grief now ... to behold the sharp decline in the quality of care of persons undergoing the acute episode. There is ever less funding, and therefore

little patience at the administrative level, for innovative programs that keep persons in a facility for more than a few days. Conveniently for the profession, this can be rationalised plausibly enough by an explanation for the occurrence of such episodes in terms of faulty brain chemistry to be corrected by a counter-chemistry. A blind eye and deaf ear are given to the obvious fact that no one hears the persons, their problems or their processes, or even seems to have time or inclination to relate to them. In this way, a lifetime of rejection becomes repeated where one is most poignantly needful of its opposite, a caring reception and affirmation.[313]

As acknowledged earlier, on one level the growing range of atypical neuroleptics that are now available promises to materially improve the quality of the medical aspects of schizophrenia treatment. Psychiatry's latest "pharmaceutical revolution" has nevertheless cast a shadow which has tended to obscure the lessons of the past. Despite the fact that Dr Loren Mosher and his colleagues took great care to document their findings in a rigorous scientific manner, the clinical implications of this work have largely been ignored, even though their essential validity has been confirmed by Professor Ciompi's more recent research. Soteria was finally forced to close in 1983. In a recent review of his work, Dr Mosher reflected on its fate:

> Despite many publications (37 in all), without an active treatment facility Soteria disappeared from the consciousness of American psychiatry. Its message was difficult for the field to acknowledge, assimilate, and use. It did not fit into the emerging scientific,

descriptive, biomedical character of American psychiatry, and, in fact, called nearly every one of its tenets into question. In particular, it demedicalised, dehospitalised, deprofessionalised, and deneurolepticised what Szasz has called "psychiatry's sacred cow" – schizophrenia. As far as mainstream American psychiatry is concerned, it is, to this day, an experiment that appears to be the object of studied neglect.[314]

It would appear that the prospect of a drug-mediated quick fix has become so tantalising that contemporary psychiatry has chosen to overlook the fact that a substantial body of research has demonstrated the powerful anti-psychotic effect of quiet, supportive, low-stimulus environments. In this context it is timely to remember that the term "asylum" was given to forerunners of modern psychiatric hospitals precisely because one of their simple purposes was to provide their disturbed (and sometimes disturbing) occupants with a place of safety, refuge, and sanctuary.

Many people feel frustrated with the present lack of Soteria-style therapeutic households or even of hospital wards that embody a truly holistic spirit. It is difficult to see this state of affairs changing without a groundswell of popular support from those who would potentially use or work in such facilities.* At the clinical

---

* A number of facilities based on the Soteria model have been established in Europe. Researchers in Finland have reported good outcomes with comprehensive psychosocial programmes involving minimal or no use of neuroleptic drugs. See Lehtinen, V. et al. (2000) 'Two-Year Outcome In First-Episode Psychosis Treated According To An Integrated Model. Is Immediate Neuroleptisation Always Needed?' *European Psychiatry*, Vol. 15, Issue 5, pp. 312-320. In the USA, Windhorse Associates is pioneering a whole-person approach to recovery from psychiatric disorders. See www. windhorseassociates.org for information.

level, progress toward developing more effective ways of helping people who experience acute psychosis, may depend on the collective willingness of the mental health professions to give open-minded consideration to the import of Dr Mosher's pioneering research. The Soteria community's decidedly low-tech approach provided the residents with a safe space in which to recover at their own pace and in their own way. As well as raising challenging questions about the nature and causes of psychosis, the positive results of the innovative research described in this chapter point toward a profoundly important possibility: that the human psyche possesses an innate self-healing capacity, and that recovery from certain kinds of acute psychosis is largely an autonomous process that can be fostered by the timely provision of sensitive support and empathic understanding. This theme is explored further in the final chapter of this book. In the meanwhile, the complex and challenging issue of long-term treatment must be addressed.

Chapter Six

MAINTENANCE NEUROLEPTIC TREATMENT

Maintenance regimes are now common practice in psychiatry but it is clear that not all patients benefit equally: there are those who relapse in spite of medication and those who remain well without medication.

Max Birchwood et al.[315]

PEOPLE DIAGNOSED WITH SCHIZOPHRENIA are now routinely advised to take neuroleptic medication on a long-term basis in order to maximise their chances of achieving and maintaining psychological and emotional stability. The recommended duration of such treatment varies considerably. Typically it ranges anywhere from a minimum of one or two years for those who have recently experienced their first psychotic episode, through to very much longer periods. Many people are eventually told they will need to take medication indefinitely, possibly for the rest of their life. Psychiatrists make no claim that this "maintenance treatment" will result in a cure. Rather, long-term administration of neuroleptic medication is often likened to giving insulin to people with diabetes to help control the symptoms of a life-long illness.

Many diagnosed individuals question their need for long-term medication, especially those who are told they will always need it. People who, for various reasons, do not believe medication is really necessary or helpful, are often understandably reluctant to continue taking it, particularly when troublesome side effects are involved. Medication non-compliance is consequently a major issue in the mental health field and a frequent cause of disagreement between prescribers and those they treat. Similar conflicts also occur in families, often because the diagnosed person and his or her relatives disagree about the need for or value of on-going treatment. Medication non-compliance or outright refusal is often ascribed to the diagnosed person's "lack of insight" and may lead to use of various coercive measures, such as enforced administration of neuroleptics by long-acting injection. Such measures are undoubtedly justified in *certain* circumstances, e.g. when the safety and/or wellbeing of the diagnosed person and others is clearly endangered, and the threat cannot reasonably be dealt with in less coercive ways. Such exceptional situations notwithstanding, there are nevertheless good reasons to question the psychiatric status quo regarding the role of maintenance neuroleptic treatment. Indeed, as this chapter will show, a substantial body of scientific research challenges the idea that most diagnosed people require long-term medical treatment if they are to have any hope of recovering and remaining well.

Frequently Asked Questions

Neuroleptic medication is given on an on-going or maintenance basis for two principal reasons:

- Its *therapeutic* effects, i.e. to alleviate persistent positive and negative symptoms
- Its *prophylactic* effects, i.e. to prevent relapse into further acute psychotic episodes

Some of the questions most frequently asked about neuroleptics – such as what these drugs actually do and what their side effects are – were addressed in earlier chapters. People receiving long-term treatment (and their relatives and friends) also often ask the following questions:

1. How long will I have to continue taking this medication?
2. What dosage do I need? Will it always remain the same?
3. Will I ever be able to safely stop taking this medication?

For various reasons it is difficult to provide specific answers to these important questions. Not the least of these is the fact that people vary tremendously, both in terms of what led to them being diagnosed with schizophrenia in the first place, and in regard to the nature and severity of their on-going difficulties. As research summarised in the previous chapter made clear, at least in the case of those acute psychotic episodes which are manifestations of a profound life crisis, the use of medication can be kept to a minimum – and possibly even avoided altogether – if appropriate emotional support is provided, in the context of a low-stress, home-like therapeutic environment. By contrast, some people continue to experience "positive" psychotic symptoms, such as hostile or intrusive voices (auditory hallucinations), irrational or reality-distorting beliefs (delusions), and distressing feelings, long after an acute psychotic episode has ended. (Interestingly, many people are entirely free of such symptoms between episodes.) Many diagnosed people also have persistent difficulties related to negative symptoms such as lack of motivation, severely reduced emotional responsiveness, and social isolation.

When discussing maintenance neuroleptic treatment it is important to appreciate that the needs of individuals who have only had a single psychotic episode are bound to be rather different from those of people who have experienced several or, in some cases, *many* such episodes. Most importantly, those who have not previously experienced psychosis have no clear "track record" on which clinicians can base predictions about their future, nor do they have an established history of individual medication responsiveness. These considerations mean that decisions about on-going treatment can only be made on an empirical basis, i.e. experimenting to find out what works best. In recent years a great deal of energy has been devoted to trying to determine the most appropriate strategies for the medical management of what is known as "first-episode" or "early" psychosis. Although considerable differences of opinion still exist, a number of general principles have begun to emerge from this important research.

Treatment of "Early" Psychosis

It has long been known that at least 25% of people diagnosed with schizophrenia only experience one psychotic
episode.[316] While neuroleptics may be helpful during a
period of psychotic turmoil (assuming Soteria-style care is
not available), such individuals do *not* require long-term
medication to ensure their psychological stability or to prevent them becoming psychotic again. At present it is not
easy to readily differentiate those who have had a one-off
experience from those who may be susceptible to further
psychotic episodes. Currently, the only practical way to
determine whether or not a newly diagnosed individual
might benefit from on-going medication, is to observe
what occurs when they stop taking it. One psychiatrist
widely regarded as an authority on schizophrenia, Dr Fuller
Torrey, has recommended that, within a few weeks of
symptomatic recovery, everyone who has experienced
psychosis for the first time should have their medication
slowly reduced and then stopped, in order to determine
whether or not they actually need such treatment on an on-
going basis. Only those who develop psychotic symptoms
during such a trial should be re-commenced on medication.[317] Dr Torrey suggests that these individuals should
remain on medication for several months, before another
drug-free trial is attempted. In his opinion, those whose
symptoms recur on this second occasion may need long-
term neuroleptic treatment (for at least several years).

In earlier times, when psychiatric hospital admissions
were measured in months rather than days, such an experiment could have been carried out easily and safely. Most
newly diagnosed people would have received in-patient
care for some time after their psychotic symptoms abated,

and would therefore have been under constant professional observation and supervision. Although long hospital stays are now relatively unusual, if adequate support can be made available, it should be possible to carry out this type of experiment outside a hospital without too much difficulty. Something of this kind was done in a study published in the *British Journal of Psychiatry* in 1986, which described the treatment of 120 people experiencing their first admission for schizophrenia. After first being stabilised on medication in hospital, these people all continued taking neuroleptic drugs for one month after discharge. Subsequently, half continued on medication while the others were gradually switched to inactive placebo. Neither the patients nor those treating them knew who was receiving active drugs and who had received placebo. The researchers reported that during the two-year follow-up period, 58% of those on active medication experienced a relapse, compared to 70% of those whose neuroleptic treatment had been stopped.[318] These findings suggest that while remaining on medication can reduce the overall likelihood of re-experiencing psychosis, a sizeable proportion of newly diagnosed people will *not* relapse, even if they do not take neuroleptic drugs. In the above study, almost one third (30%) of the drug-free patients did *not* experience relapse. On the other hand, 58% of those who remained on medication *did* relapse, thus demonstrating that the prophylactic effect of these drugs is limited.

When a more detailed analysis of the above study was done some years later, a number of unexpected findings emerged. It was noted, for example, that those who had received the placebo treatment had accrued a significantly greater number of life achievements than those given drugs. In particular, it was found that the occupational functioning of those who had had symptoms for less than a year before commencing neuroleptic treatment had been significantly *better* when they were receiving placebo. In a report in the *British Journal of Psychiatry* in 1990, the researchers commented that this observation highlights the need to be wary of indiscriminate use of neuroleptic medication among those experiencing their first psychotic episode:

> It suggests the disquieting conclusion that the benefits of active neuroleptics in reducing relapse may exact a price in occupational terms. This emphasises the need to find more effective means of predicting which patients derive benefit from maintenance neuroleptics and which do not.[319]

Most reputable authorities now believe that schizophrenia is actually a *group* of somewhat similar conditions, among which is a sub-group with an inherently favourable prognosis. Those who experience what is known as "reactive" or "good-prognosis" schizophrenia would generally be expected to recover relatively quickly and remain well *without the long-term use of medication*.[320] No reliable guidelines have yet been formulated which would allow such persons to be confidently identified among all those who have experienced psychosis for the first time. Since it is impossible to predict what anyone's future may hold, many clinicians tend to err on the side of caution and advise that, as a precautionary measure, *all* newly diagnosed people should remain on neuroleptic medication for some time after their first psychotic episode has ended. Some psychiatrists feel that a few months is sufficient (see Dr Torrey's recommendations above), whereas others favour a substantially longer period before a reduction in dosage is considered. The Royal Australian and New Zealand College of Psychiatrists has recently recommended continuing medication for at least 12 months following a first psychotic episode, and only attempting a gradual reduction thereafter if the treated person is completely symptom free.[321] It should be noted that while a more conservative approach may result in a generally lower incidence of subsequent relapse, it comes at the cost of exposing a substantial number of people to prolonged drug treatment they probably do not need.

Treatment of Persistent Symptoms

People with persistent positive symptoms (hallucinations, delusions) are often given neuroleptic medications on an on-going basis, possibly indefinitely, in the hope that it will help alleviate these frequently distressing and sometimes even disabling experiences. This medication *does* sometimes help to ameliorate such symptoms, an effect that is doubtless partly due to its ability to induce a state of psychic indifference. Rather than completely eradicating the symptoms, however, what the drugs often do is to reduce their intensity or frequency somewhat, so that they become more tolerable and less problematic. For instance, some people continue hearing voices while taking medication, but find that the voices become quieter or less intrusive. Likewise, delusional beliefs may lose some of their intensity and tend to fade into the background. Dampened-down symptoms tend to cause less anxiety and distress, thus making it easier for an affected person to ignore them and focus their energy and attention on other things.

While some unfortunate people are severely troubled by persistent positive symptoms, these are often far less of a concern in the long-term than are negative symptoms, since the latter, even when relatively mild, can seriously compromise social and occupational functioning. It is not clear to what extent drugs can realistically be expected to help with negative symptoms since a host of emotional and psychological factors play a major role in the development and persistence of these difficulties.[322] The psychological and emotional consequences of poor self-esteem, loss of self-confidence, demoralisation, and absence of a clear sense of meaning and purpose in life are far more problematic for many people than are delusions, hallucinations and other kinds of symptoms for which neuroleptics may be helpful. Psychiatrist Edward Podvoll believes one of the primary complaints of many people living in the community is a stultifying boredom that is often more problematic than are psychotic symptoms. In his view, excessive sleeping and abuse of stimulants and other mind-altering drugs is often the result of deeply felt boredom and frustration.[323] As one person with first-hand experience of this situation commented wryly: "Chronic schizophrenia is not delusions and hallucinations – it's daytime television".

Though it is now often claimed that atypical neuroleptics provide effective treatment for negative symptoms, in reality their effectiveness in this regard is rather modest. As explained in *Chapter Three*, the fact that the newer drugs do sometimes appear to help with these problems is in large part due to the fact that they tend to cause fewer negative symptom-mimicking side effects like sedation, lethargy, and akinesia. It should be pointed out that neuroleptic medication may help to ameliorate "secondary" negative symptoms that have developed as a response to stress, anxiety, or distressing positive symptoms. For instance, people who have used various degrees of social withdrawal or emotional "shut-down" to help them cope with hostile, attacking voices or anxiety-provoking persecutory beliefs (delusions), may feel less need to protect themselves in this way if the distress provoked by these painful experiences has been muted by drugs.

In summarising what is known about the post-acute therapeutic effects of neuroleptics, Dr Nina Schooler, a world authority on medical treatment of schizophrenia, has stated that "In general, overall improvement continues up to six months in drug-treated patients, although the increments in improvement are smaller with succeeding weeks."[324] While many people feel that neuroleptic medication does help to alleviate their symptoms, it is nevertheless clear that many people do *not* gain much benefit from this treatment. Clinical research has established that at least 30% of people gain only limited therapeutic benefit from these drugs, while 20% or more experience no beneficial effects whatever. It has been estimated that over 50% of diagnosed people continue to experience some persistent positive symptoms despite taking neuroleptics, and that these drugs are unlikely to have further ameliorative effects on any symptoms, positive or negative, still present after a year of treatment.[325] It is worth emphasising that, even if long-term medication does not completely eradicate persistent symptoms, it may nevertheless help keep them in check, e.g. by reducing their intensity or frequency.

To the extent that it helps to prevent such symptoms from becoming worse, maintenance treatment can play a role in helping to forestall relapse.

As explained in *Chapter Four*, it is now clear that some diagnosed people are able to utilise various *non-drug* strategies and techniques to successfully prevent or control disturbing voices and other persistent positive symptoms.[326] A wide range of similar strategies may also help to prevent or reduce negative symptoms.[237] In some instances, these methods have been used as an adjunct to regular medication, while in others they have proven effective on their own. However, as David Healy has noted, in the medication-oriented climate of contemporary psychiatry, very little interest has been shown in exploring the full potential of non-drug self-help techniques:

> In recent years there have been hints of a growing awareness on the part of some researchers that many people with schizophrenia have been handling their illness quite successfully for years, often without the aid of the caring professions. Surveys have been done on the management of hallucinations, delusions and basic disturbances by a number of groups, with findings that suggest that many patients have worked out strategies for the management of these difficulties. But evidence from patients as to what works is accorded very low priority. It should be possible to work towards a management package ... such a therapeutic approach would lead to a handing back of control of these illnesses to those who are affected. [328]

Relapse Prevention

Even if they do not have symptoms which persist between acute episodes, most diagnosed people are advised to remain on medication to reduce their risk of experiencing a recurrence of psychosis. Indeed, the main reason neuroleptic medication is given to people who are stable ("in remission") is to prevent symptom exacerbation or relapse. It is not uncommon for those who feel okay to conclude (and some may even insist) that, since they are well, there is no need for them to continue taking medication. Often they are met with statements such as, "You are only well *because* of the medication and if you stop taking it you will get sick again". As with many other issues pertaining to schizophrenia treatment, the reality is rather more complex than such simplistic interpretations would suggest. In fact, diagnosed people who believe they no longer need medication in order to stay well are *sometimes* quite correct. On the other hand, some who stop medication are likely to experience a significantly increased risk of becoming psychotic again. As is the case with early psychosis, trying to predict who will do well without long-term medication and who may be at risk if they stop taking it, is fraught with difficulty.

For various reasons, statements about maintenance neuroleptic treatment tend to emphasise its effectiveness in reducing the likelihood of relapse. It is clear, however, that not all people are at equal risk in this regard, nor do all benefit equally from long-term treatment. Indeed, it has been found that some people diagnosed as "chronic schizophrenics" are able to manage well without medication, while others will experience relapse despite taking it exactly as recommended. Though the facts surrounding

these issues are complex, they have such important implications for long-term treatment that they are worth
considering in some detail.

Since neuroleptics were introduced in the early 1950s,
psychiatrists have wanted to know how long people need
to remain on these medications to ensure their on-going
stability. In an effort to provide definitive answers to the
question of what happens when diagnosed individuals stop
the medication, researchers recently analysed the findings
of 66 studies carried out between 1958 and 1993. These
compared the relapse rates of people whose medication
had been withdrawn with those who remained on maintenance treatment. This research, based on studies of 4,365
patients (most of whom had long treatment histories), is
arguably the most comprehensive review of this subject
ever undertaken. *Table One* shows cumulative relapse
rates as reported in the highly regarded journal, *Archives of
General Psychiatry*, in 1995.[329]

TABLE ONE

Time Elapsed in months	Neuroleptic Withdrawal: Percent relapsed	Neuroleptic Maintenance: Percent relapsed
3	44%	6%
6	49%	11%
9	52%	14%
12	54%	17%
18	57%	22%
24	59%	27%

Source: Jeste et al. 1995[330]

If it is assumed that these findings are broadly applicable to everyone diagnosed with schizophrenia, it seems clear that, on the whole, those who remain on neuroleptic medication are significantly less likely to experience relapse than those who do not. For example, according to these figures, almost one in every two people (49%) who stop medication will experience a relapse within six months, while just over one in ten (11%) who stay on medication will do so in the same period. Those who have not had medication for 12 months are more than three times as likely to experience relapse as those who have remained on it (54% versus 17%). Almost 60% of people will relapse within two years of stopping their medication, while just over one quarter (27%) of those who continue taking it will do so. Judging by this data the benefits of neuroleptic maintenance seem quite clear, as do the risks of stopping treatment. Indeed, statements to this effect are glibly reported in numerous professional publications and reiterated *ad infinitum* in a host of educational materials aimed at lay audiences such as psychiatric clients and their families. For various complex reasons, many people choose to accept the validity these pronouncements without question. Those who are prepared to look a little more deeply into these matters will discover that there are important though usually overlooked facts which cast them in a rather different light.

(a) Statistics can be misleading
It is important to understand that statistics can be highly misleading. Research such as that cited above is based on the analysis of large amounts of data and, with this type of inquiry, the larger the number of subjects involved in a

particular study, the more reliable the findings are considered to be. It should be remembered that studies of relapse rates can do no more than reveal broad patterns and general trends. This information needs to be interpreted with great care since research participants rarely conform to a stereotypical "average" or "statistical norm". It must be understood that the data summarised in *Table One* refer to groups as a whole and *not to specific individuals*. For example, while it has been stated that 59% of people diagnosed with chronic schizophrenia will relapse within two years if they stop medication, this does not mean that *every* such individual has exactly the same chance of experiencing relapse. In fact, variations in personal characteristics and individual circumstances (some of which are discussed later), could mean that some people will have a much *greater* than 59% chance of relapsing without medication, while others have a much *smaller* risk than this. Since every human being is a unique individual whose life is shaped by a host of interacting influences – some of which are far too subtle to measure – statistical analyses of relapse rates can provide little reliable information about specific individuals and their likely future prospects.

(b) The concept of relapse is poorly defined

Researchers have long been interested in trying to discover how effective neuroleptic drugs are at preventing relapse and how long they should be taken to attain maximum benefit. Answering these questions is not a straightforward matter, however. For a start, a great deal depends on how relapse is defined. Some studies have defined relapse in terms of re-hospitalisation, i.e. a diagnosed person is considered to have relapsed if they have been readmitted to hospital. In others, a substantial exacerbation of symptoms is deemed to qualify as a relapse. The fact that researchers have often been referring to rather different things when discussing "relapse" means that a considerable degree of uncertainty pervades this entire body of psychiatric knowledge. Furthermore, the mere presence or absence of relapse is a very crude way of measuring the success or failure of treatment. It is conceivable, for instance, that a diagnosed person who has stopped medication might subsequently relapse but do so after experiencing an extended period of mental stability and satisfactory social functioning. Such a person might be discharged from hospital after a brief stay and return to their previous level of functioning relatively quickly. On the other hand, it is possible that some people who have remained on maintenance medication *without* experiencing relapse are deemed to be treatment successes despite doing poorly in certain regards. In this group it is not uncommon to find individuals with a low level of social and occupational functioning, severe and persistent negative symptoms, and various other forms of disability and dysfunction.

(c) Estimated relapse rates may be inaccurate

While the information set out in *Table One* was gleaned from a large number of studies conducted by competent researchers, there is reason to believe that it is neither entirely accurate nor totally reliable. Indeed, some critics have recently argued that many studies of relapse (and other aspects of neuroleptic treatment) have employed methodology that fails to meet basic standards of scientific research, thus leaving their findings open to question.[331] After reviewing 2,000 published reports on schizophrenia treatment conducted over the last 50 years, two investigators commented in the *British Medical Journal* in 1998: "The consistently poor quality of reporting is likely to have resulted in an over-optimistic estimation of the effects of treatments."[332]

Most importantly, a number of highly regarded authorities believe that the relapse rates for people who remain on neuroleptic maintenance are significantly higher than those shown in *Table One,* and that diagnosed individuals who have stopped taking medication may not necessarily be at as great a risk of relapse as these figures would appear to indicate.

In a report published in the *Journal of Psychiatric Research* in 1998, researchers Gerard Hogarty and Richard Ulrich pointed out that a re-appraisal of published studies indicates that, in the absence of formal psychosocial treatment, at least 40% of people who have previously had five or more psychotic episodes are likely to experience a relapse within one year of leaving hospital, even if they receive continuous neuroleptic treatment.[333] Likelihood of relapse increases to over 50% if such people live in stressful households – some studies have found that more than 80% may relapse within two years of discharge if they remain in stressful environments.[334] Comparable findings were reported in the *Schizophrenia Bulletin* in 1995, in a study involving 257,446 individuals who had experienced multiple psychotic episodes and been treated as outpatients under what the authors described as optimal medication conditions: "compliant patients taking optimal doses of depot neuroleptics". Comprehensive analysis revealed the relapse rate to be 3.5% per month. Assuming this rate was constant, more than 40% of these patients would have experienced a relapse within a year and over 80% by the end of two years – despite them having received what was considered to be optimal medical treatment.[335]

These estimated relapse rates *for people receiving maintenance neuroleptic treatment* are much higher than those shown in *Table One*. Relapse rates for those who have only experienced one psychotic episode are lower than for those with a history of multiple episodes but are still relatively high. For example, research published in the *British Journal of Psychiatry* in 1986 reporting on people experiencing their first psychotic episode, indicated that 58% had relapsed by the end of the two year follow-up period, despite remaining on medication – a rate significantly higher than the 27% reported in *Table One*. (This research was discussed earlier under the heading, "Treatment of Early Psychosis".) By contrast, internationally regarded experts such as Professor Manfred Bleuler, Professor Luc Ciompi, and Professor Courtenay Harding, all report that, even *without* maintenance neuroleptic treatment, people with long-standing chronic schizophrenia manage to remain stable and avoid relapse far more often than is generally believed possible or likely (see *Chapter Seven*).

(d) Abrupt medication withdrawal increases relapse risk

The figures in *Table One* indicate that 44% of diagnosed people who stop neuroleptic medication are likely to experience relapse within the next three months, while only 6% of those who remain on it will relapse in the same period. At first glance these figures would appear to decisively lay to rest any lingering doubts regarding the prophylactic value of maintenance neuroleptic treatment. However, a closer examination of the facts shows that these widely-accepted statistics are actually quite misleading when taken at face value. The fact that excessive stress can trigger the onset of relapse in predisposed individuals is now well known. For this reason diagnosed people are advised to avoid stress and take advantage of the stress-buffering effects of neuroleptic medication. One particular kind of stress, which has received relatively little attention from researchers, is related to the physiological changes which occur when medication dosages are reduced quickly. Some authorities, such as Dr Richard Wyatt, a highly regarded research psychopharmacologist with the US National Institute of Mental Health, believe that *rapid* reduction in medication dosage can induce a particular kind of stress – referred to as *pharmacological stress* – which may itself be sufficient to precipitate a psychotic episode:

> Abrupt withdrawal of medications that affect both normal and abnormal systems is likely to disrupt these systems, produce internal stress, and perhaps in itself cause a relapse. The majority of the patients in the studies reviewed [*Table One*] experienced a relatively abrupt withdrawal of their medications ... If medications were tapered over months to years, I predict that breakthroughs [exacerbation of psychotic symptoms] would be less severe and relapses more easily treated.[336]

Dr Ross Baldessarini, an international authority on psychiatric drugs, has suggested that pharmacological stress, though often overlooked, plays an important role in relapse such that those whose medication is stopped quickly are more likely to relapse than those who are weaned off it more gradually.* Dr Baldessarini has noted that the majority of studies from which the relapse statistics in *Table One* were derived involved very rapid withdrawal of medication: treatment was stopped in a *single day* in 42 of the 66 studies (prior to this the individuals concerned had received continuous neuroleptic treatment, often for many years). In the others, medication was withdrawn over periods ranging from 2 to 60 days. Rapid withdrawal of neuroleptic medication, he has found, is associated with a monthly relapse rate *three times greater* than occurs when it is discontinued gradually (over periods ranging from 2 weeks to 2 months).[337] Other authorities have suggested that rapid medication reduction may be associated with relapse rates more than *six times* greater than occurs when it is reduced gradually. One group of researchers recently reported finding that 50% of people undergoing rapid neuroleptic withdrawal (over 2 weeks) experienced relapse within the following 6 months, while only 6% of those whose medication was withdrawn more gradually (over an 8-week period) had relapsed during this same time.[338]

Many mental health professionals are unaware of the crucially important role played by pharmacological stress. Nevertheless, the facts discussed above strongly suggest that the figures in *Table One* do not provide an accurate

---

* The phenomenon of pharmacological stress has important implications for drug trials. Studies in which research subjects are **abruptly** switched from active medication to placebo are likely to artificially inflate the drug/placebo difference in favour of the experimental drug. If a process of gradual withdrawal was used the drug advantage would likely be considerably smaller. See: Baldessarini, R. and Viguera, A. (1995) "Neuroleptic Withdrawal in Schizophrenic Patients". *Archives of General Psychiatry,* Vol. 52, p. 191.

indication of the relapse risk for *all* diagnosed people who stop taking medication. Rather, they refer more specifically to the risk for those who have stopped it relatively *abruptly*. On the whole, those who reduce or stop neuroleptic treatment very gradually are likely to experience a smaller risk of relapse than *Table One* suggests. Although it is often assumed that most people with a long-standing history of schizophrenia will eventually relapse if they stop taking medication – *regardless of whether they do so quickly or slowly* – Dr Baldessarini and others have concluded that, rather than simply delaying relapse, reducing the medication dosage gradually may actually help *prevent* some of the risk. In a recent report specifically examining the differential effects of abrupt and gradual withdrawal of maintenance neuroleptic treatment, Dr Baldessarini and his colleagues studied the incidence of relapse among 1,210 people diagnosed with schizophrenia. Their key findings, described in an article published in the *Archives of General Psychiatry* in 1997, include the following:

- There is a high risk of relapse soon after *abrupt* discontinuation of oral neuroleptic treatment, with up to 50% of people experiencing relapse within 30 weeks if they stop the medication quickly (a relapse rate similar to that shown in *Table One*)
- Inpatients are significantly more likely to relapse than outpatients when medication is withdrawn: 50% of inpatients relapsed within 18 weeks of stopping medication, while only 40.8% of outpatients had experienced a relapse during the following 3.69 years
- When neuroleptic medication was withdrawn

gradually, only 35% of people relapsed during the next 14 weeks, while the majority remained relapse-free off medication

- Most people who have remained stable for 6 months after stopping their medication will continue to do so for long periods, without maintenance neuroleptic treatment

These researchers specifically noted that "there were remarkably few additional relapses after the first six months without medication". While *Table One* suggests that 59% of diagnosed people will relapse within two years of stopping neuroleptic maintenance, Dr Baldessarini's research indicated that a substantially smaller number (around 40%) had relapsed in this time:

There was a high early risk of exacerbation of psychotic symptoms soon after the abrupt interruption of on-going oral neuroleptic maintenance ... Among patients whose conditions remained stable during the first several months after they stopped taking neuroleptic drugs, the later risk of relapsing was remarkably limited – particularly in outpatients, only 40% of whom relapsed within 2 years.[339]

If Dr Baldessarini's findings can be generalised to all diagnosed people, they suggest that a significant proportion, possibly as many as 60%, will experience a low risk of relapse if they gradually stop maintenance neuroleptic treatment. Furthermore, those who relapse are most likely to do so quite soon – usually within the first 3 months or so of going off medication – with the risk being significantly greater if treatment is stopped abruptly. Since none of the research upon which these estimates were based took relevant non-pharmacological influences into account, it would be reasonable to assume that in optimal social circumstances (low-stress environment, good coping skills, and adequate support), the risk of relapse could well be *even lower* than 40%, despite the absence of on-going medication.

(e) What if people had never received medication in the first place?

All the studies referred to thus far have involved large groups of people treated with neuroleptics for various lengths of time before treatment was eventually stopped. As the preceding discussion indicated – and in distinct contrast to what many people have come to expect – a substantial number of these people did *not* experience relapse after their medication was withdrawn. Of those who *did*, the question could be asked: what would have happened if they had never been given any neuroleptic drugs in the first place?

Because it is now increasingly rare to find diagnosed people who have never been treated with psychotropic medications, it is actually quite difficult to answer this question. Nevertheless, a number of sources provide thought-provoking clues. For example, the World Health Organisation (WHO) conducted research in the 1970s which led to the unexpected discovery that psychotic individuals in a range of developing countries were actually *more* likely to recover and go on to do well than were similar people in Western countries. This is despite the fact that the former had never had access to anti-psychotic drugs or, for that matter, any kind of modern psychiatric treatment.[340] After conducting a thorough analysis of this and related research, psychiatrist and anthropologist Dr Richard Warner commented:

> Up to four billion dollars was spent on the treatment of schizophrenia in the United States in 1971 – about 0.5 per cent of the gross national product ... Such a substantial investment should surely have yielded Americans significantly better rates of recovery than in less affluent parts of the world. By contrast, psychiatric care is very low on the list of priorities in developing countries. Despite this fact, the evidence points overwhelmingly to much better outcome from schizophrenia in the Third World ... There are numerous reports that psychoses have a briefer duration in the Third World, and virtually none to indicate that such illnesses have a worse outcome anywhere outside the Western world.[341]

The WHO research led some authorities to suspect that neuroleptic treatment could itself be one of the factors (among many others) responsible for poorer outcomes in Western countries. In particular, it has been suggested that these drugs could inadvertently be contributing to creating a situation in which treated individuals become *more* prone to experiencing relapse if they eventually stop treatment – especially if they do so abruptly – than they would have been if they had never had neuroleptics in the first place. Some of the findings discussed in *Chapter Five* lend support to this hypothesis. Thus, research conducted by Drs Carpenter, McGlashan and Strauss, of the US National Institute of Mental Health, Dr Rappaport at Agnews State

Hospital, and Dr Loren Mosher's Soteria Project, led to the observation that people diagnosed with acute schizophrenia who never received medication (neuroleptic-naïve individuals) tended to relapse *less* often and *less* severely, in the years following discharge, than did those given standard drug treatment.

Some authorities believe that neuroleptic-treated individuals experience a heightened risk of relapse upon withdrawal of medication as a direct result of the fact that prolonged exposure to these drugs can result in various changes in the treated person's brain. Some commentators believe that one of these changes, *dopamine-receptor supersensitivity*, may play an especially important role in this regard (see *Chapter Two*). Dr Baldessarini and his colleagues have recently concurred with these suggestions. In attempting to account for the fact that rapid discontinuation of maintenance neuroleptic treatment is associated with a 50% risk of relapse within 30 weeks, these medication experts stated in the *Archives of General Psychiatry* in 1997:

> An essential question is whether the observed early morbidity [relapse] merely reflects the natural history of untreated severe psychotic illness that re-emerges without protective medication ... However, an early relapse risk may well exceed the natural course of psychotic illness. This early risk may be related to the stress of removing treatment, which may reflect pharmacodynamic adaptations [brain changes] associated with prolonged drug treatment. Such changes include the induction of dopaminergic supersensitivity in the forebrain; this requires 4 to 6 weeks to return to basal levels even after a single dose of a neuroleptic drug in

animals, or longer after repeated dosing, and so may be congruent with [the] high relapse risk after the abrupt interruption of clinical treatment.[342]

Proponents of the supersensitivity hypothesis argue that, rather than being a resurgence of schizophrenia symptoms no longer adequately controlled with medication, relapse which occurs soon after abrupt cessation of neuroleptic treatment may actually be a withdrawal phenomenon.[343] In line with this view, it has been suggested that the substantially lower relapse rate associated with very slow medication reduction is due to the fact that this gradual approach allows supersensitive receptors time to adjust and begin returning to normal. The fact that there is a "remarkably limited" risk of relapse six months after medication is stopped, as Dr Baldessarini and his colleagues noted, is consistent with this possibility.

Note: Medication withdrawal phenomena are discussed in detail in Chapter Ten.

(f) Failure to consider psychosocial influences

Most research on psychiatric treatment tends to focus almost exclusively on quantifying the various effects of drugs on a diagnosed person's symptoms (i.e. their "clinical response"). Critics argue that this narrow focus can be misleading, as it fails to provide relevant information about non-specific effects such as how a particular drug makes a person feel, or whether or not it actually helps them manage their life more satisfactorily (quality of life issues). It has also been suggested that drugs may have various effects in the highly artificial setting of clinical trials which are quite different to their effects in the real world. Furthermore, since various factors *other* than medication can significantly influence the results of treatment for better or worse, there is little doubt that a diagnosed person's mental health and wellbeing, present and future, will be determined by many things *other* than the medications they take. None of the 66 studies summarised in *Table One* took psychosocial influences into account, despite the fact that it has long been known that "a large proportion of outcome variance [in schizophrenia treatment] is explained by characteristics of the social environment to which the patient returns."[344]

It is clear that a wide range of influences, apart from medication, have a significant bearing on whether or not a given individual is likely to experience relapse. Indeed, researchers have found that relapse rates can be reduced by as much as 50% when various kinds of psychosocial treatment are added to maintenance drug therapy.[345] As important as non-pharmacological influences are, they are rarely taken into account, an oversight which raises serious doubts about the validity of much of the published research pertaining to relapse. The various factors discussed below warrant careful consideration by anyone with a serious interest in evaluating the role of prophylactic neuroleptic treatment.

1. Self-fulfilling Prophecies

People who have been taking medication for some time are often exhorted to remain on it, possibly indefinitely. In *some* instances this is probably sound advice, especially for those who have a clear history of relapses following cessation of treatment. Those who question this recommendation often encounter dire predictions about the terrible consequences of non-compliance. While such responses are understandable, they may nevertheless have various untoward effects. It is now well known that what people believe about medication and their expectations regarding its likely effects can strongly influence how they will respond to it. The placebo effect is powerful testimony to the important role beliefs and expectations play in shaping a person's responses to medications. Even if it is well intended, the use of scaremongering to encourage medication compliance can plant seeds of fear and doubt in a highly sensitive person's mind which may be sufficiently stressful that it increases the likelihood that the predicted "disaster" will eventually occur! Professor Ciompi's research led him to conclude that a diagnosed person's prospects are, indeed, strongly influenced by his or her expectations, together with those of significant others, such as treating professionals and family members.[346]

2. Relapsing on Medication

When people with an established history of schizophrenia experience relapse, it is often assumed that this is probably due to the fact that they were not taking maintenance neuroleptic medication as advised. However, as Dr Nina Schooler has pointed out, in some cases it is likely that the reverse sequence of events has taken place:

> Some patients do experience a relapse or symptom exacerbation while receiving neuroleptic medication. Medication discontinuation does not always precede symptom exacerbation. For some patients, the process of relapse may begin while they are taking medication and their failure to continue to take medication

is a consequence of the relapse process rather than its cause.[347]

In other words, a diagnosed person who has been taking medication regularly may start to become psychotic and subsequently stop taking it (as *Table One* indicated, even if they remain on neuroleptics more than one in four diagnosed people are likely to experience relapse over a two-year period). Reasons for non-compliance in such cases could include growing suspicion about possible negative effects of the medication, reduced understanding of the need for it (often referred to as "lack of insight"), or simply forgetting about it as a result of becoming increasingly distracted and preoccupied with other things.

3. Stress

It is now recognised that being exposed to excessive stress can significantly increase the likelihood that a diagnosed person will experience an exacerbation of symptoms or even a full-blown relapse. A person's social circumstances can have a marked influence on their liability to relapse and thus on their need for the protective stress-buffering effect of neuroleptic medications. This fact was clearly illustrated in the study cited in *Chapter Four* which showed that, over a nine-month period, people living in high-stress home environments were nearly four times more likely to experience relapse than were a comparable group living in low-stress homes. This study showed that, even if they stop taking medication, diagnosed people living in low-stress family environments are still much less likely to relapse than are those in more stressful environments. Though stress is known to be one of the major influences determining whether a diagnosed person will do well or poorly over time, this independent variable is rarely taken into account in drug trials. In other words, it is usually simply *assumed* that every person receiving a particular drug treatment will be exposed to similar amounts of stress during a given period. In actual fact, there may be vast differences in this regard between one group or individual and another. It is particularly significant that not one of the 66 studies summarised in *Table One* took environmental stress into account.

4. Social Supports and Coping Abilities

It is often assumed that the longer a diagnosed person has been unwell, the more likely they are to require neuroleptic medication on an indefinite basis, and the greater the likelihood that they will relapse without it. While the experiences of certain individuals would appear to support this view, there is evidence to suggest that things are not actually quite so straightforward. For example, a study published in the *Archives of General Psychiatry* in 1972 reported on what took place when long-term hospitalised patients had their medication reduced. Interestingly, despite the fact that the individuals concerned were a "hard-core long-term group" with an average of 17 years continuous hospitalisation, withdrawal of low-dose maintenance medication had no deleterious effects, so long as the individuals concerned were able to participate in a supportive psychosocial treatment programme. Summarising their unexpected findings, the researchers commented:

> The combined findings clearly indicate that withdrawal of low-dose maintenance psychotropic drugs as prescribed in practice with hard-core long-term mental patients failed to have deleterious effects when

patients were concurrently exposed to positive social-environmental programs ... suggesting that progressive social-environments may render maintenance by low-dosage psychotropic drugs essentially superfluous.[348]

An article entitled "Sustained Remission in Drug-Free Schizophrenic Patients", published in the *American Journal of Psychiatry* in 1987, noted that, after a period of in-patient treatment, a "definite proportion" of individuals diagnosed with chronic schizophrenia achieve a sustained good outcome, *without* maintenance neuroleptic treatment. The authors concluded that duration of illness did not in itself predict how likely a person was to relapse without medication. Rather, they felt, "what appeared important was the extent to which, at any time before becoming ill, the patient had acquired skills allowing him or her to embark on a meaningful life path".[349] In the opinion of these researchers, the best guide to assessing relapse risk is the extent to which a person possesses the skills and abilities necessary to meet the demands of their living situation. These and similar findings leave little doubt that acquiring life skills and developing coping abilities can significantly reduce a person's risk of relapse, even if they have a long history of schizophrenia.

5. Withdrawal-Emergent Side Effects

Many people who take neuroleptic medications experience extrapyramidal side effects (EPS) such as akathisia (restless agitation) and dyskinesia (abnormal involuntary movements), these problems being especially common with the older-type drugs. While reducing the dosage may alleviate such side effects this frequently recommended strategy is not always effective. In fact, EPS may appear for the first time or, if already present, become *worse* when medication dosages are being reduced. A condition termed *withdrawal-emergent dyskinesia* sometimes begins in the first few weeks after a person stops taking neuroleptics and may be severely distressing to the individual concerned and others. Some researchers have noted that a crisis may sometimes ensue which, if not recognised for what it actually is – a drug withdrawal phenomenon – may be misinterpreted as an imminent relapse precipitated by medication discontinuation. A report in the *American Journal of Psychiatry* described this type of situation as follows:

> Some patients who appear to deteriorate within a few weeks of drug withdrawal may in fact be developing dyskinesia rather than adverse clinical change … newly appearing dyskinetic movements after anti-psychotic withdrawal can be assumed to [be] a covert form of persistent dyskinesia, previously suppressed by drugs and made overt by drug discontinuance … some patients appeared to react to a relatively sudden increase in dyskinesia with agitation, psychosomatic complaints, and miscellaneous symptoms seemingly unrelated to movement disorders. To observers such as family, foster parents, aftercare staff, or even physicians, these behavioural changes may have indicated clinical deterioration … We believe that at least some relapses, especially during the first 4 to 6 weeks after anti-psychotic withdrawal, are attributable to withdrawal emergent dyskinesia rather than to psychotic decompensation.[350]

The fact that neuroleptic-induced akathisia can also be mistaken for incipient psychosis was discussed in *Chapter Two*.

Researchers have noted that akathisia sometimes occurs for the first time or becomes *worse* when a person's neuroleptic medication dose is being reduced or treatment has been stopped.[351] As with other severe withdrawal–emergent side effects, tardive (late onset) akathisia could very easily be incorrectly interpreted as imminent or actual relapse.

6. Social and Illicit Substance Use

Many diagnosed people ingest various psychoactive drugs in addition to those prescribed for them. These include social drugs such as caffeine (in tea, coffee, cola drinks), nicotine (tobacco), and alcohol, as well as illicit (street) drugs like marijuana ("dope", "pot"), amphetamines ("speed") and hallucinogens such as LSD ("acid"), psilocybin ("magic mushrooms"), and MDMA ("ecstasy"). These substances can have range of detrimental effects on a diagnosed person's psychological and emotional state which could, in certain circumstances, result in a substantially increased risk of relapse.

Illicit Drugs: While there is considerable controversy regarding the question of whether substance abuse can *cause* schizophrenia, there is little doubt that illicit drug use can have various deleterious consequences. As well as tending to be poorly compliant with their prescribed medications, people diagnosed with chronic schizophrenia who abuse street drugs such as marijuana, amphetamines and hallucinogens, frequently exhibit erratic disruptive behaviour, poor self–care, and significantly increased rate of re–hospitalisation.[352] Some diagnosed people use illicit drugs to help them relax, to alleviate anxiety and depression, and to facilitate socialisation.[353] While some claim these drugs have a beneficial effect on their symptoms (e.g. decreasing the intensity of hallucinations), it has been noted that even quite small amounts of drugs such as marijuana can sometimes exacerbate psychotic symptoms, or even trigger the onset of an acute psychotic episode, in people previously well-stabilised on neuroleptic medication.[354]

Caffeine: While moderate caffeine consumption generally has few adverse effects there is evidence that *excessive* intake can cause anxiety and lead to an exacerbation of psychotic symptoms. Some studies have suggested that caffeine can interfere with the absorption of neuroleptic drugs, with the result that heavy users may require larger dosages of medication to ensure their stability.[355] Some researchers believe that certain diagnosed individuals are hypersensitive to the effects of caffeine and can deteriorate dramatically under its influence.[356]

Alcohol: Neuroleptic drugs can accentuate the effects of alcohol with the result that people on these medications can become intoxicated relatively easily. Of greater concern is the fact that excessive alcohol consumption can accentuate akathisia.[357] Furthermore, some research has suggested that long-term alcohol abuse can induce dopaminergic hypersensitivity.[358]

Nicotine: Nicotine is a potent psychoactive drug that has a stimulating effect on dopamine activity in the human brain. It has recently been suggested that the dopamine-stimulating effect of cigarette smoking may lead to its use as a form of self-medication against negative symptoms such as apathy and lack of motivation.[359] Although the evidence is rather contradictory, some researchers believe that nicotine may decrease the effectiveness of some neuroleptic medications.[360] Research has established that nicotine can lead to a decrease in the blood levels of some neuroleptics, due to its activating effect on the enzymes responsible for eliminating these drugs from the body.[361] It has been found, for example, that smoking stimulates the metabolism of olanzapine (Zyprexa), with the result that this drug is cleared from the body 33% more rapidly in those who smoke. Olanzapine is known to remain in the body of a non-smoker 21% longer than it does in that of a smoker.[362] On the whole, diagnosed people who smoke tend to receive higher doses of neuroleptic drugs (though they also tend to experience fewer parkinsonian side effects, suggesting that cigarette smoking may sometimes help to alleviate these side effects).[363]

Although cigarette smoking, caffeine consumption, and illicit drug use have generally been ignored in studies concerning medication and relapse, many authorities now feel their influence is far more significant than has previously been appreciated. Many diagnosed people consume these potent psychoactive substances in amounts sufficiently large to negatively affect their physical and mental health.* Furthermore, reducing or stopping cigarette smoking after prolonged heavy consumption is likely to result in a

---

* Some diagnosed people complain vociferously about having to take prescribed psychotropic medications which they consider "toxic" and therefore dangerous to their health. Ironically, these same people sometimes consume large quantities of social and street drugs without experiencing the slightest concern about the possible negative consequences of doing so, despite the fact that some of these substances (e.g. tobacco, alcohol, marijuana) are known to have a wide range of potentially serious deleterious effects on physical and mental health.

withdrawal syndrome characterised by anxiety, restlessness, irritability, anger, difficulty concentrating, and insomnia. Researchers have noted that people often tend to increase their consumption of caffeine while withdrawing from nicotine, and that stopping smoking causes blood caffeine levels to increase. It is not difficult to imagine that the resulting state, which could involve a combination of nicotine-withdrawal symptoms and caffeine toxicity (characterised by agitation, anxiety, tremors, rapid breathing, and insomnia) could sometimes be misinterpreted as an incipient relapse — if it does not actually trigger the onset of an acute psychotic episode.

Conclusion

It is now common to hear or read simplistic statements regarding the relationship between relapse risk and maintenance treatment. Indeed, the information in *Table One* is frequently cited as though it were fact. Accordingly, it is said that about 60% of people with long-standing schizophrenia will relapse within two years of stopping neuroleptic medication, while fewer than 30% of those who remain on it will do so during the same period. For the reasons outlined above, depending on their specific situation and circumstances, the actual likelihood of a diagnosed person relapsing without medication may, in many cases, be substantially *lower* than this estimate. On the other hand, many *more* people who remain on maintenance medication may experience relapse than the usual clinical predictions would suggest. At the very least, scientific research summarised in this chapter highlights the limited effectiveness of neuroleptic drugs in preventing relapse, *especially when they are used on their own.*

Even if the estimates shown in *Table One* are accepted, it must be remembered that they only apply to groups as a whole. Reliable assessment of a specific individual's relapse risk requires a sensitive evaluation of his or her total circumstances. Many factors other than medication can influence the likelihood of future relapse with some, such as effective stress management, helping to reduce it while others, such as substance abuse, may increase it substantially. To illustrate this point, consider the following scenarios involving two people with similar psychiatric histories and several hospital admissions for schizophrenia. The first person has been "stabilised" on neuroleptic medication and lives in a supportive, low-stress environment. He has a network of friends and relatives, has rewarding part-time employment, and sustains a healthy lifestyle involving moderate caffeine consumption, no cigarette smoking, and no illicit drug use. Although keen to minimise his maintenance medication, he has agreed to reduce it gradually with the guidance of his psychiatrist and support from his case manager and other helpers. The second person leads a rather isolated, aimless life with few stable friendships and intermittent contact with health services. He smokes heavily, drinks copious quantities of coffee, and regularly abuses marijuana and any other street drugs he can get hold of. He hates "psych drugs" and abruptly stops taking them as soon as he is able to without getting caught. Question: which of these two people is more likely to require large dosages of medication to forestall relapse? Which of the two is more likely to relapse some time during the coming year, with or without maintenance neuroleptic medication?

Apart from being administered as a precaution against relapse, maintenance neuroleptics are also used therapeutically to alleviate or control persistent positive and negative symptoms, although their actual effectiveness in this regard is highly variable. Nevertheless, many diagnosed people do find that, as well as helping to reduce anxiety, the stress-buffering effect of medication makes them less prone to becoming emotionally overwhelmed in situations that expose them to excessive stimulation and potential information overload. It is now known that various non-drug strategies and techniques can often be extremely helpful in this regard as well.

Despite its limited effectiveness in preventing relapse, many authorities believe that, rather than stopping neuroleptic medication completely, many diagnosed people would be better advised to continue using it, but to avoid the kind of long-term, high-dose maintenance treatment that has been standard psychiatric practice until quite recently. Possible alternative strategies could include reducing the dosage to the lowest possible level necessary to maintain stability, replacing some or all of it with non-neuroleptic drugs, or only using neuroleptics on an "as needed" or intermittent basis (see *Chapter Nine*). Research has demonstrated that these strategies can be just as effective as continuous neuroleptic treatment for many people, while at the same time entailing a significantly reduced risk of immediate and long-term side effects.

Many mental health clinicians accept that around 60% of diagnosed people will experience a psychotic relapse within two years of stopping their maintenance treatment. While this estimate appears to be impressive testimony to the prophylactic value of neuroleptic medication, it can be looked at in another way: this same prediction suggests that nearly 40% of people on long-term maintenance medication will probably *not* experience relapse if they stop taking it, an outcome that is even more likely if the medication is reduced slowly in the context of adequate support and good coping skills. This suggests that as many as four out of every ten people who receive neuroleptic drugs on a long-term basis may not actually need them. Although there is currently no simple way to determine in advance who can safely do without medication and who should probably remain on it, it is heartening to know that a substantial proportion of people diagnosed with schizophrenia can do well without having to take neuroleptic drugs indefinitely.

Chapter Seven

CHRONIC SCHIZOPHRENIA: TREATMENT AND RECOVERY

It is never safe, in schizophrenia, to talk of permanent disability.

John Wing[364]

A CLINICAL RULE OF THUMB, employed by many psychiatrists, says that diagnosed people who have had three or more psychotic episodes are suffering from an enduring condition often referred to simply as *chronic schizophrenia*. Since those who experience recurrent psychosis have usually received medication for extended periods, a great deal is known about the benefits and limitations of such treatment for this particular group. In spite of this accumulated knowledge, a considerable amount of uncertainty still exists regarding the role of neuroleptic drugs in treating those who have a long history of schizophrenia. For all practical purposes, many mental health clinicians come to simply assume that most "chronic schizophrenics" will eventually become "sick" again if they stop taking their medications. Consequently, they generally encourage such people to remain on these drugs for prolonged periods, often indefinitely. While it is certainly not difficult to find individuals who can be confidently expected to relapse if they go without medication for even a relatively short time, it is nevertheless true that many others do well *without* prolonged neuroleptic treatment. As this chapter makes clear, there are no hard and fast rules regarding long-term use of neuroleptics, even for those who are often considered the prime candidates for this type of treatment.

The Myth of "Chronic Schizophrenia"

Before proceeding, it should be noted that the number of diagnosed people who go on to improve significantly or eventually recover has long tended to be under-estimated. A variety of factors have served to perpetuate this tendency. One of the most important is the fact that psychiatrists and their clinical colleagues are often required to spend considerable amounts of time working with the neediest clients. This is particularly true in the public health systems in which medical personnel and other clinicians generally receive their initial training. The fact that the most severely disabled individuals tend to accumulate and remain in clinical caseloads contributes to a phenomenon that has been termed "the clinician's illusion".[365] As a result, the lasting impression may be created in the minds of direct care workers that, of all their clients, those diagnosed with schizophrenia tend to fare the worst and remain in need of care the longest. Since clinicians generally lose contact with clients who stop attending their mental health service, such negative impressions may never be adjusted in light of more recent information. Professor Courtenay Harding and her colleagues have commented on this important phenomenon:

> Perhaps only a certain segment of the entire population of people who once were diagnosed as schizophrenic continues to need and receive care over the long term, a possibility that is rarely noted. The group that clinicians continue to see and treat appears to them to represent the entire picture of schizophrenia ... If a marginally functioning patient drops out of a clinician's caseload, the busy clinician often assumes that the patient has simply transferred to another clinician's caseload across town or is living a marginal existence ... Rarely does the clinician assume that the patient has made a forward movement toward better functioning and reintegration into the community. There is no built-in systematic feedback to clinicians about eventual outcome successes. They receive only the negative messages signalled by the reappearance of patients who have relapsed.[366]

Families involved in the care of diagnosed individuals are not immune to influences such as these, nor are community-based carer support groups. As a consequence, both can very easily develop biased perceptions and skewed expectations. Psychiatric researchers may also fall victim to the clinician's illusion. This can occur because research frequently involves groups of diagnosed people receiving treatment in hospital or living in the community and attending hospitals or mental health clinics as outpatients. Since those who are doing well sometimes choose not to remain in contact with any clinical mental health service, they often simply disappear from view as far as research is concerned, and are therefore not counted in statistical analyses. Two highly regarded schizophrenia researchers commented on this important phenomenon in the *American Journal of Psychiatry* in 1987, where they noted: "since drug-free patients with good outcomes did not need and/or were prone to avoid further psychiatric treatment, clinicians and researchers may have underestimated their numbers."[367]

Chronic Schizophrenia or Prolonged Schizophrenia?

For a good part of the last century psychiatrists have believed schizophrenia to be characterised by a progressive deterioration which, whether it occurs rapidly or very gradually, is an inevitable feature of this disorder. This pessimistic notion has been held in tandem with the conviction that schizophrenia itself is essentially an incurable condition (a belief sometimes crudely alluded to in sayings like "Once a schizophrenic, always a schizophrenic"). Although these ideas continue to be highly influential in certain quarters, their validity has been challenged by a steadily growing body of sound research. In particular, a range of scientific studies investigating the long-term prospects of diagnosed people have concluded that early assumptions regarding clinical deterioration have been both incorrect and unnecessarily pessimistic. Furthermore, this research has shown that, in time, a substantial proportion of diagnosed people experience significant improvement and many eventually become free of any discernible schizophrenia symptoms.[368]

In a review published in the *British Journal of Psychiatry* in 1992, Professor Harding and her colleagues stated that it is now clearly established that clinical recovery is feasible for a far greater percentage of diagnosed people than was once thought possible.[369] Indeed, all five major research studies which have assessed long-term outcome, show between half and two-thirds of people diagnosed with schizophrenia eventually recovered entirely or experienced significant improvement. The following table summarises the relevant details of these extremely important long-term studies:

TABLE TWO

Five Long-Term Studies	Number of Subjects	Length of Study (Years)	% recovered and/or significantly improved
M. Bleuler (1972)*	208	23	53-68
Huber et al (1979)	502	22	57
Ciompi & Müller (1976)	289	37	53
Tsuang et al (1979)	186	35	46
Harding et al (1987)	118	32	62-68

Source: Harding et al. 1992[370]

---

* Professor Bleuler found that 68% of those experiencing their first admission went on to recover or improve significantly during the course of his study, while 53% of *all* the diagnosed individuals he observed (including those with long histories of institutionalisation and "chronic" schizophrenia) eventually did so.

In light of these and related findings Professor Harding's group concluded that the phenomenon of *chronicity*, characterised by severe deterioration in self-care, social relations, and occupational functioning, is *not* as an inherent aspect of schizophrenia, as has long been believed. Rather, they feel, it is best understood as the result of prolonged exposure to a multitude of negative extraneous influences, prominent among which are the following:

- Effects of institutionalisation
- Socialisation into a "mental-patient" role
- Lack of opportunities for rehabilitation
- Enforced poverty and social isolation
- Stigmatisation and discrimination
- Loss of hope and demoralisation
- Lack of expectations of improvement
- Self-fulfilling prophecies
- Medication side effects

While it is true that many diagnosed individuals do eventually attain a "chronic" status, scientific research has demonstrated that this fate is *not* an inevitable consequence of schizophrenia, nor is it necessarily a permanent state:

The possible causes of chronicity may be viewed as having less to do with any inherent natural outcome of the disorder and more to do with a myriad of environmental and other psychosocial factors interacting with the person and the illness ...The substantial list of psychosocial artifacts that create chronicity, over and above illness factors, has contributed a large segment of patients for whom chronicity could have been avoided. The current state of the art is such that clinicians are unable to predict who will remain truly chronic and who does not have to remain at that level ... Given a more complete picture, the number of patients who significantly improve or recover is much greater than is now expected by most clinicians.[371]

In view of the realisation that substantial numbers of supposedly chronic individuals will eventually improve, Professors Harding, Zubin, and Strauss have urged their psychiatric colleagues to abandon the use of terms such as "chronic schizophrenia" altogether. An appropriate alternative, they suggest, might be *prolonged schizophrenia*, since this term "does not have the implications of relentless progressive deterioration, residual symptoms, deficits in functioning, and hopelessness that are commonly associated with the term 'chronic' [and thus] might be more in keeping with the recent studies on outcome we have described."[372]

Manfred Bleuler's Unique Perspective

Because he spent his entire professional life as a psychiatrist working closely with, learning from, and treating people diagnosed with schizophrenia, the views of Professor Manfred Bleuler deserve special consideration. The fact that he was able to maintain continuous contact with his patients over long periods granted Bleuler a perspective impossible to achieve in contemporary health care systems whose increasingly economically driven agenda prizes rapid "throughput". Bleuler's views, by contrast, were based on 23 years of continuous observation of 208 diagnosed individuals whom he treated personally and whose long-term progress he was able to monitor and assess at first-hand. In addition, he studied the experiences of many others in Europe and the USA. In summarising his sixty years of intensive experience and research involving 1,158 diagnosed individuals observed over long periods, Bleuler was especially keen to challenge the pessimistic views held by many of his psychiatric colleagues regarding the long-term course of schizophrenia:

> I have found the prognosis of schizophrenia to be much more hopeful than it has long been considered to be ... The old assumption that schizophrenia is usually a progressive disease which leads to an increasingly severe dementia, is incorrect.[373]

Among his many important observations, Professor Bleuler especially emphasised the following:

(a) On average, after a duration of about five years, schizophrenia does not progress any further but tends rather to improve

Somewhat unexpectedly, rather than remaining in an unchanging, permanently deteriorated state, even those individuals considered to be very chronic are subject to substantial change over time. These changes, Bleuler noted, were more often than not in the direction of improvement:

> The closer we live together with the patients, the more astonished we are at fluctuations in the condition even of very chronic patients. And it is even more astonishing that *the great majority of the alterations are clearly in*

the direction of improvement and that further impairment is much less frequent. In my study the proportion of improvement to impairment in the late phase of seemingly chronic psychoses was 6:1. The improvements are manifold: some of the patients who had hardly ever uttered coherent sentences start to speak normally on certain occasions; others behave suddenly in a normal way when on leave, during hospital entertainments, or while they are suffering from a physical disease. Other patients suddenly take up social activities when they have been apathetic for many years. I have repeatedly watched improvement after a chronic psychosis of 40 years' duration. In many patients the cause of improvement is an enigma.[374]

(b) At least 25% of diagnosed people eventually recover entirely and remain recovered for good

Bleuler's criteria for full recovery include the absence of psychotic symptoms, the ability to work, and normal social integration.[375] Interestingly, he noted that many who eventually go on to recover had earlier appeared to be severely chronic:

> The symptomatology of patients who later recover can for a long period not always be distinguished from the symptomatology of those patients who remain permanently deteriorated.[376]

(c) In the long-term at least 20% of diagnosed people can be considered cured

Those Bleuler considered cured had once been afflicted with schizophrenia but had been fully functioning for at least five years and were no longer seen as mentally ill by their families. About 35% of diagnosed individuals, he noted, "appear cured and almost cured for long periods" (though some remain vulnerable to experiencing further acute psychotic episodes).[377] It is noteworthy that many of those whom Bleuler considered cured had experienced *several* acute psychotic episodes earlier in their lives.[378]

(d) A normal life continues behind the psychosis

In distinct contrast to what many believe, Bleuler was adamant that schizophrenia is only ever one aspect of a diagnosed person's being and that "hidden behind the psychotic manifestations there are an intact personality, intact intellectual abilities, and very human and warm feelings."[379] A sensitive observer, he felt, would recognise the on-going existence of these concealed aspects:

> The obvious symptomatology is but one level of the schizophrenic's personality. A healthy life exists buried beneath this confusion. Somewhere deep within himself the schizophrenic is in touch with reality despite his hallucinations. He has common sense in spite of his delusions and confused thinking. He hides a warm and human heart behind his sometimes shocking affective behaviour.[380]

It was Bleuler's conviction that even those most severely affected by schizophrenia retain a healthy and intact inner life: "Even the most chronically and severely sick patients always show signs of normal psychological life existing behind their psychotic behaviour."[381]

Bleuler felt that as well as raising important questions about the nature of schizophrenia, the realisation that "so much of the inner life of the schizophrenic remains human, natural, and healthy" highlights the value and importance of appropriate care and ought to encourage therapeutic endeavours.

Like Professor Harding and her colleagues, Bleuler was firmly of the opinion that social influences play a crucial role in shaping long-term outcomes for better or worse. In his view, good outcomes were mainly due to spontaneous remissions or the benevolent effect of non-specific therapeutic factors: "success is not due mainly to one treatment method but to an overall improvement and activation of therapy and care for the patients."[382] Unlike many psychiatrists, Bleuler felt that those who are diagnosed with schizophrenia benefit from essentially the same influences that promote the development of mentally well individuals:

> In respect to therapy we can now make a remarkable statement … *What is effective in the treatment of most schizophrenic patients is also effective, and decisive, in the development of the healthy individual*: clear and steady personal relations; activity in accordance with one's talents, interests, and strengths; confrontation with responsibilities and even dangers; and, at the right time and in the right rhythm, rest and relaxation. Exactly the same influences that form and stamp the healthy personality, the ego, from babyhood on and restrain pre-logical, unrealistic, disordered, and autistic mental life from overflowing are effective in the treatment of schizophrenia, in the treatment of the disrupted ego – and hardly anything else is.[383]

Bleuler's findings regarding the long-term course of schizophrenia have been substantially corroborated by other investigators (*Table Two*). Professor Ciompi and his team found that around three-fifths of the 289 individuals they studied over 37 years had favourable outcomes, described as recovery or definite improvement.[384] Ciompi, too, noted that social influences play a major role in shaping the long-term course which, he concluded, "is as vulnerable to change as life itself."[385] Like Bleuler, Professor Ciompi challenged the long-standing idea that schizophrenia is necessarily a deteriorating condition. He summarised his conclusions with this statement in the *British Journal of Psychiatry* in 1980:

> Doubtless, the potential for improvement of schizophrenia has for a long time been grossly under-estimated. In the light of long-term investigations, what is called "the course of schizophrenia" more closely resembles a life process open to a great variety of influences of all kinds than an illness with a given course.[386]

On the basis of their long-term research, professors Bleuler and Ciompi were both inclined to the view that poor outcomes, as reflected in failure to improve over time or recover, often seem to be largely attributable to unfavourable circumstances. Indeed, it was Bleuler's opinion that "the most severe cases are usually the result of bad treatment or unfavourable psychological factors".[387]

A Neuroleptic "Stolen Generation"?

Introduction of atypical or second-generation neuroleptics is widely hailed as a major advance in the pharmacological treatment of schizophrenia. If these drugs do produce fewer distressing or disabling extrapyramidal side effects, as has been claimed, their widespread use may prove a boon, particularly to those who have in the past experienced debilitating neurological symptoms such as akinesia, akathisia, dystonia, and tardive dyskinesia (TD), as a result of their psychiatric treatment. Cleaner medications together with routine use of low-dose, or intermittent-treatment strategies, could indeed herald a far more hopeful era for many diagnosed people and those who care for them. In the optimistic glow of this dawning new era, little attention has been paid to one rather obvious fact: if the newer drugs are "better", the older ones must have been "worse". It is worth reflecting on this fact and sobering to think about some of the negative consequences of treatments that were widely administered until recently. (The older drugs are *still* frequently used, particularly in the form of long-acting medications administered by injection.) Professor Patrick McGorry has alluded to what might be considered psychiatry's neuroleptic "dark age", an epoch whose terrible legacy is rarely acknowledged, even though it is still being felt:

> In the past decade we have begun to emerge from something of a dark age in which anti-psychotics have been widely used in the treatment of psychotic illnesses in seriously excessive doses. There has been little regard for the subjective experiences of patients or evidence on [optimal] dosages which has been available for some time … Many found themselves marooned on excessive doses which produced distressing and disabling side effects … This has created a huge backlog of problems …[388]

An entire generation of diagnosed people were treated with the original neuroleptic drugs, in many cases for extremely long periods, and often with dosages that would now be considered grossly excessive. The earliest scientific descriptions of the effects of these drugs highlighted the fact that they not only modified outward behaviour, but could also have a profound inhibiting effect on the treated person's inner psychological state. The clinical responses of hospitalised psychotic patients to chlorpromazine, the first neuroleptic to be used in psychiatry, were described in a series of reports that appeared in professional journals beginning in the early 1950s:

Chlorpromazine induced in patients a profound indifference. They felt separated from the world "as if by an invisible wall" … Other European psychiatrists soon found it useful for the same reason. Chlorpromazine, they announced, produced a "vegetative syndrome" in patients. Psychotic patients on chlorpromazine became "completely immobile" and could be "moved about like puppets". British psychiatrist D. Anton-Stephens found that drugged patients "couldn't care less" about anything around them and would lie "quietly in bed, staring ahead" − a bother to no one in this drugged state. The first psychiatrist in North America to test chlorpromazine was Heinz Lehmann … Like his European peers, Lehmann speculated that it "may prove to be a pharmacological substitute for lobotomy". Medicated patients became "sluggish", "apathetic", "disinclined to walk", less "alert", and had an empty look − a "vacuity of expression" − on their faces. They spoke in "slow monotones". Many complained that chlorpromazine made them feel "empty" inside, Lehmann noted. "Some patients dislike the treatment and complain of their drowsiness and weakness. Some state that they feel 'washed out', as after an exhausting illness, a complaint which is indeed in keeping with their appearance."[389]

It should be understood that these observations were made at a time when relatively *small* amounts of medication were still being used: patients typically received chlorpromazine in dosages of 100 mg to 200 mg per day. In subsequent decades very much larger quantities gradually became the norm, with daily doses of 800 mg to 1200 mg or more being common by the 1970s. As routine dosages gradually climbed, so did the incidence of debilitating side effects, a problem that was to be greatly magnified with the eventual introduction of neuroleptics substantially more potent than chlorpromazine. One commonly prescribed high-potency neuroleptic, haloperidol, was notorious for its propensity to cause severe extrapyramidal side effects (EPS) such as akathisia and dystonia. Introduced in the late 1960s, the typical dosage of haloperidol for hospitalised psychotic patients rose to 25 mg a day between 1978 and 1983 (with a daily maximum of 100 mg in the US). Recent research, published in the prestigious *Archives of General Psychiatry,* concluded that oral dosages of 20 mg of haloperidol per day can have substantial "psychotoxic" effects by the second week of treatment, with many people experiencing marked anxiety, dysphoria, apathy, withdrawal, akinesia, and intolerable akathisia, leading to non-compliance or treatment refusal.[390] Furthermore, when the older neuroleptics were in routine use people on maintenance medication were frequently given anti-parkinsonian drugs (APs) in the hope of preventing or counteracting neurological side effects. These drugs, too, were often administered for prolonged periods. As explained in *Appendix B*, it is now known that such side-effect medications can cause memory impairment and may also contribute to akathisia and tardive dyskinesia.

Commenting on neuroleptic prescribing practices medical journalist Robert Whitaker recently noted how "American psychiatrists, for more than thirty years, prescribed such drugs at virulent doses."[391] In Professor Richard Bentall's view, this cavalier approach has had terrible consequences: "Over-zealous use of neuroleptic medication has led to a world-wide epidemic of avoidable iatrogenic disease, causing unnecessary distress to countless vulnerable people."[392] Surveys have repeatedly produced incontrovertible evidence of the negative effects on treated individuals of such practices. For example, the majority of respondents to a recent Australian survey spoke of feeling stupefied, numb, slowed down, unable to interact in a normal fashion or undertake even modest activities, and of having a constant desire to sleep or lie down.[393] As well as being forced to struggle under the oppressive yoke of debilitating side effects, many members of the "pre-Clozapine generation" were further harmed by the stultifying effects of long periods of incarceration in under-stimulating institutional environments.

Widespread general ignorance about mental illness, together with unenlightened attitudes toward mental patients in the broader community, only served to amplify the corrosive effects of institutionalisation. While not suggesting that medication was itself *entirely* to blame, it is not at all unreasonable to ask whether some members of this generation may have had their capacity to recover seriously compromised – if they did not lose it altogether – as a consequence of the very treatments that were supposed to be helping them. It is not hard to imagine how the young man who said, "When I take my medication, I feel as though I am walking with lead in my shoes", may have answered this question. One cannot help wondering what fate befell another young person who said in despair, "I want to stop my medication. I want to dream my own dreams, however frightening they may be, and not waste my life in the empty sleep of drugs."[394]

Almost as if to add insult to injury, the fact that many members of this generation failed to recover has routinely been attributed to the severe and intractable nature of their psychotic "illness" rather than to iatrogenic factors such as institutionalisation and debilitating neuroleptic side effects. This belief has had very far-reaching consequences in terms of how a majority of mental health professionals have tended to think about schizophrenia. In particular, it has caused a general aura of hopelessness and pessimism to become inextricably linked with this diagnosis in the minds of many clinicians, feelings which have imbued their views about treatment and which they inevitably pass on (often unwittingly) to patients and their families. Samuel Taylor Coleridge has said, "In the treatment of nervous cases, he is the best physician who is the most ingenious inspirer of hope". If such sentiments are true, the consequences of a fundamental *lack* of hope on the part of treating professionals are tragically obvious. Professor Luc Ciompi's research led him to conclude that the future prospects of diagnosed individuals are indeed strongly influenced by their own expectations, together with those of others, a view he summarised thus: "Among the most important determining factors are the expectations of the family, the professionals, and the patients themselves; at least in part, these seem to act as self-fulfilling prophecies."[395]

It might be argued that treatment of schizophrenia prior to the introduction of neuroleptics with fewer debilitating side effects was as good as it could possibly have been, given the obvious limitations of the medications then available. This argument has some merit, but only up to a point. Many *other* useful and effective therapeutic tools – such as various types of milieu therapy, stress management, counselling, and family therapy – have long been available to mental health clinicians and could certainly have been used in conjunction with the older drugs to a far greater extent than they were. As early as the 1970s (heyday of the first neuroleptic era), warnings were already being heard within the psychiatric professions about the danger of becoming overly reliant on medication, and of the negative consequences of excluding other treatment modalities. Evidence had by then become available from carefully conducted research, like the Soteria Project, regarding the effectiveness of low-dose or medication-free treatment, when it is provided in the context of a genuinely supportive environment. In 1974, psychiatrist John Perry, clinical director of Diabasis, a Jungian-style therapeutic community, commented that people experiencing the turmoil of acute psychosis are "in desperate need of the human response of empathy, for which drugs are so poor a substitute as to amount to a mockery".[396] Though these words largely fell on deaf ears, they reflect a view about the proper role of psychiatric medications with which many people would doubtless still agree.

Medication and Long-Term Improvement

It is often assumed that the main reason many diagnosed people do better in the long-term than was once thought possible is because neuroleptic medications have helped them achieve and maintain stability. However, while it may be true that short-term use of neuroleptics can be helpful during acute psychotic crises, and that long-term medication may be necessary for *some* people, research has shown that prolonged maintenance medication plays a rather equivocal role. After personally monitoring the progress of large numbers of diagnosed people for many years, Professor Bleuler concluded that, for the majority, long-term neuroleptic treatment had *not* played a key role in their eventual improvement or recovery:

> Of all my numerous patients who had long-standing remissions or who had even reached a stable recovery lasting throughout the observation period, not a single one has been on long-standing neuroleptic medication. Many of them were given neuroleptics during active phases of the psychosis, but not for longer than a few weeks after they had recovered. This should be remembered when we consider the value of continuing neuroleptic medication after recovery. Like every psychiatrist, I have certainly come across some recovered schizophrenics (outside my group of 208 closely studied patients) who need long-standing medication, because they become psychotic again

when the medication is stopped. I know, however, many more recovered schizophrenics who do well for many years without it. It is good to know that it is not necessary to give neuroleptics to all recovered schizophrenics, as long-standing medication so frequently has unpleasant side-effects.[397]

In Bleuler's opinion, on-going maintenance medication is only warranted if experience has *proven* that relapse inevitably occurs without it. The majority of diagnosed people, he believes, can eventually reach a point where neuroleptic medication is no longer necessary:

For many patients these drugs had their beneficial effect not only in the acute phases, but also in chronic states over extended periods of time ... But most of these patients sooner or later reached a state in which they fared as well or better without the drugs than with them. Many requested that medication be stopped because of undesirable side-effects or for the sake of convenience, and many others did not take their prescribed medications for the same reasons ... Like all clinicians, I am acquainted with other schizophrenics who often suffered relapses after the cessation of neuroleptic drugs, but who can be maintained outside the clinic with long-term medication ... I am reluctant to advise against the prescription of long-term medication with neuroleptics for prophylactic purposes in every case of schizophrenic remission. Nevertheless, my experiences ... are a clear indication that the value of any – and particularly of prophylactic – long-term maintenance with neuroleptics of remitted or partially remitted schizophrenics must not be overestimated. The assumption that the majority of improved schizophrenics would remain improved only under neuroleptics for any length of time is an error.[398]

Bleuler noted, furthermore, that, "not one of the permanently cured patients has during the last few years been under continuous medication."[399] On the other hand, he pointed out that some people may require continuous neuroleptic treatment in order to remain stable, though he stressed that, in his experience, this only applies to a *small minority* of diagnosed individuals:

We can dispense with permanent administration of drugs more frequently than usual. However, there are some patients in whom new acute [psychotic episodes] can only be prevented by medication lasting many years. In other instances a chronic psychosis can only be kept under a certain control with permanent medication.[400]

Professor Ciompi reached similar conclusions to Manfred Bleuler regarding the role of maintenance medication. "As 96% of our 289 subjects were hospitalised and treated long before the neuroleptic era," he noted, "the great majority of observed remissions and recoveries took place without neuroleptics."[401]

Medication, Rehabilitation, and Recovery

A closer examination of the findings which emerged from the long-term research conducted by Professor Harding's group (*Table Two*), throws further light on the role played by medication over extended periods. Participants in this study, originally residents of Vermont State Hospital, were described as being "very chronic" and "treatment resistant", having been unwell for an average of 16 years, totally disabled for an average of 10 years, and continuously hospitalised for 6 years. Despite the severity of their disabilities, these individuals were discharged from hospital in the 1950s to attend a comprehensive community-based rehabilitation programme. When re-assessed in the 1980s, rather than exhibiting the expected uniformly poor outcome, one-half to two-thirds of this initially very severely disabled group were found to have evolved into "various degrees of productivity, social involvement, wellness, and competent functioning". Unexpectedly, a sizeable majority (68%) were found to have no schizophrenia symptoms, either positive or negative, and almost half (45%) had no psychiatric symptoms of *any* kind. While many would no doubt be inclined to attribute the substantial improvements experienced by these "chronic schizophrenics" to prolonged neuroleptic treatment, the researchers had reason to question this assumption. They eventually discovered that, although the vast majority (84%) of study participants with a diagnosis of schizophrenia had once been prescribed medication, many did not take it regularly, while others never took it at all:

> Seventy-five percent of the subjects stated they were complying with their [drug] regimes, but field interviewers were eventually told, after hours of interview time had elapsed, that the actual compliance pattern was closer to the following: 25% of the subjects always

took their medications, another 25% self-medicated when they had symptoms, and the remaining 34% used none of their medications. Adding the 34% who were non-compliers to the 16% who were currently not receiving any prescriptions for psychotropics means that 50% of [this group] was not using such medication.[402]

As well as underscoring Professor Bleuler's findings, the results of this study highlight the fact that different medication regimes suit different people. Thus, while some people seem to do best if they remain on continuous medication, others manage well in the long term without it. It is clear, furthermore, that some people benefit from using neuroleptics on an "as-needed" basis, as at least 25% of participants in Professor Harding's study reported doing (the use of medication on an intermittent basis is discussed in *Chapter Nine*).

Aging, Neural Plasticity, and Medication

The widely held assumption that *all* people diagnosed with chronic schizophrenia must remain on medication indefinitely if they wish to avoid relapse, has been proven erroneous by long-term research. Indeed, the realisation that substantial numbers of such people will eventually improve or recover – and that many will do so without continuous maintenance treatment – is itself powerful testimony to the fact that growth and change remain an ever-present possibility, even for those with very long histories of schizophrenia. As Professor Bleuler noted, "even the apparently dullest, most rigid, inert schizophrenics are internally alive and somehow developing".[403]

No one has yet been able to satisfactorily account

for the frequent occurrence of long-term improvement, although it has been noted that aging itself often seems to have a salutary effect. As Professor Ciompi observed: "the latter half of life often exerts a levelling, smoothing and calming influence on schizophrenia".[404] Psychiatrist Fuller Torrey recently opined that medication dosages can generally be reduced as diagnosed individuals get older: "Many can do so in their forties or fifties, and most can do so by their sixties. Usually the older a person gets, the lower the required dose of anti-psychotic medication."[405]

A growing appreciation of the human brain's remarkable capacity to change and adapt – the phenomenon of neural plasticity – has led eminent researchers such as Professor Harding to reject the old idea that progressive deterioration is the norm for people living with schizophrenia. In fact, she recently suggested that, in optimal circumstances, a range of compensatory mechanisms may be mobilised in a diagnosed person's brain and body which lead to improved adaptation:

> many components of aging that were once considered the natural biological expression of advancing years, have been found to be due primarily to the "disuse and abuse" of the body and can be delayed or prevented altogether. Brain research is also reporting significant alterations in cell structure and neurochemistry when the brain is subjected to impoverished or enriched environments ... considerable evidence indicates that the brain is in dynamic interaction with environmental influences ... aging brain and body are more resilient, plastic, and modifiable than previously assumed ... Persons with repeated episodes of schizophrenia show

a wide variety of outcome trajectories, not just the expected chronic course. Associated neurochemical and structural brain anomalies may not remain as permanent deficits but, rather, may be alterable over time. The person with delayed adult development has the potential to reconstitute lost skills, improve his or her level of function, and develop further.[406]

In addition to whatever natural healing processes may occur in the brain over time, people who have lived with schizophrenia for an extended period have also had numerous opportunities to learn from experience, develop and consolidate practical coping skills, and undertake activities that contribute to their growth and development as human beings.

Long-Term Medication: Who Needs It and Who Doesn't?

Since their individual characteristics and specific circumstances vary so greatly, it is impossible to make any absolute statements regarding the long-term treatment of those diagnosed with chronic schizophrenia. Nevertheless, a substantial body of carefully conducted scientific research, together with extensive clinical experience, supports the following general conclusions:

(a) The need for neuroleptic drugs tends to diminish over time

Research has clearly demonstrated that, in the long-term, many diagnosed individuals eventually go on to improve or recover without maintenance treatment. Aging itself seems to lead to a reduction in the need for medication.

It should be remembered that continuing neuroleptic treatment when it is no longer necessary not only carries the risk of avoidable side effects, but may also interfere with rehabilitation and other psychosocial therapies (e.g. by reducing energy and motivation, adversely affecting memory, impairing learning ability, and inducing various psychological side effects).

(b) Some people may require continuous long-term medication

Some people tend to experience relapse or a substantial worsening in the severity of their persistent symptoms if they go without neuroleptic medication for even a relatively short time. In Professor Bleuler's experience only a "small minority" of diagnosed individuals belong in this category (see above). In order to reduce the risk of relapse and/or keep their persistent symptoms under control, such individuals may need to remain on continuous medication over prolonged periods. (It is most important to understand that some people who appear to relapse when they stop their neuroleptic treatment, may actually be experiencing a medication-withdrawal reaction rather than a flare up of inadequately controlled schizophrenia – see the discussion in *Chapter Ten*).

(c) Medication is not the only thing that helps

Active psychosocial treatment and rehabilitation can enhance the beneficial effects of maintenance medication. Research has demonstrated that appropriate psychosocial therapies can reduce the need for long-term medication and may, in some instances, render it unnecessary.[407] As explained in *Chapter Four*, a wide variety of non-drug factors can exert a beneficial influence on long-term outcome. This realisation led Professor Bleuler to comment: "The dispensing of medication was by no means the only help nor even the most important one that could be given to chronic patients."[408]

(d) Some people do not benefit from neuroleptic treatment

Some diagnosed individuals either do not benefit from neuroleptic medication (a fact that is now often attributed to treatment resistance) or are actually made *worse* by it (e.g. due to experiencing disabling side effects) and are therefore probably better off − or at least no worse off − without it. Professor Bleuler estimated that about 10% of people diagnosed with chronic schizophrenia may remain permanently and actively psychotic despite prolonged neuroleptic treatment.[409]*

(e) Placebo maintenance treatment is sometimes effective

It has been estimated that as many as 20%-30% of people diagnosed with "chronic" schizophrenia are placebo responders who remain well without neuroleptic medication as long as they receive some kind of placebo medication in its place.[410] Such people often appear to be better off taking placebo pills than nothing at all, and some may actually experience an increased risk of relapse if their placebo treatment is stopped.[411] (The fact that some people may do

---

* Medications are sometimes continued even when it is fairly obvious they are of questionable benefit to those being treated. In some cases this happens because of the fear that deterioration will occur without it. In others, the primary motivation is the desire of treating personnel and carers to "do something" which might help the diagnosed person. In cases of this kind, it might not be unreasonable to suggest that medication is sometimes given for the benefit of persons other than the ones receiving it.

just as well on placebo as on active medication gives rise to a challenging ethical dilemma. Thus, if a particular person is known to be a placebo responder, it might be feasible for them to remain on placebo maintenance indefinitely, rather than having to take neuroleptic medication. However, since the placebo effect depends on the diagnosed person believing they are taking "real medication", it may not be possible for those providing this treatment to gain informed consent from those they wish to help.)

(f) Medication may sometimes be required to control behaviour

Great care should be exercised when contemplating making changes to an established medication regime if the person concerned has a demonstrated tendency to experience rapid relapse, especially if this is accompanied by substantial loss of "insight" into their condition. Similar precautions apply when there is an established history of self-harm (including attempted suicide), or where the person concerned has previously exhibited serious anti-social, violent, and/ or aggressive behaviour. In cases such as these, even if on-going medication is not especially effective in ameliorating schizophrenia symptoms, it may nevertheless help to control socially undesirable behaviours. (Medication used in this way is sometimes disparagingly referred to as a "chemical straitjacket".) Counselling and other forms of psychological therapy (such as those aimed at behaviour modification) can often make a valuable contribution to risk reduction.

Conclusion

Long-term research conducted by several of the world's foremost authorities on schizophrenia has prompted a reappraisal of many of psychiatry's cherished beliefs about this enigmatic condition. As Professor Luc Ciompi noted, "Practically none of the old and seemingly secure dogmas about this illness hold when we look at them closely and long enough."[412] It is now known that a far greater number of diagnosed people will go on to improve or recover than was once thought possible, and that earlier ideas regarding the inevitability of deterioration were incorrect. Furthermore, many of those who improve over time either do so without long-term medication, or eventually reach a point when it is no longer necessary. Sadly, it is still often the case that those who are labelled as "chronic schizophrenics" rarely receive sufficient assistance of a kind that would truly help them actualise their potentials. Instead, many find themselves profoundly isolated, with little more than medication and occasional brief contact with a clinician whose principle task is to monitor their "maintenance" treatment (a role that often revolves around making sure they are actually taking the medication). The common expectation that improvement is unlikely for those with a history of prolonged schizophrenia, Professor Harding and her colleagues believe, very often leads to the creation of a self-fulfilling prophecy. In the view of these experts, other outcomes are possible:

> Unfortunately, treatment systems are set up for either acute or chronic status without much attention to persons with prolonged illness who eventually get better. The irony is that just as the illness begins to lift after several years, and patients begin to regroup their energies toward development of work and relationships, the system, families, and often the patients themselves become discouraged and resigned to permanent chronicity. We suggest that if increased

programmatic intervention can occur at this juncture in the long-term trajectory, such an effort might interrupt the possibility of a self-fulfilling prophecy and contribute to a significant improvement in functioning and quality of life for many patients.[413]

In the context of long-term treatment, medication might contribute to improvement, have little effect one way or another, or, in some cases, possibly hinder progress. There is little doubt that neuroleptic medication helps *some* diagnosed people feel less anxious and preoccupied, less chaotic, more in control, and less prone to becoming overwhelmed and irritable (effects which are largely attributable to its stress-buffering properties). Any treatment which helps people remain calm by alleviating their mental and emotional anguish may be an invaluable aid to recovery. On the other hand, research has demonstrated that some people with long-standing schizophrenia who have been on maintenance treatment for extended periods, seem to *improve* when their neuroleptic dosages are reduced. For example, a study published in the *Archives of General Psychiatry* in 1994 reported that, when a group of sixteen chronically psychotic hospital patients had their neuroleptic medication slowly reduced by up to 60%, their symptoms improved significantly during the course of the next ten months.[414]

In summarising some of the main issues associated with long-term maintenance treatment, a review article published in the *American Journal of Psychiatry* pointed out that the only practical way to determine whether or not a given individual needs to remain on medication, is to observe what occurs when it is gradually withdrawn. In the opinion of the senior psychiatrists who authored this review,

up to one half of all people diagnosed with chronic schizophrenia may be better off without long-term medication:

> The question arises of what proportion of chronic
> schizophrenic outpatients may not need to be on anti-
> psychotics, either because they would do well without
> medication or because they would not do well on
> drugs for reasons including failure to find optimal drug
> or dose level, non-compliance, or toxicity. Judging
> by this review, the proportion of such patients may
> be as high as 50% ... *The major principle we wish to
> stress is that every chronic schizophrenia outpatient main-
> tained on anti-psychotic medication should have the benefit
> of an adequate trial without drugs* ... Our review of drug
> discontinuance studies in outpatient schizophrenics
> maintained on anti-psychotics suggested that perhaps
> as many as 50% of such patients might not be worse
> off if their medications were withdrawn. In view of
> the long-term complications of anti-psychotic drug
> therapy – primarily tardive dyskinesia – an attempt
> should be made to determine the feasibility of drug
> discontinuance in every patient.[415]

How often should long-term maintenance medication
regimes be altered? A conservative view is that if someone's
medication has been stopped or the dosage substantially
reduced in the past with negative results (e.g. psychotic
symptoms became worse, relapse occurred), then it can be
assumed that further experiments of this kind are also likely
to fail. However, while this may be a reasonable assumption for *some* people, it leaves little room for the possibility
that circumstances may have changed for the better since

the last time the dosage was adjusted. In the case of those who have been on medication for a very long time, a more adventurous approach would be to carry out such a trial at least once every few years, *as long as the person's psychological state and social circumstances are such that there is a reasonable chance of a successful outcome.* The aim of such an experiment is to discover whether or not medication is necessary and, if it is, to determine the lowest effective dose. It does *not* necessarily mean stopping medication completely, though as the research described in the chapter makes clear, this is certainly feasible for some people.

It must be emphasised that the manner in which this kind of experimentation is conducted can materially affect the outcome for better or worse. It is now known, for instance, that there is a significantly greater risk of relapse when neuroleptic medications are stopped or reduced *abruptly* than occurs if the dosage is decreased very gradually. By adhering to the guidelines outlined in the next chapter, diagnosed people and their helpers can greatly improve their chances of successfully working out an appropriate medication regime.

Chapter Eight

USING MEDICATION WISELY

*One must cease to regard all patients as replicas, and honour
each one with individual attention, attention to how he is doing,
to his individual reactions and propensities; and, in this way
one may find therapeutic ways which are better than other ways,
tactics which can be modified as occasion requires.*

Oliver Sacks[416]

LEARNING TO USE PSYCHIATRIC medication wisely is both
an art and a science and, as with any complex undertaking,
experience is undoubtedly the best teacher. The task of finding ways to maximise the potential benefits of neuroleptic
and other psychotherapeutic drugs, while at the same time
minimising their possible detrimental effects, calls for genuine collaboration between prescribers and those receiving
treatment. Creative application of their combined knowledge and experience greatly increases the likelihood of

success. As pointed out earlier, experimentation is the only practical way to discover whether medication is necessary and, if it is, of finding which particular drug or combination of drugs will prove most beneficial. With this aim in mind, all parties concerned must be prepared to work together toward the common goal of learning what role medications might play in enhancing a diagnosed person's sense of wellbeing, promoting recovery, and improving their overall quality of life.

Two important points must be made before proceeding. First, it is essential that everyone involved – the prescribing doctor, the diagnosed person, his or her relatives, mental health support workers, and friends – have a clear understanding of what psychiatric medications can realistically be expected to do, and what they will not and cannot do. Everyone must realise that, while these drugs may be very beneficial at certain times and in certain ways, there are nevertheless very real limits to what they are capable of. It is particularly important that they not be looked upon as some kind of magical cure-all that will provide an easy solution to any problem or difficulty the treated person happens to experience. These facts are easily forgotten in today's aggressively commercial culture in which medications are promoted in ways that tend to foster unrealistic expectations on the part of doctors, patients, and their families. Writing in the *American Journal of Psychiatry*, Professor Philip May has provided a much-needed counterbalance to fanciful thinking in this regard:

> Times have changed in the treatment of schizophrenia
> ... [However] we are forced to admit that all current
> methods of treatment have serious limitations and

may produce unwanted side effects. Schizophrenia is still difficult to treat. There is no miracle cure. Nor is the patient's plight improved when treatment is determined by rote or doctrinaire prejudices rather than by thoughtful understanding of his needs and their social context ... Drugs have their limitations. They can never be all there is to the treatment of the schizophrenic person. They may be helpful in promoting restitution but they sometimes have toxic effects. Moreover, they do not enlighten the patient about his problems, inform him how to adapt, or help him to take advantage of opportunities or to accept his limitations. They do not repair self-esteem, nor do they repair the damage that the patient may have done to his friends and family. They cannot get him a job, they cannot make mothers or mothers-in-law change their minds, they don't handle traffic violations, and they cannot teach him to do something he couldn't do before.[417]

Another point worth repeating is that *all* treatments involve various kinds and degrees of risk which cannot be avoided entirely. Thus, while it is true that stopping neuroleptic medication or substantially reducing the dosage may result in a generally increased risk of experiencing relapse for some people, remaining on medication entails the risk of immediate and long-term side effects, especially if treatment involves prolonged high dosages. Rather than endeavouring to eliminate risk altogether, the art of using medication wisely involves seeking ways to maximise its potential benefits, while working to reduce the possibility of harm as much as possible.

Fourteen Principles for the Neuroleptics

Developing a rational approach to the use of neuroleptics requires a realistic appreciation of what these powerful psychoactive drugs can and cannot do, together with a sound understanding of their benefits and liabilities. The main points made in this book can be summarised as follows:

(a) Neuroleptics can be very helpful

The ability of these drugs to induce a state of psychic indifference can help to protect highly sensitive individuals from becoming hyper-stimulated and emotionally distressed, thereby reducing their tendency to "spin out" into an acute psychotic crisis. By lowering a diagnosed person's level of emotional arousal, neuroleptics can also indirectly help to reduce the intensity and frequency of positive psychotic symptoms such as hallucinations and delusions.

(b) Neuroleptics are often only partially effective

Many people experience limited benefit from neuroleptics and some do not benefit at all. Although a lack of satisfactory therapeutic response is often attributed to the diagnosed person's treatment resistance, it is in fact more likely to be a result of inherent limitations of the drugs themselves – neuroleptics are not specifically "anti-schizophrenic" nor even "anti-psychotic". It has been clearly demonstrated that, for some people, various non-drug coping strategies may be more effective than neuroleptics in preventing or ameliorating hallucinatory experiences and delusional beliefs.

(c) Neuroleptics are not a panacea

As useful as they can sometimes be, neuroleptic drugs are not multi-purpose cure-alls. Like all other human beings, those diagnosed with schizophrenia have many legitimate emotional, social, psychological, and spiritual needs which must be addressed using appropriate means. Attempting to fix everything with drugs is certain to fail – and could even cause additional problems.

(d) Neuroleptics have many side effects

Possible side effects range from relatively minor physical symptoms (dry mouth, blurred vision) to more significant problems such as reduced energy, motivation, and spontaneity (akinesia); restless psychomotor agitation (akathisia); abnormal bodily movements, including tardive dyskinesia (TD); weight gain; and even potentially fatal blood disorders (agranulocytosis). Long-term exposure may lead to the development of receptor supersensitivity. Most people treated with neuroleptic drugs will experience at least some of these or other side effects.

(e) Debilitating side effects sometimes go unrecognised

As well as experiencing the psychological and social stigma that may be associated with having to take psychiatric medications, many people also experience various "invisible" side effects. These include akinesia, akathisia, and neuroleptic-induced dysphoria. Because they can closely resemble behaviours that tend to be interpreted as manifestations of schizophrenia (e.g. negative symptoms, psychotic agitation), these side effects are sometimes misdiagnosed or unrecognised.

(f) Neuroleptic side effects can usually be minimised

It is generally possible to avoid or minimise debilitating side effects using a combination of skilful prescribing, regular assessment, a flexible individualised approach (e.g. neuro-leptic-free, low-dose or intermittent treatment), and the judicious use of atypical neuroleptics or non-neuroleptic drugs such as the benzodiazepines.

(g) Some people refuse potentially beneficial treatment

For a variety of reasons, including concerns about side effects (whether real or imagined), denial, and fear of losing control, some diagnosed people do not co-operate with recommended treatments that could be beneficial. While some who refuse medication probably lack an ability to appreciate its potential value (those in thrall to certain kinds of delusional ideas or hallucinatory experiences, for example), it would nevertheless be inappropriate to attribute *all* instances of non-compliance to lack of insight, as now often occurs.*

(h) Recovery sometimes occurs without medication

Though conclusively demonstrated by carefully conducted research (such as the Soteria Project), the fact that many diagnosed people do well without neuroleptic drugs has been all but forgotten in the heavily medication-oriented milieu of contemporary psychiatry. It is clear that, if they

---

* It is noteworthy that while mental health professionals often tend to attribute patient refusal of medication to "lack of insight" or various other *pathological* factors (e.g. unconsciously-driven resistance to treatment), surveys reveal that many would be extremely reluctant to take neurolep-tic drugs themselves. David Healy has commented that neuroleptics "are drugs that physicians are happy to give to agitated patients. In contrast, if agitated themselves they would be much more likely to prescribe a sedative for fear of exposing themselves to some of the dramatic and uncomfortable side effects that neuroleptics can have. Thus, where the prescription of neuroleptics is concerned, there is evidence of double standards." See: Healy, D. *The Suspended Revolution*, London: Faber and Faber, 1990, p. 197.

are given adequate and appropriate support, many people only require medication for a relatively short time, e.g. to facilitate stabilisation after an acute psychotic episode. Long-term studies have also shown that, among those who eventually experience substantial improvement or complete recovery, many have not required prolonged maintenance treatment.

(i) Claims regarding the effects of medication are often exaggerated

Whether helpful or not, there are tangible limits to what psychotropic drugs can do. This fact is just as easily forgotten by those who favour medication as it is by those who oppose it. It is potentially harmful to attribute *all* improvements that occur during a period of neuroleptic treatment to the effects of medication, while simultaneously dismissing the importance of the diagnosed person's own efforts and the therapeutic value of the caring, support and encouragement provided by others. On the other hand, some people make medication into a kind of scapegoat which they proceed to blame for every problem, shortcoming, or difficulty they happen to experience. Extreme views in either direction are unrealistic and lacking in perspective: medication in itself is neither all good nor all bad.

(j) The placebo effect is real and powerful

Some of the beneficial effects routinely attributed to medication are, in fact, a result of the placebo effect: the phenomenon by which instillation of hope and positive expectations stimulates natural healing mechanisms of mind and body. Holistic therapies strongly emphasise the existence of an inner healer and its vital role in restoring and preserving physical, mental, and emotional health and wellbeing.

(k) Medication is only one component of holistic treatment
Schizophrenia is a complex, multifaceted condition that involves psychological, social, emotional and spiritual dimensions as well as biological ones. A genuinely holistic approach recognises the interconnectedness of these facets and endeavours to address them in totality. While medications of various kinds may sometimes play a useful role, they are insufficient on their own to bring about true healing.

(l) Medication requirements may change over time
Since all living human beings are subject to a process of constant change, it follows that a person's need for and response to psychiatric medications is also bound to change over time. Schizophrenia is known to gradually diminish in severity as people age, with a consequent reduction in the amount of medication that tends to be required. As their condition becomes milder and they learn to use coping strategies more effectively, some diagnosed individuals may eventually use their accumulated life experience to grow beyond the need for medication. Others who once needed continuous neuroleptic treatment may reach a point at which low dose or intermittent medication is sufficient to ensure their stability and prevent the occurrence of relapse.

(m) Beneficial effects of medication do not prove schizophrenia is a biological illness
It is often assumed that, since neuroleptics work by blocking various neurotransmitters in the brain, the underlying cause of schizophrenia must be related to some kind of

disturbance in the activity of these substances, i.e. to a chemical imbalance. Although this hypothesis is now widely promoted, it is conceivable that the reverse sequence occurs and that changes in brain chemistry are actually a *consequence* of severe mental distress rather than its primary cause. Despite its logical plausibility this proposition (which raises the proverbial "chicken and egg" question) is rarely considered.

(n) Lack of medication is not responsible for everything that goes wrong

It is not wise to assume, as many people now do, that if anything undesirable happens to someone who has stopped taking neuroleptics, absence of medication must be directly responsible. Whether or not a person has been diagnosed with schizophrenia, things can go wrong in their life that have nothing at all to do with medication. The fact that certain behaviours (e.g. social withdrawal, anger, hostility, preoccupation, self-harm) can sometimes be curtailed by re-instating medication does not necessarily prove that such behaviours were manifestations of schizophrenia (or any other type of psychiatric disorder) since tranquillising drugs are likely to reduce the incidence of such behaviours in *anyone* to whom they are given.*

---

* A practice for which the Soviet Union became notorious during the 1970s involved the use of powerful tranquillising drugs to suppress behaviours deemed to be socially unacceptable and politically incorrect. Thus, many dissidents found themselves imprisoned in psychiatric hospitals under the pretext of being given treatment for a mental illness referred to as "sluggish schizophrenia", a characteristic symptom of which was said to be an unhealthy and dangerous preoccupation with "reformist delusions" and other ideas threatening to the state-sanctioned political status quo.

Guidelines for Using Medication Wisely

Wise use of psychotropic medications is guided by the following general principles:

(a) Correct Diagnosis and Regular Assessment

Neuroleptics are powerful psychotropic drugs which should only be used to treat specific types of mental disorder. In order to safeguard against inappropriate use of these medications, it is essential that people are diagnosed correctly. Since this aspect of psychiatric practice is still far from being an exact science, people sometimes receive incorrect diagnoses. The likelihood of this happening is increased by the fact that mental illnesses are not, in reality, the neatly circumscribed and clearly identifiable entities that are portrayed in diagnostic handbooks such as the American Psychiatric Association's highly influential *Diagnostic and Statistical Manual of Mental Disorders* (*DSM-IV*). Furthermore, medical practitioners who have limited experience dealing with mental health issues sometimes prescribe neuroleptics and other psychiatric drugs inappropriately or incorrectly.

Although it is highly desirable that a correct diagnosis be made *prior* to commencing drug treatment, in actual practice this is not always easy to do, especially if it is the first time someone has experienced psychosis. First-episode psychosis may be associated with a number of diagnoses other than schizophrenia (e.g. drug-induced psychosis, schizophreniform psychosis, brief psychotic disorder, schizoaffective disorder, and psychotic disorders occurring as a result of various medical conditions). Some acute psychotic episodes that are diagnosed as schizophrenia are probably better understood as manifestations of profound psychospiritual crises, which have been termed "spiritual emergencies" (see later in this chapter). The realisation that a range of mental disorders can mimic schizophrenia has caused many psychiatrists to exercise greater caution when assigning diagnoses, especially to those with no prior treatment history. Holding off on assigning a diagnosis until the clinical picture is clearer reduces the likelihood that neuroleptic or other psychotropic drugs will be given inappropriately. Nevertheless, Richard Warner believes that the phenomenon of "treatment resistance" is partly due to the fact that some people given neuroleptic drugs have been *incorrectly* diagnosed with schizophrenia.[418]

Where a diagnosis of schizophrenia *has* been firmly established, people should still have the benefit of a regular assessment of their psychiatric status and medication responses. From time to time everyone who takes neuroleptic or other psychotropic drugs should be thoroughly assessed by a competent and experienced psychiatric clinician, in order to determine whether or not they still have a genuine ongoing need for these drugs and, if they do, what type and dose of medication is likely to be most beneficial.

(b) Respect for Individuality

Psychiatrists in clinical practice follow a range of general guidelines when prescribing neuroleptic medications. As useful as these guidelines may be, it is important to appreciate that they are based on statistical analyses of large groups and are, therefore, not necessarily applicable to every recipient of treatment. It is imperative that treatment be individualised. Each diagnosed person is a unique individual with his or her own pattern of symptoms (both positive and negative), specific set of past and present life circumstances, and highly idiosyncratic physiological and biochemical sensitivities.[419]

Psychiatrists have long been interested in finding ways to predict how their patients will fare in the long-term and, in particular, how they are likely to respond to the various treatments they receive. In an effort to determine the likely prognosis of people diagnosed with schizophrenia, researchers have considered a wide range of factors including age, race, sex, intelligence, marital status, and the type, severity, and duration of their symptoms. It is now widely accepted that none of these factors are reliable indicators of how well or poorly a given individual can be expected to do in the long-term.[420] It is noteworthy that, in their desire to be objective, researchers have tended to pay scant attention to what diagnosed people themselves have had to say about their treatment. Nevertheless, there is good reason to believe that subjective responses to neuroleptic medication – in particular, *how these drugs make a person feel* – provide a very useful indicator as to the likely success, or otherwise, of such treatment.

It has been found that a person's initial response to the drugs they are given can sometimes predict whether or not they will benefit from them in the long-term. Researchers have noted that some people experience an unpleasant subjective reaction – termed a *dysphoric response* – when they are given a neuroleptic for the first time.[421] People use a wide variety of words to describe this drug-induced state, e.g. "tired", "drowsy", "goofy", "lazy", "dull", "fuzzy", "zombified", "drugged", "slowed down", and "like a hangover without a headache". By contrast, those who have a positive response may say the medication makes them feel "calmer", "more relaxed", "less worried", or "less fearful".[422] From the very beginning, dysphoric responders may complain that their treatment is making them worse. (It should be noted that people who experience an unpleasant reaction may sometimes *not* suspect that the medication could be responsible. As David Healy has pointed out, most patients tend to assume that the treatment they are given will not have a negative effect: "My doctor wouldn't have prescribed something that could make me feel worse"[423].)

Clinical research has established that the dysphoric response is often persistent, i.e. it tends *not* to diminish, even if a treated person has had time to get used to the medication. Those whose initial reaction to the drugs is negative tend to respond poorly to on-going treatment and some may even deteriorate on neuroleptic therapy.[424] Richard Warner summarises these observations:

> Interestingly enough, it may be possible to predict which schizophrenics will respond poorly to treatment with the neuroleptics. Different groups of researchers have independently shown that patients who find the first dose of these drugs particularly unpleasant are most likely to show little benefit from their use and to relapse early. Such "dysphoric responders" react to a small amount of the drug with depression, anxiety, suspiciousness and immobilisation – symptoms which are not alleviated … by the usual antidotes to the extrapyramidal side effects of the neuroleptics.[425]

An individual's subjective response to neuroleptic medications is determined by a complex combination of physical and psychological factors. The actual physiological effects of a given drug undoubtedly play an important role, with some research suggesting that neurological side effects such as akathisia and akinesia often contribute to the dysphoric response.[426] The diagnosed person's feelings and beliefs about the medication are also likely to influence his or her responses to it. For instance, those who value autonomy and fear loss of control may interpret even relatively minor side effects as evidence that they are being taken over, manipulated, or perhaps even poisoned. Likewise, while some people may feel that a degree of neuroleptic-induced psychic indifference provides a desirable respite from stress, anxiety, and over-stimulation, others may experience it as imposing intrusive and unwelcome constraints on their individuality, creativity, and sensitivity. Like dysphoric responders generally, those belonging to the latter group are likely to refuse medication altogether or to become non-compliant at the earliest opportunity:

> Both old and new [neuroleptic] drug treatments may cause a vague dysphoria, a sense of unease, a feeling that things are not quite right in the brain. Because of the difficulty in defining it precisely, this dysphoria does not always emerge in the lists of the side effects of the drugs, but conversations with patients make it clear that this is one of the main reasons why so many people stop treatment.[427]

As well as endeavouring to ensure that people are treated with the most appropriate drug, i.e. one which elicits a beneficial response, care must also be taken to ensure that they receive the correct amount of it. This can only be determined by a process of experimentation.

While it is possible to specify "average" daily doses for each of the neuroleptics, there is still considerable variability in the way particular individuals respond to these and other psychoactive drugs. This phenomenon is well known to pharmacologists:

> The dose of a drug that produces a specific response varies considerably between individuals. Inter-patient variability can result from differences in rates of drug absorption and metabolism, previous experience with drug use, various physical, psychological, and emotional states, and so on … any population of individuals will have a few subjects who are remarkably sensitive to the effects (and side effects) of a drug, while a few will exhibit remarkable drug tolerance, requiring quite large doses to produce therapeutic results … although the average dose required to elicit a given response can be calculated easily, some individuals respond at doses that are very much lower than the average, and others respond only at doses that are very much higher. Thus, it is extremely important that the dose of all drugs be individualised. Generalisations about "average doses" are risky at best.[428]

Though there still tends to be something of a production-line mentality in some quarters, many mental health clinicians now recognise that there needs to be a range of different approaches to the way neuroleptics are used. In particular, research has demonstrated that *individually tailored medication strategies* are not only more effective therapeutically but also help reduce the incidence of problematic side effects. The Soteria Project (described in

Chapter Five) demonstrated that, in a calming, genuinely supportive therapeutic environment, acutely psychotic individuals can often be successfully treated with substantially reduced amounts of medication.

(c) Openness to Change

Every diagnosed person is a living human being and therefore subject to continual change. Indeed, successful recovery *depends* on people exercising their capacity to change, grow, and develop over time in a wide variety of different ways. Recent neuroscientific research has even established that, rather than being an inert mass of tissue, the human brain constantly changes in response to inner and outer stimulation – the phenomenon of neural plasticity. Changes to a diagnosed person's inner state and outer circumstances are liable to be accompanied by changes in their need for and response to psychiatric drugs. For example, since low self-esteem, demoralisation, and lack of direction and purpose are major sources of stress for many diagnosed people, it follows that positive changes in these areas may reduce a person's need for the protective stress-buffering effect of neuroleptic medication. A similar effect could be expected when changing from a highly stressful living situation to a less stressful, more supportive one.

When thinking about the role of medication it is important to understand that something which is helpful at one point in time may not necessarily be helpful later on. The calming effect of neuroleptics may be extremely beneficial during the psychological upheaval and emotional turmoil of an acute psychotic crisis. However, positive symptoms like hallucinations and delusions often become less prominent over time, while negative symptoms, such as withdrawal and reduced motivation, often tend to become more pronounced. Since neuroleptics are not generally useful for problems of the latter kind – and may even tend to exacerbate them – it follows that dosages can often be lowered during the maintenance phase of treatment. It is known that schizophrenia itself tends to become milder with age so that, in general, the older a diagnosed person becomes the less medication they will usually require.

The fact that medication requirements may change over time has not been well recognised until relatively recently. As a result, diagnosed people have frequently been kept on fixed and often quite large dosages of drugs over extended periods, a scenario that used to be particularly common among those labelled as "chronic schizophrenics". Indeed, it is still possible to find people who have been on large doses of neuroleptics for many years, possibly for decades on end, with little if any variation (this was a common "management" strategy in old-style mental hospitals, prior to the era of de-institutionalisation). The assumption that people with long histories of schizophrenia will necessarily require constant high doses of maintenance medication to ensure their mental stability has been challenged by a substantial body of research. As a consequence, it is now understood that everyone receiving long-term treatment should have their medication needs carefully assessed on a regular basis. It is especially important that all concerned – treating professionals, diagnosed people themselves, their family and friends – at least remain open to the *possibility* of change. While this may sound simple enough, past experience shows how easy it can be to fall into the trap of assuming that certain people are no longer capable of growing or developing as human beings.

(d) Responsible Experimentation

The very first time a person takes a neuroleptic medication – and each time they alter the dosage or switch to a different drug – they are participating in an experiment. This is so because nobody can predict exactly how a given individual will respond to a particular medication or dosage or, indeed, what might occur if the treatment is stopped. People given psychiatric drugs sometimes complain that they are being "treated like guinea pigs". It should be remembered that a great deal of medical prescribing is based on a process of trial-and-error. Thus, it is often necessary for a patient to take a particular drug for a while and for the prescribing doctor to observe their specific responses, both positive and negative, over a reasonable period, before deciding whether or not the drug is having the desired effect, while at the same time not causing unacceptable side effects.

Finding the optimal medication regime (which for some people may mean no medication) requires close collaboration between the prescribing doctor, diagnosed person, and other helpers. In this endeavour it is vital that the *subjective* responses of the person receiving the medication – especially how the drugs make them feel – are taken into account. As an internationally recognised authority on psychotropic drugs, David Healy believes that when neuroleptics are administered for the first time, a period of experimentation based on a process of *test dosing* is highly desirable since individual responsiveness to these drugs is so variable:

> Whether an individual will settle with a particular neuroleptic or not is something they (the patient) can

often tell after the first day – sometimes after the first dose. Current evidence is that those who from the start like what they get do well – those who do not like the effects of the drug they are put on do not do as well. This suggests that test dosing and a willingness to switch around neuroleptics until the right one is found for each individual should be standard practice.[429]

Individual psychiatrists and their clients vary considerably in terms of how they interpret and apply medication guidelines. While some are inclined to err on the side of caution, others may be far more willing to experiment. Those belonging to the former group may feel rather reluctant to consider changing anything once an acceptable degree of stability has been achieved. While this is an understandable attitude in many instances, it is nevertheless vital to avoid becoming excessively rigid. In keeping with the principle outlined above regarding the importance of remaining open to change, it is highly desirable to develop a *flexible* attitude toward medication.

At certain times during the course of their treatment many diagnosed people may wish to alter their medication regime in some way. As explained earlier, substantial changes should ideally be made with the support and guidance of the prescribing doctor. Even then, a degree of risk may still exist due to the inherently unpredictable nature of the situation. It is good to remember that, while experimenting with medication may sometimes result in undesirable outcomes (such as an increased risk of relapse), it may, on the other hand, open up the possibility of significant positive change, e.g. increased energy, fewer side effects, enhanced sense of autonomy. *The crucial point to understand is that there is a huge difference between reckless, ill-considered experimentation, and experimentation based on careful consideration of the facts and a willingness to exercise due care and a high level of personal responsibility.* The process of adjusting medication dosages, changing drugs, or stopping treatment can be approached with an irresponsible, devil-may-care attitude, or with patience, intelligence, and thoughtful adherence to appropriate guidelines.

After being on a particular drug or dosage for a long time it can take considerable courage to gradually reduce the dose or switch to a different medication, even when there is good reason to believe it might be advantageous to do so. Furthermore, just as some people reduce or stop their medication in unwise ways, e.g. suddenly refusing to take it any more, there are those who become excessively cautious and who resist any kind of change due to a fear of upsetting the applecart. As understandable as this attitude may be, progress in recovery requires having the courage to take sensible risks from time to time, a point Emma Pierce strongly emphasises:

Many people are trapped in a half way recovered situation, afraid to go past where they are at, bluffed by past memories ... when you are almost "out the other side" and fearful memories hold you trapped, fighting to stay where you are at, but never really succeeding because you are a living being. You cannot stay where you are at. If you have not been going forward, you have been going backward ... There is a time when you simply have to take your courage in your hands and go forward, risking the possibility of another breakdown. At no other time in your growth process is the courage to make a mistake so utterly vital ... many people never get past a certain point on the way to full recovery because they are so desperately afraid that they will lose the amount of progress they have made. They are too afraid of being crazy again to risk the possibility that it might happen again.[430]

When contemplating medication changes, it is good to remember that the overall goal of treatment should not simply be to control symptoms or reduce the risk of relapse – as important as these may be. Rather, the broader aim should be for the treated person to experience a heightened sense of wellbeing and a genuinely improved quality of life. A trade-off must sometimes be made between symptom control and quality of life. For example, some people may prefer to put up with having a few symptoms, or be willing to live with an increased likelihood of experiencing relapse, in return for a greater sense of self-determination or fewer side effects (including adverse social and psychological effects).

(e) Active Participation
Diagnosed people and others (such as their families) sometimes develop highly unrealistic beliefs about medication, e.g. expecting that it will fix all of their problems or possibly even cure them. While such expectations tend to be more prevalent among those with limited experience, it is a fact that some people cling for years to the chimerical hope that a new wonder drug will eventually be discovered that will finally do the trick. Magical beliefs regarding the power of drugs can have the unfortunate effect of discouraging self-responsibility

and self-help, to the extent that some people may come to expect medications to do all the work for them.* A passive stance is disempowering and inimical to real progress. By contrast, many people eventually discover that adopting an active stance – in particular, learning to *use* the medication rather than simply taking it and remaining passively compliant – represents a decisive step in their journey of recovery.

A key aspect of this healing attitude involves understanding that, while medication may be helpful, it is necessarily limited in what it can do. Anyone who desires a satisfactory quality of life must take responsibility for doing all they can to care for themselves. Simon Champ's views on this issue have been echoed by many others. Thus, while he found medication to be a useful aid in his own recovery, many years of experience taught him that far more than medication is involved:

> I have become increasingly concerned that, with the dominance of biochemical and physiological explanations of the schizophrenias ... there is an increasing assumption that all you need to do for a person is to find the appropriate medication. My own journey

---

* Such expectations are sometimes fostered by exaggerated claims in both lay and professional media touting "revolutionary new developments" or "radical breakthroughs" in available treatments. It is sobering to reflect on the fact that the history of psychiatry is replete with examples of supposedly wondrous new treatments which were eventually abandoned as worthless or possibly even harmful. In his recent book, *Mad In America*, (Cambridge, MA: Perseus Books, 2002) Robert Whitaker provides a thought-provoking overview of three centuries of psychiatric treatment. It is noteworthy that advent of second-generation neuroleptics has recently led to calls for use of the older neuroleptics to be abandoned, despite the fact that these very same drugs were once seen as a godsend.

with a whole range of different medications has taught me that medication is only one tool in recovery, that no one really recovers by medication alone. Real recovery requires counselling or therapy in addition to medication … Real recovery is far from a simple matter of accepting diagnosis and learning facts about the illness and medication. Instead, it is a deep searching and questioning, a journey through unfamiliar feeling to embrace new concepts and a wider view of self. It is not an event but a process. For many, I believe it is a lifelong journey.[431]

In order to be in a position to use medications wisely, diagnosed people must be prepared to take responsibility for learning as much as possible about them. This will entail undertaking a personal research project, both practical and theoretical, which could extend over a considerable period. *Warning*: while written information about neuroleptic and other psychotropic drugs is now readily available in the form of books, pamphlets, education kits, audiovisual materials, and so on, it is necessary to exercise a great deal of caution when researching this subject. Identifying sources which are accurate, up-to-date, reliable, and free of bias, can be very difficult. Many organisations and individuals have a vested interest in promoting a particular point of view, while others may have their own personal axe to grind on this subject. The advent of the Internet has made it possible for anybody to say anything they like on any subject, with the result that sorting wheat from chaff can be a formidable challenge. In recent years pharmaceutical manufacturers have become actively engaged in advising and funding a wide range of supposedly independent initiatives (e.g. various "illness awareness" campaigns and lay support groups) whose stated purpose is to provide unbiased information, but whose real agenda is to foster demand for their products.[432] Gaining more than a superficial knowledge of psychiatric drugs requires considerable personal effort and a willingness to not simply accept without question everything one is told (see *Chapter Eleven*).

In gathering information about medication it can be very helpful to speak with others who are knowledgeable and experienced in this area. Such people may include mental health clinicians, other diagnosed persons, relatives, and support workers. In this undertaking, diagnosed individuals must be assertive enough to ask questions and make their own views heard, while at the same time being willing to listen to the views and opinions of others. As valuable as external sources of information can be, in the end, firsthand experience with various medications is undoubtedly the best teacher. Published information can indicate, in a fairly general way, how various drugs tend to affect people. However, it cannot predict with certainty how a particular drug will affect a specific individual: at most it provides a broad indication of a drug's *possible* benefits and risks. Thus, there can be no substitute for actually taking a medication over a period of time and experiencing, for oneself, its various effects – both positive and negative.

As well as educating themselves about medications, diagnosed people have an important role to play in terms of educating others, e.g. by providing them with feedback about the effects of the various prescription drugs they have taken. Rather than sitting back and allowing others to take all the responsibility for making decisions about medications, people can participate more actively in their own treatment by informing mental health professionals about the effects and side effects of drugs they have had in the past, as well as those of any current medications. This kind of active participation is especially important in regard to neuroleptics since these drugs can have a range of *subjective* effects which are invisible even to experienced clinicians. Thus, for example, while side effects such as tremor or shuffling gait may be readily obvious to others, it is impossible for an external observer to perceive inner experiences such as diminished spontaneity, mental dullness, or dampening of creativity.[433] As a consequence, clinicians are only able to assess the full extent of a drug's impact if their clients provide them with adequate information.

It is impossible for anyone to take medications without having an attitude toward them and a set of beliefs about their likely effects. Such beliefs – whether positive (e.g. "I believe I need these drugs and that they help me"), or negative (e.g. "I don't like taking these drugs and I don't believe they help") – can significantly influence a drug's effects and even its side effects. (Researchers are aware of this and use procedures such as the double-blind protocol in an effort to minimise the extent to which trial results are affected by the expectations of the investigators and experimental subjects.) These facts are highly relevant to diagnosed people, since they highlight the extent to which their own beliefs and feelings about medication – and even their feelings about those who prescribe it – can influence the way it affects them. It is possible for people to resist and fight the effects of a drug just as it is possible to accept and co-operate with it. In some instances this could contribute to a self-fulfilling prophecy for better or worse, since the effects a person expects a drug to have are somewhat more likely to occur than are unexpected ones. Research has demonstrated that people are likely to gain the most benefit from medication when they trust and have confidence in those responsible for prescribing it.

Those intent on recovery must be prepared to re-examine their attitude toward medication from time to time. This is vital because people take medications – or refuse them – for a variety of reasons, some of which they may only be partially aware of. For example, while people sometimes have good reasons for refusing medication, at times such refusal may be a manifestation of denial, unwillingness to accept responsibility, rebelliousness, or hostility, all of which may be largely unconscious. Deciding to stop medication against advice could be motivated by a wide range of unconscious or partly conscious factors. By contrast, some people are only too willing to comply with medication but may have questionable motives for doing so. Prescription drugs, like social and illicit ones, can be abused or even used as a means of avoidance.

(f) A Holistic Perspective

In order to maximise the potential benefits of treatment, while simultaneously reducing the risk of adverse effects, it is imperative that psychoactive drugs are employed in the context of a holistic approach (outlined in *Chapter Four*). Although the validity of this basic principle is supported by an abundance of scientific and clinical evidence, it is still very common for these medications to be used excessively or aggressively in pursuit of a quick fix. Such an approach may have numerous untoward consequences, as psychiatrist Edward Podvoll explains:

The early situation of psychosis is usually very fragile and flickers back and forth between clarity and confusion. The amount of this flickering is often conditioned by *who* one is with and *how* one is being treated. When the environment is a safe one, with healthy friendships and patience, the psychosis may resolve itself in short order. On the other hand, when a psychosis that might naturally last only several hours or days is overreacted to by others in an attempt to suppress it as quickly as possible (as with over-medicating or other subjugating techniques), the disoriented one often fights against the effects of what he feels is an intrusion and a punishing abuse of his already-fragile mind. Such situations commonly lead to months or years of aggravated struggle with oneself and with psychiatric and legal authorities (while the psychosis worsens).[434]

Excessive reliance on psychotropic drugs is encouraged by exaggerated claims regarding their therapeutic efficacy. Wise use, on the other hand, is predicated on a clear understanding of what they can and cannot do. Dr Podvoll elaborates this important principle as follows:

By this time, it is well known that medications are not a "cure" for psychosis, that they do not specifically affect voices, visions, or delusions. Primarily, they have been given to control behaviour. But at times, they do lower the "amplitude" of outrageous sensory phenomena, or they lower the excitement and panic caused when the senses are in disarray ... They may give a patient an opportunity to live with some relatively quiet moments, when the sensory phenomena are not so imperious, and when one can turn away from the hallucinatory demands to live in "two places at once". There may be some precious spare time to relax, to begin to approximate reality, and to gain some semblance of dignity by not appearing to others as continuously distracted and forgetful.[435]

It is crucial, Dr Podvoll adds, that these potent drugs be used with great skill and care: "that is, when they are given in as small a dose as possible, and when they are incrementally withdrawn as soon as their therapeutic effect is achieved."[436]

It has been conclusively demonstrated that favourable social circumstances – particularly those which help to allay stress and anxiety – can exert a powerful therapeutic influence. Professor Ciompi's research, together with that of many others, has made it quite clear that less medication is generally required when adequate and appropriate support is provided:

> Medication represents a potentially useful tool that is best employed when a patient's total social and personal situation is taken into account. The results from the Soteria Project indicate that drug therapy can become unnecessary even for acute schizophrenics if other conditions for therapy are particularly favourable.[437]

The likelihood that medication will be utilised excessively increases greatly when the main (or only) goal of treatment is the suppression or eradication of symptoms. By contrast, medication is likely to be used more sparingly when its principle purpose is to aid containment, i.e. when it is used to help people deal more effectively with their difficulties by reducing anxiety and agitation, thus rendering distressing, distracting, or overwhelming experiences more manageable. The latter approach is founded on the understanding that the beneficial effects of medication are enhanced by benign social, psychological, and spiritual influences of many kinds. Excessive or inappropriate use of medication, on the other hand, can inhibit or even undermine the therapeutic effectiveness of positive psychosocial influences.

(g) Awareness of Contraindications

In most contemporary treatment settings it is routine procedure to give neuroleptic drugs to people experiencing psychosis. Indeed, such treatment often commences automatically, once a preliminary assessment has established the presence of psychotic symptoms. A long-accepted medical principle emphasises that it is just as important to know when *not* to give a person medication as it is to know when it may be beneficial to do so. Very little effort has yet been devoted to developing criteria which would allow neuroleptics to be used more selectively. Nevertheless, it is evident that people vary tremendously in the way they respond to these drugs, with some either not benefiting at all or even being adversely affected by them:

> The introduction of chlorpromazine in the early 1950s ushered in a new era of more effective management of schizophrenia and made the community psychiatry movement possible ... It soon became clear, however, that not all schizophrenic patients benefit equally from medications, and some may not benefit at all. Some

investigators have questioned whether a subgroup of schizophrenic patients not only fails to derive any benefit from neuroleptic therapy but may even deteriorate in psychosocial functioning. In addition, all neuroleptics can produce a wide range of side effects that may prove disabling to many schizophrenic patients and lead to non-compliance with medications and a less favourable outcome.[438]

People who do not respond to neuroleptic therapy in ways that are considered satisfactory are these days likely to be deemed "treatment resistant" and an attempt will usually be made to find drugs to which they *will* respond. It is likely, in fact, that some diagnosed people either do not need this type of medication, react badly to it, or are unresponsive for a range of possible reasons.[439] The following circumstances may be especially relevant in this regard:

1. Misdiagnosis

Since a number of psychiatric disorders can resemble schizophrenia in various ways, some people given this label are likely to have been misdiagnosed. Conditions sometimes incorrectly identified as schizophrenia include: brain disorders which give rise to psychotic-like symptoms, drug-induced psychosis, states of drug intoxication and/or withdrawal, severe depression, manic and hypomanic states, post-partum psychosis, conversion disorders (*hysteria*), borderline personality disorder, and dissociative identity disorder (formerly called multiple personality disorder). The fact that it is quite common for people to have been given a number of different diagnoses during an extended period of psychiatric treatment suggests that some of them may have been inappropriate. Most authorities now agree that people experiencing non-psychotic disorders should generally *not* be treated with neuroleptic drugs.

2. Full or partial recovery

Some diagnosed individuals who only experience mild or occasional symptoms are able to manage satisfactorily without routine medication and may prefer to do so. Such people include those who have learnt to ignore or put up with their symptoms, as well as those who have managed to acquire a repertoire of effective non-drug strategies for dealing with them if they become problematic (see *Chapter Four*). Some people in this situation may have required neuroleptic treatment earlier (e.g. during the first few years after being diagnosed), but have gradually grown beyond the need for continuous medication.

3. Severe adverse reactions

Some people experience such problematic side effects with neuroleptic medication that the cost of this kind of treatment outweighs any benefits they might gain from it.[440] Included in this group are those who experience a severe dysphoric response to these drugs, as well as those who are prone to disabling psychological and social side effects (e.g. stigmatisation, demoralisation).

4. Psychospiritual crises

Mainstream psychiatry's view of psychosis as a biological illness that must be treated medically overlooks the possibility that *some* acute psychotic episodes may be better understood as profound psychological or psychospiritual crises which contain the potential for healing and trans-formation. One particular form such crises can take has been referred to by psychiatrist Stanislav Grof and others as a "spiritual emergency".[441] As explained in *Chapter Five*, episodes of this kind tend to be time-limited if responded to in an appropriately supportive manner, i.e. they will gradually come to an end without the use of suppressive measures.[442] Indeed, over-zealous administration of drugs to people experiencing this type of crisis may inhibit the operation of innate self-healing mechanisms. As a result, the treated individual may become "frozen" in the psychosis, unable to move forward toward the person they might become nor backward to the person they once were:

> Insofar as the psychotic break contains potential for helping the patient alter pathological conflicts within himself and establish a more adaptive equilibrium with his environment, our present-day practice of imme-diate and massive pharmacological intervention may be exacting a price in terms of producing "recovered" patients with greater rigidity of character structure who are less able to cope with subsequent life stresses.[443]

Observations from a variety of sources suggest that potentially transformative psychotic episodes, for which standard psychiatric treatment is contraindicated, tend to be distinguished by the following characteristics:[444]

- Abrupt onset, often with identifiable psychosocial stressors acting as a trigger
- A satisfactory level of social and occupational functioning prior to the episode

- Content of psychotic symptoms (delusions, hallucinations) involves "universal" or "cosmic" themes, e.g. meaning of life, search for ultimate purpose and identity
- Absence of paranoid symptoms (suspicion, persecutory feelings, hostile voices)
- Expression of feelings (e.g. excitement, anxiety, anger, perplexity) during episode as opposed to a distinct lack of emotion (blunted or flattened affect)
- Some awareness of intrapsychic nature of process, i.e. affected person understands psychosis to be a subjective, inner experience (i.e. absence of projection, blaming)
- Ability to relate to and cooperate with others (able to trust, willing to accept help)

Writing in the *Schizophrenia Bulletin* in 1982, psychiatrist Peter Buckley noted the existence of a number of similarities between psychotic crises centred on psychospiritual themes and the mystical experience. Medication may become unnecessary, he concluded, if people undergoing such crises possess psychological characteristics which enable them to cope with, and even benefit from, these potentially life-changing experiences:

> Their psychological coping mechanisms and self-observing capacities appear to be more resilient than those of other groups of schizophrenic patients, and these same psychological attributes may have an anti-psychotic effect that obviates the use of medication.[445]

Conclusion

The fundamental questions that must be asked of any type of treatment are firstly, "Does it help?" and secondly, "Is it feasible?". Experimentation is the only reliable way to discover whether or not a particular treatment will actually prove to be helpful. The second question can be somewhat more difficult to answer. There is a lot more to using medication wisely than deciding which pills to take and how often to take them. These important decisions are made within the broader context of a set of beliefs and attitudes about the drugs and about what is being treated and why. Medications can be extremely useful – a point that has been emphasised repeatedly throughout this book – but there is no room for complacency. The power of psychotropic drugs to alleviate psychological distress can be a boon if it is used to help people move forward in their lives. On the other hand, these very same drugs can be used as a means of avoidance or escape. It is so much easier to take a few pills than it is to face and deal with difficult personal problems! Psychiatric drugs can be used in ways that facilitate personal growth and development. They can also become a ready substitute for constructive action and genuine self-responsibility. While acknowledging the potential value of psychotropic medications, those who adopt a holistic approach to mental health know that true healing cannot occur unless appropriate attention is also paid to the social, psychological, and spiritual aspects of the treated person's life.

Chapter Nine

INDIVIDUALISED MEDICATION STRATEGIES

There is no single "100% correct way" that can be recommended dogmatically for treating all schizophrenic patients. In other words, treatment must be individualised.

Patricia Gilbert et al.[446]

A GREAT DEAL OF RESEARCH has shown that it is possible – and advisable – to employ medication in a flexible way, with the specific drug, administration schedule, and dosage being carefully tailored to suit the diagnosed person's individual needs and circumstances. It has become quite clear that, for the majority of people, the old practice of administering large dosages of maintenance neuroleptic medication for an indefinitely extended period is not the most helpful or beneficial way of utilising these drugs. Several possible alternatives to continuous high-dose neuroleptic treatment have been extensively investigated in recent years. An obvious advantage of these regimes is that they entail a significantly reduced risk of short and long-term adverse effects. Furthermore, they might actually prove *more* beneficial than standard forms of neuroleptic therapy for many people. The specific medication regimes discussed in this chapter include the following:

- Low-dose neuroleptic treatment
- Intermittent neuroleptic treatment
- Use of non-neuroleptic medications

As recommended previously, before commencing any new medication regime its appropriateness, potential advantages, and possible disadvantages should be carefully assessed in consultation with knowledgeable and experienced mental health clinicians.

Low-Dose Neuroleptic Treatment

It used to be common practice, when people were admitted to hospital in a floridly psychotic state, for them to be immediately given large doses of neuroleptic medication, the aim being to achieve control of symptoms as quickly and completely as possible. This often led to the administration of large – sometimes *very* large – quantities of tranquillising drugs, with these doses frequently being continued for extended periods. It is now known that such practices were based on faulty premises, in particular the belief that, if a little bit of medication is good, more must be even better. *It is now known that the notion "more is better" does not generally apply to neuroleptic treatment.* In fact, findings resulting from the Soteria Project and other research has demonstrated that, if a calm and genuinely supportive setting is provided, many people will recover from an acute psychotic episode relatively quickly with minimal or no use of medication. Although contemporary clinical settings are unable to emulate the home-like therapeutic milieu that characterised Soteria, it is now known that far less medication can often be used than was once thought necessary.

A substantial body of clinical research has demonstrated that many diagnosed people can be successfully "maintained" on far smaller medication dosages than were once routinely used.[447] In its recently formulated practice guidelines for the treatment of schizophrenia, the American Psychiatric Association noted that "An international consensus conference made the reasonable recommendation of a reduction in anti-psychotic dose of approximately 20% every six months until a minimal maintenance level is reached."[448] Anecdotal evidence indicates that some people do well on *extremely* small doses, the merest "kiss" of medication being all that certain individuals require to allow them to maintain their balance and stability. There is also a growing appreciation of the fact that, due to their generally lower body weight, women tend to require less medication than men. Some very recent research has suggested that female hormones can influence neuroleptic responsiveness and that women with higher oestrogen levels may require somewhat smaller medication dosages.[449]

It has been found that young people experiencing their first psychotic episode are often especially sensitive to neuroleptics and may only require very small doses to produce a substantial therapeutic response. In line with this understanding, better treatment facilities employ an approach reflected in the motto, "start low and go slow". In other words, if medication is required, it is given in very small doses initially which are subsequently increased *only* if this proves truly necessary. Recent research has shown that for so-called "neuroleptic naïve" individuals (those who have never previously been exposed to these drugs), doses of haloperidol as low as 2 mg per day can result in satisfactory therapeutic responses with minimal side effects.[450]*

Similar trends toward the use of less medication also apply to those with an established history of schizophrenia. Thus, for example, after conducting a comprehensive review of relevant research, the American Psychiatric Association concluded that dosages of the frequently prescribed depot medication fluphenazine decanoate (Modecate), in the range of 5-10 mg per fortnight, may be just as effective as dosages in the order of 25-50 mg per fortnight, though the latter have tended to be far more common in clinical practice.[451] Similar considerations apply to other neuroleptics that are often utilised in maintenance-treatment regimes.

The phenomenon referred to as "treatment resistance" still occurs, despite the advent of atypical neuroleptics. One result is that diagnosed people sometimes have their medication dosages increased to a high level in an attempt to overcome it. While some individuals *do* seem to require unusually large dosages of neuroleptics before

---

* Compare these findings with recommendations made during the late 1970s and early 1980s when the now discredited technique known as "rapid neuroleptisation" was in vogue. This involved giving repeated large doses of neuroleptics during the first few days of treatment in the belief that gaining rapid control of psychotic symptoms would be therapeutically more effective than giving smaller doses over a longer period. One regime involved starting treatment with injections of 10 mg of haloperidol and repeating these every 30 minutes until patients received a total of 120 mg in a day (Source: Searle Laboratories, 1981, product information leaflet).

they experience any worthwhile therapeutic benefit, in most cases large amounts of medication will not necessarily result in better symptom control. In fact, persisting with this approach may tend to exacerbate negative symptoms such as apathy, loss of motivation, and blunting of affect, as well as increasing the risk of inducing debilitating extrapyramidal and other side effects (e.g. sedation, weight gain). The belated realisation that large amounts of medication are not necessarily required to achieve satisfactory symptom control has led to a trend toward the use of much lower dosages of neuroleptics in the maintenance treatment of schizophrenia.[452] This new understanding was summarised in a recent review article in the *Journal of Clinical Psychopharmacology*:

> Major trends in the pharmacotherapy [drug treatment] of schizophrenia point toward the use of lower neuroleptic dosages. No advantages of higher neuroleptic doses over low dose strategies have been demonstrated, either in the treatment of acute exacerbation or in maintenance treatment of schizophrenia ... about 50% of schizophrenic patients could benefit from generally low neuroleptic threshold doses [about 3mg for haloperidol and 150mg for chlorpromazine] ... Recent reports support the advantages of low-dose neuroleptic treatment ... a substantial proportion of schizophrenic patients can be managed with very low doses.[453]

It has long been known that some people are extremely sensitive to neuroleptics and will experience significant therapeutic responses with very small doses. It has been found that, for many diagnosed people, quite small amounts of medication are actually just as effective – and sometimes even *more* effective – than substantially larger ones. Recent research has demonstrated that substantial blockade of receptors is achieved with relatively small amounts of neuroleptic medication: 70-90% of dopamine receptors are blocked with low doses and this percentage does not increase very much as dosages are increased.[454] Interestingly, people who exhibit treatment resistance have been found to have 80-85% of their dopamine receptors blocked, well within the range of those who *do* respond to medication.[455] Once receptor saturation has occurred, increasing the dose cannot possibly improve therapeutic response and will only cause more side effects.

These facts have important practical implications. For example, a recent report described a person who was receiving 12 mg of haloperidol per day, a dose which controlled the symptoms but caused akathisia.[456] Researchers were able to determine that this dose resulted in 86% of his dopamine receptors being blocked. When the haloperidol was reduced to 8 mg per day, this person's symptoms were still well controlled but akathisia no longer occurred. Dopamine receptor blockade was 84% on the lower dosage – virtually the same as had occurred at the higher, side-effect-inducing dose. It has been found that good response to neuroleptic therapy occurs when 65-85% of dopamine receptors are blocked, a level that has been shown to occur on neuroleptic dosages equivalent to 80-400 mg of chlorpromazine per day.[457]

It might seem reasonable to assume that, while low-dose maintenance medication may suit some people, this approach would surely not be appropriate for those whose functional level is relatively poor and who have severe, long-standing symptoms. Surprising as it may seem, various pieces of research have challenged even this assumption. Thus, while it has been common for those with treatment-resistant symptoms to be given ever-increasing amounts of medication, research has shown that some persistently psychotic individuals experience general *improvement* when their medication dosage is *reduced*.[458] For example, a recent study cited the case of Mr. K, a 55-year-old man with multiple hospital admissions who, despite taking large amounts of neuroleptics, felt the TV and radio were continually talking about him, that he was getting messages from passing cars, and that he was on a mission from God. Mr. K had minimal tardive dyskinesia (TD) and moderate to severe parkinsonism. His maintenance treatment consisted of fortnightly injections of 50 mg of fluphenazine decanoate (Modecate), and 400 mg of chlorpromazine (Largactil) tablets daily. This was gradually reduced to 10 mg of Modecate fortnightly and 80 mg of Largactil per day – one fifth of its original level. As a result, Mr. K's symptoms temporarily became somewhat worse before he gradually regained his stability. His mental condition and overall quality of life was reported to be significantly improved on the lower medication dosage:

> During the early weeks of the drug-reduction period, Mr. K's delusions increased, and loose associations appeared. By the fourth week these symptoms subsided and he returned to his normal mental status. After six months at the reduced neuroleptic dose, his mental status was unchanged. Mr. K's tardive dyskinesia continued to be minimal, and his parkinsonism improved substantially. Mr. K stated that he had more energy and had "not felt

better in years". He increased his work as a carpenter's helper from two to seven hours daily.[459]

It is very important to understand that, when neuroleptic doses are being reduced, there may be a transitional period during which a person's symptoms temporarily become worse while a new level of stability is gradually established. Appropriate care must be exercised during this time since it can be difficult to ascertain whether what is occurring is part of a withdrawal syndrome, an incipient relapse, or simply part of a necessary adjustment process. The likelihood of untoward consequences can be minimised by reducing neuroleptic dosages gradually. It is good to remember that the dosage can always be increased if necessary until things have settled down again. Adopting a flexible attitude is crucial to the success of low-dose therapies. For those receiving this type of treatment over an extended period (i.e. months or years), being willing to *temporarily* increase the dosage during stressful periods or when emotional stability is threatened, may be sufficient to prevent the occurrence of relapse and thus avoid having to return to continuous high dose treatment.

It should be noted that compared to those whose treatment involves much larger amounts of medication, people on low-dose regimes have considerably less leeway in terms of altering their daily intake. Thus, people who take tens or hundreds of milligrams of neuroleptic drugs every day could conceivably miss a dose or two without necessarily experiencing any significant negative consequences. By contrast, missing a single dose (whether deliberately or inadvertently) could have a far greater effect on the equilibrium of someone who routinely takes a very small dose of medication. In short, because they only take very small amounts to begin with, people on low-dose regimes must pay particular attention to the issue of compliance.

Note: Appendix A contains information regarding the optimal dosage ranges of some commonly prescribed neuroleptic medications.

Intermittent Neuroleptic Treatment

For many diagnosed individuals, maintenance neuroleptic treatment has a primarily prophylactic function. In other words, rather than having a specific therapeutic effect in terms of ameliorating or abolishing positive symptoms such as hallucinations and delusions, its main function is to reduce the likelihood of relapse.[460] This is especially so for those who only experience severe symptoms during episodes of acute psychosis and who are relatively free of them at other times, as well as for people whose persistent symptoms are not alleviated by medication. This fact raises an important question: do *all* diagnosed people need to take neuroleptic drugs on a continuous basis (every day) or can some stop this medication and recommence it only if and when relapse appears imminent? A large body of carefully conducted clinical research suggests that such intermittent treatment may indeed be a feasible option for a substantial number of people.

Intermittent treatment has been referred to as "early intervention, time-limited, targeted pharmacotherapy" because it involves only using neuroleptic medication for a limited duration at specific times.[461] In general, this approach involves recommencing medication at the first signs of a possible impending relapse. Fortunately, for the majority of people, onset of a psychotic episode is *not* sudden but tends instead to develop in a series of identifiable stages which gradually unfold over a period which can last anywhere from around one week to a month or considerably longer.[462] A range of subtle changes in feelings, thinking, perception, and behaviour tend to occur very early on, which diagnosed people and others can learn to recognise and use as indicators that they may be at risk of becoming psychotic.[463] Researchers have found that about 70% of diagnosed people are able to identify such changes – referred to as *prodromal symptoms* – while their relatives are even *more* likely to notice them, with over 90% indicating they have observed such changes in a family member when he or she was first starting to become unstable.[464] The practical value of prodromal symptoms is that they can act as *personal warning signals* which indicate the need to take steps to avert the possible development of a full-blown psychotic episode.

Researchers have studied large numbers of people in order to learn more about prodromal symptoms. As a result, it is possible to specify the kinds of changes that diagnosed people typically experience when they are beginning to move into a state which could eventually culminate in an acute psychotic episode.[465] Some of the most common prodromal symptoms are listed below. It is worth noting that, while those on the right could be described as resembling mild psychotic symptoms, those on the left are similar to what *most* human beings might experience when they are stressed.

Common Prodromal Symptoms:

Feeling tense and nervous	Preoccupation with one or two things
Anxiety and restlessness	Feeling laughed at or talked about
Trouble concentrating	Increased religious thinking
Trouble sleeping	Talking in a nonsensical way
Enjoying things less	Sense of being controlled
Seeing friends less	Hearing voices and/or seeing things
Depression	Same thoughts over and over

As well as experiencing the more common kinds of prodromal symptoms, some people may think, feel, or act, in ways that are highly idiosyncratic when they are excessively stressed. For example, one young man noticed that he became hypersensitive and was easily upset by the music which he ordinarily enjoyed listening to. Another example involved a woman who said she could always tell when her son was becoming troubled because he took to wearing sunglasses indoors together with a hat which he pulled down to conceal his face. Neurologist Oliver Sacks has pointed out that the earliest indication that all is not well often comes, not in the form of specific symptoms, but rather as a subjective feeling which may be difficult to express in words:

> The first symptom ... is *the sense* that something is going wrong ... The patient does not experience a precisely formulated and neatly tabulated list of symptoms, but an intuitive, unmistakable sense that "there is something the matter". It is not reasonable to expect

him to be able to define exactly what is the matter, for it is the indefinable sense of "wrongness" that indicates to him, and to us, the *general* nature of his malaise: the sense of wrongness which he experiences is, so to speak, the first glimpse of a *wrong world.*[466]

Though it is difficult to define precisely, the subjective sense that "something is not quite right" is an experience most people are familiar with since this kind of feeling also occurs as a very early prelude to the onset of common physical illnesses such as colds or flu.

The potential usefulness of prodromal symptoms as early warning signals is enhanced by the fact that many people seem to experience a fairly similar pattern of such symptoms each time they are at risk of becoming psychotic. In fact, some researchers believe that diagnosed people tend to develop a characteristic pattern of prodromal symptoms which can be seen as their uniquely individual "relapse signature". In this view, each time relapse occurs it provides a diagnosed person and his or her helpers with an opportunity to learn more about this potentially invaluable, highly individualised "early-warning system":

It may be more appropriate to think of each patient's prodrome as a personalised *relapse signature* which includes core or common symptoms together with features unique to each patient. If an individual's relapse signature can be identified, then it might be expected that the overall predictive power of "prodromal" symptoms will be increased. Identifying the unique characteristics of a relapse signature can only be achieved once a relapse has taken place: with each successive relapse further information becomes available to build a more accurate image of the signature. This kind of learning process has been acknowledged by patients and could be adapted and developed by professionals and carers as well.[467]

It is important to understand that the development of prodromal symptoms indicates only that a relapse *may* be imminent, not that one is necessarily *going* to occur. One of the challenges associated with using intermittent medication involves learning to differentiate between prodromal symptoms which suggest the possible beginnings of a psychotic episode, and those which simply indicate that the person concerned is going through a stressful period and experiencing what *anybody* might at such times. In either case, of course, it is advisable to take steps to minimise stress and increase the amount and quality of support available. If such measures are taken soon enough and they prove adequate, the likelihood that a "prodromal episode" will evolve into a florid psychotic state can be substantially reduced.

Marcia Lovejoy has provided a practical illustration of some of the key principles upon which successful intermittent treatment is based. Experiencing a number of relapses taught her that her symptoms tend to develop in a series of recognisable stages, each involving particular kinds of feelings and thoughts. Most importantly, she learnt that each successive stage could be somewhat more engrossing than the previous one. The first stage in this unfolding process involved a number of subtle changes in feelings and perception, these being her characteristic prodromal symptoms. At first she questioned the validity of these experiences, but if she reached the final stage she found herself becoming overwhelmed by an influx of chaotic impressions:

> My symptoms return in a series of stages, each with a corresponding physical and emotive component ... In the first stage, I feel just a bit estranged from myself. From my eyes the world seems brighter and more sharply defined, and my voice seems to echo a bit. I start to feel uncomfortable being around people, and also uncomfortable in sharing my changing feelings. In the second stage, everything appears a bit clouded. This cloudiness increases as does my confusion and fear, especially fear of letting others know what is happening to me ... Songs on the radio begin to have greater meaning, and people seem to be looking at me strangely and laughing, giving me subtle messages I can't understand. I start to misinterpret people's actions toward me, which increases my fear of losing control. In the third stage, I believe I am beginning to understand why terrible things are happening to me: others are the cause of it ... I carry on an argument with myself as to whether these things are true: "Is the FBI or the devil causing this? ... No, that's crazy thinking. I wonder why people are making me crazy." In the fourth and last stage, I become chaotic and see, hear, and believe all manner of things. I no longer question my beliefs, but act on them.[468]

Experience taught Marcia Lovejoy that certain kinds of stressful situations tended to bring on her prodromal symptoms. She also discovered that she needed to take *prompt* action, as soon as she became aware of these symptoms, in order to prevent things from getting out of hand. As well as implementing practical stress-reducing strategies (e.g. relaxing, getting more sleep), she emphasised the importance of seeking the support of trusted helpers:

> The first stage is the most important; if I do not take appropriate steps to gain control here, each successive stage is more difficult ... The first stage can appear easily, after I become overly tired or have been exposed to large groups of demanding folks with whom I feel uncomfortable. I have learned to watch for this stage and then to examine my recent environment ... more sleep, in conjunction with some quiet, and a low-sugar diet seem to aid in restoring the peace ... It is very important that I talk to others, people who have helped in earlier crises and can remind me of things I can do to regain control. Sometimes it really helps for people just to acknowledge that I'm feeling uncomfortable, and even though they believe it will pass they have empathy for what I'm feeling; they don't try to argue me out of my feelings but comfort and guide me.[469]

The concept of intermittent treatment is based on the idea that relapse can generally be prevented if appropriate steps are taken during the early prodromal phase. The kinds of measures that are likely to prove effective can vary greatly from one individual to another. Some people may be able to avoid an impending crisis by employing non-drug stress-reducing coping strategies, e.g. temporary social withdrawal ("time out"), counselling or therapy, relaxation, physical exercise. In an emergency, taking medication may be the quickest way to reduce distress and restore a sense of calmness and stability (remember the principle effect of neuroleptics is the induction of a state of "psychic indifference" or a "who cares?" feeling).* Short-term use of anxiety-reducing drugs, such as those belonging to the benzodiazepine family (see next section), may be an effective alternative to neuroleptics for some people. A study recently published in the *American Journal of Psychiatry* reported on the successful use of diazepam (Valium) to prevent relapse among diagnosed people experiencing prodromal symptoms.[470] The individuals in this study were given 10 mg of diazepam three times per day when they first started experiencing warning signals. This treatment regime was continued for four weeks, reduced to two tablets per day for another week, then one tablet per day for a week before the medication was stopped. Gradual dose reduction minimises the risk of withdrawal reactions. People on intermittent treatment sometimes keep a supply of medication on hand at all times so that they are able to take a pre-determined amount as soon as they need to. Once psychological and emotional stability has been securely re-established, the dose can be slowly reduced by those who wish to continue their treatment on an intermittent basis.

Mental health clinicians who favour intermittent treatment

---

* In the 1950s researchers realised it was sometimes possible to prevent psychotic episodes from occurring by short-term administration of neuroleptics during the prodromal phase: "In a few cases we had the impression that the immediate administration of the drug [chlorpromazine] for three or four days prevented a psychotic breakdown in patients with a history of one or more psychotic episodes who were exhibiting their typical prodromal symptoms." See: Lehmann, H. and Hanrahan, G. (1954) "Chlorpromazine: New Inhibiting Agent for Psychomotor Excitement and Manic States", *Archives of Neurology and Psychiatry*, Vol. 71, p. 232.

emphasise that it is *not* suitable for every person diagnosed with schizophrenia. Some general guidelines have been worked out to help identify those who may benefit from this approach and those for whom it is less likely to be successful.

Good candidates for intermittent treatment:
- Remain stable when gradually weaned off neuroleptic medication
- Experience a phase of clearly identifiable prodromal symptoms (warning signals)
- Retain insight and are able to take appropriate steps if they begin experiencing characteristic prodromal symptoms
- Have a network of supports and are willing to collaborate with lay and professional helpers (e.g. prodromal-symptom monitoring, using others to assist with a personal "reality check" if and when this is necessary)
- Willingly accept responsibility for actively participating in treatment
- Respond favourably to neuroleptic medication (i.e. are not treatment resistant and do not experience severe and/or debilitating side effects)

Poor candidates for intermittent treatment:
- Deteriorate significantly when medication is reduced (such individuals may require continuous neuroleptic treatment to control persistent symptoms)
- Experience an *abrupt* onset of florid psychotic symptoms (i.e. prodromal phase is relatively brief or prodromal symptoms not readily identifiable)

- Tend to quickly lose insight and become uncooperative (e.g. suspicious, hostile, avoidant, aloof, negativistic, disruptive, impulsive, paranoid)
- Have an established history of antisocial behaviour (e.g. violence, aggression)
- Have a recent history of self-harming behaviour (including suicide attempts)
- Lack adequate support and regular monitoring, due to their social isolation
- Unwilling or unable to accept responsibility for participating in treatment
- Habitually abuse street drugs and/or alcohol (may trigger *abrupt* relapse)

The above restrictions notwithstanding, it appears that many people might benefit from intermittent treatment. Indeed, even quite conservative psychiatrists have suggested that up to 50% of people diagnosed with schizophrenia might be able to successfully use medication on an intermittent basis if appropriate supports were available.[471] Professional recognition of the viability of intermittent treatment is quite recent. Nevertheless, it is a fact that many diagnosed people choose to use their medication this way, regardless of what their prescribing doctor recommends. Professor Courtenay Harding and her colleagues discovered that at least 25% of the people they interviewed as part of their long-term research project only took medication when they felt they needed it (this finding was discussed in *Chapter Seven*). Professor Marvin Herz and his colleagues, whose pioneering research established the viability of intermittent treatment, made the following remarks in a recent article in the *British Journal of Psychiatry*:

> Most patients retain enough reality testing during prodromal episodes to enable them to co-operate in treatment. Families have been found to be very helpful in the collaborative process of managing the patient, both in calling attention to early prodromal symptoms and during the prodromal episodes themselves ... Not all stable schizophrenic out-patients can be treated with an intermittent approach, but as we learn more, there is a good possibility that we will be able to identify a substantial group of patients for whom this approach will be the treatment of choice. In the meantime since the procedure is relatively safe, it can be used by experienced clinicians on a case-by-case basis with little risk.[472]

As well as contributing to a significantly reduced risk of both immediate and long-term side effects, intermittent treatment can have important psychological benefits. Learning to use this strategy successfully invariably enhances a diagnosed person's sense of control, self-determination, and autonomy. The knowledge that they are playing an active role in their own treatment can itself provide a significant boost to self-confidence and self-esteem.

A unique feature of an intermittent approach is that it might prove acceptable to people who would otherwise not cooperate with psychiatric treatment. Thus, some diagnosed individuals who adamantly refuse to take medication on a continuous basis might agree to take it for a limited time "when they need it". In such cases, it may not even be necessary for the individual concerned to accept that they have an illness called schizophrenia. In fact, all that may be required is for them to understand that their experiences and behaviour sometimes get them into trouble, and that it may be possible for them to avoid unpleasant situations by using medication to help them remain more in control:

> Some patients, who find taking medication everyday regardless of how they feel unacceptable, enthusiastically embrace the idea of using medicine only at times of identifiable need ... Patients must accept at some level, however basic or tentative, that they are subject to a disruptive inner process that, when left untreated, leads to undesirable consequences. Instilling this level of awareness is an achievable objective for most patients. For example, patients who do not question the validity of delusional beliefs can frequently understand that the anxiety engendered by these beliefs and the urge to act on them can cause both personal discomfort and difficulty with others. Such a narrow consensus between patient and therapist can be enough to build a needed framework for cooperation.[473]

In cases such as this, clear instruction must be provided regarding the importance of early recognition of personal warning signals, and the necessity of taking appropriate action as soon as they appear must be strongly emphasised.

Use of Non-Neuroleptic Medications

Neuroleptics have been the principal medical treatment of schizophrenia for half a century. In recent years the potential value of a range of other drugs – used on their own or in combination with neuroleptics – has been the subject of considerable interest. Many clinicians believe the adjunctive use of non-neuroleptic medications may provide a way of augmenting treatment effectiveness. Using such drug combinations has a number of specific therapeutic goals:[474]

- To achieve a more rapid therapeutic response (neuroleptics on their own can take weeks or months to reach maximum effectiveness)
- To achieve a more satisfactory therapeutic response (many people respond only partially or not at all to neuroleptic treatment)
- To alleviate symptoms that have failed to respond satisfactorily to neuroleptics, e.g. negative symptoms, persistent positive symptoms, mood disturbances (anxiety, depression, impulsivity, mood-swings)
- To allow for the use of lower dosages of neuroleptics (thus helping to avoid or minimise problematic and/or debilitating side effects)
- To help alleviate certain neuroleptic side effects (e.g. akathisia)

Before discussing some of the drugs now often used in combination with neuroleptics, an important therapeutic principle should be emphasised. Since neuroleptics currently provide the foundation of schizophrenia treatment, it is vital to ensure that they are being used correctly before any other medications are prescribed. Giving people *additional* drugs when the initial ones are not appropriate, are not being used correctly (e.g. doses too high or too low), or are causing intolerable side effects, may result in even more problems. As explained earlier, rather than giving extra drugs, it is often possible to devise a neuroleptic-only regime (*neuroleptic monotherapy*) which will prove more effective and more acceptable than continuous high-dose neuroleptic treatment. Clinicians and researchers have investigated a very wide range of drugs and drug combinations in an attempt to improve the effectiveness of schizophrenia treatment. The following are some of the drugs now often used in this way:

(a) Benzodiazepines

Though long considered to have no useful role in treating schizophrenia, a large group of drugs known collectively as *benzodiazepines* have recently experienced something of a renaissance in this regard. Sometimes referred to as "minor tranquillisers" or "benzos", these drugs have been the pharmacological treatment of choice for stress-related anxiety and insomnia since being introduced to psychiatry in the 1960s. Well-known members of the benzodiazepine family include diazepam (Valium), chlordiazepoxide (Librium), temazepam (Euhypnos), oxazepam (Serepax), clonazepam (Rivotril), and alprazolam (Xanax). A substantial body of clinical research has shown that benzodiazepines, either alone or in combination with neuroleptics, can be helpful in a number of different ways. Researchers estimate that between 30% and 50% of diagnosed people may respond favourably.[475] It is important to note that clinical response to these drugs is remarkably varied, i.e. while they may help some people, others experience no worthwhile benefits or are possibly even adversely affected by them. The following are among some of their possible uses:

1. Stress and anxiety

Benzodiazepines are highly effective anxiolytic (anti-anxiety) medications. Since diagnosed people are often particularly sensitive to the destructive impact of stress and anxiety, drugs which have a stress-reducing effect can be very beneficial at times (the stress-buffering effect of neuroleptics was discussed in *Chapter One*). Research indicates that benzodiazepines can be particularly useful when used as adjunctive medication (i.e. in addition to neuroleptics) for people who are prone to on-going symptoms of anxiety, tension, panic, hostility, and PTSD.[476] Since high levels of stress, agitation, and anxiety commonly occur during acute psychotic episodes, benzodiazepines might be especially beneficial at such times. As noted in the previous section, timely administration of an anxiety-reducing drug when a person is developing the prodromal symptoms which warn that a psychotic episode could be imminent, may be sufficient to prevent the development of a full-blown relapse.[477]

2. Psychotic agitation

People experiencing psychosis (whether for the first time or during relapse) often become agitated, excited, hyperactive, highly anxious, and distressed. The anxiolytic effect of benzodiazepines can be extremely beneficial at such times and, in adequate dosages, can dramatically reduce a disturbed person's level of agitation. In some cases it may be sufficient to administer benzodiazepines on their own, while in others they may be given in combination with neuroleptic drugs (in which case it may be possible to use a somewhat smaller dosage of the neuroleptic than would otherwise have been required).[478] A review published in the

American Journal of Psychiatry in 1989 reported the same over-all degree of improvement in a group of acutely psychotic individuals given diazepam (Valium) as occurred in those receiving neuroleptic drugs.[479] Midazolam (Hypnovel) is a potent, short-acting benzodiazepine administered by intra-muscular injection to induce a state of profound sedation in individuals who, in the throes of acute psychosis, are highly agitated, aggressive, or hostile (see *Chapter One*).

3. Positive symptoms

The use of benzodiazepines in the treatment of psychotic disorders has tended to be overlooked because these drugs have gained a reputation of having anti-anxiety but not anti-psychotic effects. This impression may be erroneous. Indeed, there is evidence that as well as alleviating non-specific symptoms such as anxiety, tension, and agitation, benzodiazepines may also help ameliorate core psychotic symptoms such as hallucinations, delusions, and thought disorder in some people.[480] It is possible the anti-psychotic effect of benzodiazepines is related to their ability to block the release of dopamine in certain parts of the brain.[481] It is important to note that in some studies these drugs either did *not* help ameliorate psychotic symptoms or even appeared to reduce the effectiveness of the concomitant neuroleptic medications.[482] The wide variability of benzo-diazepine responsiveness seems especially evident in regard to their effect on psychotic symptoms.

4. Negative symptoms

Negative symptoms of schizophrenia such as loss of motivation, lack of emotional responsiveness, and social withdrawal often respond poorly, if at all, to neuroleptic treatment. As surprising as it may seem, several studies have suggested that, for some people at least, benzodiazepines can help to ameliorate symptoms such as blunted affect, emotional withdrawal, and lack of spontaneity.[483] Indeed, it has long been known that individuals experiencing catatonic stupor can often be released from this most extreme state of withdrawal as a result of administering (by injection) diazepam or another benzodiazepine.[484] The fact that benzodiazepines sometimes help to ameliorate negative symptoms appears to support the notion that certain of these behavioural patterns are, at least in part, self-protective measures. In this view, hypersensitive individuals use emotional "shut-down" and social withdrawal to prevent themselves from being overwhelmed by an onslaught of stimuli from inner and outer sources.[485] The following anecdote, concerning the experiences of a young woman admitted to hospital in a catatonic-like state, illustrates the potential effectiveness (albeit temporary) of anxiolytic treatment in such cases:

Apparently overwhelmed by auditory hallucinations and environmental stimuli competing for her attention, she stands in one spot all day, immobilised. She is unable to answer simple questions, each hesitant phrase trailing off unfinished. She appears frightened, highly aroused and her pupils are widely dilated. Within one hour of taking a moderate dose (5 to 10 milligrams) of diazepam (Valium) she has completely returned to her normal self – capable, outgoing and calm. After a few hours the effect of the drug wears off and the patient is again extremely psychotic. Taking the drug regularly, the patient's psychosis is well controlled but, after a week, tolerance to the anti-psychotic effect of the drug develops and higher doses are required to achieve the same benefit. The effectiveness of the benzodiazepines in this case and in other psychotics may be due to a reduction in the patient's level of arousal.[486]

Researchers have indeed been able to demonstrate that the most withdrawn, unresponsive "chronic" individuals are often experiencing the highest levels of internal arousal.[487] Drugs such as benzodiazepines, which help lower arousal and induce a state of calm relaxation, might therefore be expected to reduce a diagnosed person's need to resort to tortoise-like withdrawal and isolation as strategies for coping with stress and anxiety.

5. Extrapyramidal side effects

As discussed in *Chapter Two*, people taking neuroleptic medications frequently experience a range of neurological side effects known as extrapyramidal symptoms (EPS). While these are especially common with the older drugs, they can also occur during treatment with atypical neuroleptics. The most problematic EPS are akathisia (restless agitation), dystonia (muscle spasms), and dyskinesia (abnormal involuntary movements). Clinical research has shown that benzodiazepines may help alleviate EPS, especially neuroleptic-induced akathisia.[488] Long-term use of benzodiazepines for this purpose should only be considered if other measures, such as reducing the neuroleptic dose or seeking a medication with fewer side effects, are either impractical or unsuccessful.

6. Long-term treatment

Even among those who acknowledge the possible benefits of benzodiazepines in treating acutely disturbed individuals, there is considerable scepticism regarding the value of these drugs in long-term maintenance treatment. Nevertheless, there is evidence that some people with "chronic" schizophrenia can also benefit, with researchers estimating that between a third and half of all such persons may be helped by the addition of a benzodiazepine to their neuroleptic regime.[489] A recent study of a group of people receiving long-term maintenance treatment compared those who were only given neuroleptics with a similar group given alprazolam (Xanax) as well.[490] The researchers reported that those receiving a neuroleptic plus alprazolam generally continued to experience the therapeutic benefits of the combination throughout the three-year trial period. Furthermore, several of those who received combination treatment were able to reduce their neuroleptic dosage, whereas none of those treated with neuroleptics alone were able to do so.

When benzodiazepine treatment is being considered, care should be taken to evaluate the potential benefits and possible risks associated with use of these drugs. The following general facts should be borne in mind:

Positive aspects:
- Benzodiazepines are highly effective anxiolytic (anxiety-reducing) medications
- They are fast acting, with beneficial effects often occurring within the first few hours, days, or weeks of treatment (neuroleptics often take much longer)
- They have relatively few side effects compared to

neuroleptics (particularly neurological side effects such as akathisia, dyskinesia, and akinesia)
- Because they work by reducing dopamine release in certain parts of the brain, rather than by blocking dopamine receptors as neuroleptics do, benzodiazepines are less likely to cause problems such as tardive dyskinesia (TD) and dopamine-receptor supersensitivity (a phenomenon discussed in *Chapter Two*).

Negative aspects:
- Possible side effects include sedation (sleepiness), lethargy, cognitive problems including impairment of memory and learning, mental confusion, and ataxia (impaired co-ordination of voluntary movement)
- Tolerance may develop, i.e. diminished therapeutic response may occur after a few weeks treatment and larger doses may be needed to achieve the same results. (This is highly variable: some people appear to gain little benefit after a few weeks, whereas others experience beneficial effects, despite years of continuous treatment)
- Concerns have been expressed about the possibility of psychological dependency and the related potential for abuse of benzodiazepines following long-term use
- Abrupt cessation of these drugs may result in a withdrawal syndrome involving anxiety ("rebound anxiety"), irritability, faintness, disturbed sleep, bizarre dreams, and temporary exacerbation of psychotic symptoms

In view of concerns about the possible development of *tolerance* and *dependency*, caution should be exercised when using benzodiazepines. Except in cases where long-term treatment has proven beneficial, prolonged administration on a regular basis should be avoided. *These drugs should be employed sparingly.* Taking the smallest effective dose on an as-needed basis (i.e. only when it is required rather than in a set daily routine), for relatively short periods, will minimise the risk of adverse consequences. Such restrictions allow for the *short-term* use of these drugs to help alleviate anxiety and tension when prodromal symptoms may be threatening to escalate into a full-blown psychotic episode (taking benzodiazepine medication for a day or two may be all that is required in some cases). Restricting exposure in this way also allows for short-term use (a few days or up to a week or two) to help diminish anxiety and agitation and promote sleep during a period of acute psychotic turmoil. The beneficial effects of benzodiazepines are likely to be enhanced when they are combined with general measures aimed at improving the social situation, such as a calm environment, reduced stimulation, and sensitive empathic support.

Clinical research suggests that benzodiazepines, alone or in combination with neuroleptics, are most likely to benefit diagnosed individuals who experience prominent anxiety, distress, and agitation, or whose negative symptoms (e.g. emotional "shut-down", withdrawal) are a secondary response to such feelings. However, since it is impossible to predict how a given individual will respond to these drugs (as is the case with neuroleptic treatment), a period of experimentation will often be necessary. Clinicians experienced in the use of benzodiazepines advise that a *two-week trial* is usually adequate, and that these drugs should be gradually discontinued if no observable therapeutic benefits have occurred within this time.[491]

(b) Mood Stabilisers

Drugs known as "mood stabilisers", including lithium and certain anti-convulsants, which are primarily used to prevent or control mood swings (depression or elation) associated with mood disorders, may sometimes be useful in treating schizophrenia.

1. Lithium

For several decades lithium has been the treatment of choice for *bipolar disorder* (formerly known as "manic depression"). More recently it has been given to people diagnosed with *schizoaffective disorder,* a condition characterised by a mixture of schizophrenia and mood-disorder symptoms. The combination of lithium and neuroleptics has mainly been used with people experiencing acute psychosis and is reported to be helpful in reducing excitement, aggression, overactivity, euphoria, and depressive symptoms.[492] It has also been claimed that some individuals with treatment-resistant "chronic" schizophrenia may improve significantly when lithium is added to their neuroleptic regime. Those who respond positively to lithium are described as improving in multiple areas including psychotic symptoms, co-operativeness, neatness, social competence, irritability, and excitement.[493] There has been little research on the long-term use of lithium in conjunction with neuroleptics, and it is not known whether the combination will allow a reduction in maintenance neuroleptic dosage. Lithium can cause memory impairment and adversely effect creativity and cognitive functioning.[494] Weight gain is common, with some reports indicating that up to 30% of people receiving long-term treatment may become frankly obese.[495] It should be noted that, as well as having its own side effects, lithium can cause an increase in extrapyramidal side effects (EPS) – possibly to an extreme degree – when combined with neuroleptics.[496] To lessen such problematic side effects some authorities recommend that neuroleptic dosages should be reduced by 10% -25% when lithium is added.[497]

2. Anti-convulsants

Among the large number of available anti-convulsant drugs, two in particular, carbamazepine (Tegretol) and sodium valproate (Epilim), have been combined with neuroleptics with variable results. Though not effective on its own, carbamazepine has been reported to reduce hyperactivity and aggression when used in combination with neuroleptics to treat acute psychosis, and to decrease anxiety, social withdrawal, and depression in individuals considered to be treatment-resistant.[498] Variable results have been reported in terms of its effect on psychotic symptoms, though some researchers claim carbamazepine treatment resulted in fewer side effects and meant less neuroleptic medication was required.[499] Carbamazepine has a wide range of side effects, some of which may become especially problematic with long-term use (e.g. agranulocytosis, liver inflammation). Carbamazepine can cause a reduction in the level of neuroleptic drugs in the bloodstream, which may explain why some diagnosed people become worse when treated with this drug.[500] A corollary to this effect is that neuroleptic blood levels may rise when carbamazepine is stopped, with a consequent increase in extrapyramidal side effects.[501] As with carbamazepine (for which it is sometimes substituted), adjunctive use of sodium valproate (or valproic acid) has had mixed results. Possible side effects can include sedation, tremor, increased appetite, weight gain, gastrointestinal disturbances (nausea, vomiting, abdominal pain), and liver-function abnormalities.

(c) Anti-depressants

It is estimated that up to 25% of people diagnosed with schizophrenia experience depression at some time (though it is acknowledged that it can be difficult to differentiate between this mood disorder and neuroleptic side effects such as akinesia, which are also characterised by reduced spontaneity, apathy, and physical and mental slowness). Treating acutely psychotic individuals with antidepressant drugs can result in exacerbation of psychotic symptoms, though this does not seem to occur in diagnosed persons well stabilised on neuroleptic medication.[502] Some authorities have suggested increasing the neuroleptic dosage if positive symptoms do become worse during anti-depressant treatment.[503] Anti-depressants belonging to the group known as Serotonin-Specific Re-Uptake Inhibitors (SSRIs) have recently been reported to improve negative symptoms, positive and negative symptoms in non-depressed persons, and obsessive-compulsive (OCD) symptoms.[504] It should be noted that such treatment is described as producing only *modest* improvement in these symptoms and that some people appear to deteriorate on these drugs. The extremely popular SSRI fluoxetine (Prozac) can cause blood levels of some neuroleptics to rise by up to 20%.[505] Combining SSRIs and neuroleptics could potentially lead to significant problems with neurological side effects such as akathisia since there is growing evidence that SSRIs can cause such EPS even when given on their own.[506] Sexual side effects of various kinds (e.g. impotence) are common among people treated with SSRIs.[507]

(d) Beta-blockers

The group of drugs known collectively as *beta-adrenergic receptor antagonists* or "beta-blockers" are primarily used to treat hypertension (high blood pressure) and cardiovascular disease. One of these drugs, propranolol (Inderal), has often been used as an adjunct to neuroleptic treatment of schizophrenia, although no consistent anti-psychotic effect has been demonstrated. Nevertheless, propranolol has been found to be an effective treatment for neuroleptic-induced akathisia (restless agitation), a condition which can mimic psychosis and, when severe, may lead to violence or even suicide. Some researchers believe the reason some people improve when given propranolol is largely a result of its ability to alleviate akathisia.[508] People treated with this drug have sometimes reported a sense of feeling "soothed and calmed".[509] A decrease in akathisia may occur within 1-3 days of treatment with 30-80 mg of propranolol per day. Side effects can include hypotension (low blood pressure) and bradycardia (slow heart beat). Propranolol treatment can result in an increase in some neuroleptic blood levels, especially with older drugs such as chlorpromazine (Largactil) and thioridazine (Mellaril).[510]

Polypharmacy or Holistic Treatment?

In psychiatry, as in other branches of medicine, an effort must constantly be made to ensure that the possible benefits of a particular treatment outweigh its costs. Schizophrenia is no exception to this rule. There is little doubt that the use of low-dose or intermittent medication may involve a higher risk of relapse for some people, and that these treatment regimes can place considerable demands on *all* concerned (monitoring prodromal symptoms involves constant vigilance, for example). On the other hand, reducing the burden of debilitating side effects like akinesia and akathisia, can contribute immeasurably to improving a diagnosed person's quality of life, quite apart from the enhanced self-confidence and self-esteem that accompany the sense that one is exercising greater control over one's own life and destiny.

While acknowledging that the adjunctive use of medications such as those described in this chapter might prove to be of considerable benefit to some diagnosed individuals, it is essential that treating professionals, their clients, and caring relatives, do not embark on an endless search for a drug or drug combination that will finally "fix" everything once and for all. This issue is especially relevant to schizophrenia as there is now a strong tendency to construe this disorder as an entirely biological phenomenon (e.g. the result of a genetically-determined chemical imbalance) for which drugs are the only effective treatment. While these simplistic notions have understandable appeal, they raise grave concerns about the potential dangers of seeking pharmaceutical solutions for every problem diagnosed people happen to experience ("a pill for every ill"). Indeed, a growing number of influential psychiatric authorities now appear to believe that *all* human problems do indeed have a biological cause for which an effective drug remedy will soon be found.

In her influential book, *The Broken Brain: The Biological*

Revolution in Psychiatry, Professor Nancy Andreasen boldly asserts that such common problems as poor self-esteem and excessive guilt can be seen as direct reflections of disturbed neurochemical processes in the brain which it will soon be possible to rectify with drugs.[511] Lay and professional literatures are replete with examples of biological reductionism, especially when discussing complex conditions such as schizophrenia. As "therapeutic polypharmacy" gains ever more clinical converts, scenarios such as the following could soon become the norm:

> Still experiencing symptoms? Let's try increasing your medication dosage a little. If that doesn't work there are other neuroleptics we haven't tried yet. Feeling a bit worried and anxious? Not a problem, we'll just pop you on an anti-anxiety drug. Been a bit down? We have antidepressants for that. Still not progressing as you'd hoped? Perhaps an anti-convulsant or a beta-blocker will help. Life seems a bit of a roller coaster ride, constantly up and down? Let's start you on a mood-stabiliser. Oh, by the way, there's a whole new class of drugs we're about to start testing. Would you like to participate in an experimental trial?

Remembering that there are limits to what medications can realistically be expected to do provides a counterbalance to this kind of thinking. It is noteworthy that experienced clinicians who have worked closely and intensively with diagnosed people invariably acknowledge the therapeutic efficacy of *non-drug* aspects of treatment. Professor Manfred Bleuler, an internationally acclaimed psychiatrist who spent his professional career working with people diagnosed with schizophrenia, certainly held such views. Summarising his findings, Professor Bleuler emphasised the therapeutic value of "calming actions and influences" which he felt could take many forms, "the best of them being talking and togetherness, and another being neuroleptic drugs".[512]

It is clear that, in certain instances, it is possible to achieve therapeutic results similar to or even better than those attributed to medications using non-drug techniques. This was illustrated by the Soteria Project described in *Chapter Five*. A report published in the journal *Psychiatry* in 1986 described use of a beta-blocker drug (see above) to treat a young man diagnosed with "chronic" schizophrenia. After observing a remarkable improvement in his condition over the next two and a half years his therapists made the following remarks:

> Beta-blockers … seem to have a soothing effect similar to a caregiver's love and support. Other, more verbal patients on beta-blockers have reported a sense of feeling soothed and calmed, much as if they were being held … *It is our hypothesis that the results we achieved through the use of beta-blockers are generalisable to any treatment modality that acts in some way to soothe the state of chronic agitation* … The patient's increased comfort in his own skin allows him to tolerate for a longer period of time stimuli perceived as potentially disorganising, and gradually to develop greater flexibility and a richer repertoire of adaptive behaviours in response to them.[513]

Working out the optimal treatment regime for a given

person, i.e. specific drug, dosage, and frequency, can take considerable time. In this search it should always be remembered that some people manage well without *any* medication, neuroleptic or otherwise. Furthermore, some diagnosed individuals who might be considered unsuitable candidates for low-dose or intermittent treatment may not necessarily always be so. One of the key principles guiding wise medication use entails remaining open to the possibility of change. Experience attests to the fact that all human beings possess an innate capacity to grow and develop over time. Those who have been diagnosed with schizophrenia are no exception.

Chapter Ten

REDUCING OR STOPPING NEUROLEPTIC MEDICATIONS

The optimal solution in a substantial proportion of cases would probably be to slowly taper the neuroleptic therapy to the lowest dose that would control the symptoms of schizophrenia to a satisfactory degree. In some patients, the lowest dose may be zero – stopping neuroleptic therapy.

Patricia Gilbert et al.[514]

THIS CHAPTER IS SPECIFICALLY intended for those who are thinking of reducing or stopping their own neuroleptic medication, or who are involved in supporting somebody else who is planning to do so. It must be emphasised at the outset that it is *not* the author's intention to encourage anyone to stop or substantially alter their medication regime in any way without first seeking advice and guidance from the prescribing physician and other helpers. Having said this, it is important to acknowledge the existence of widely differing attitudes towards medication issues within the mental health field, with some practitioners being far more conservative in this regard than others. Those who adhere to a narrow medical-model view of schizophrenia as an essentially biological disorder tend to place far greater emphasis on the role of drugs than do those who adopt a broader holistic perspective. In any event, diagnosed persons who express a desire to reduce or stop their drug treatment are often met with very simple advice: "Don't!". While this is probably sound advice in *some* cases, it is not helpful to those who might actually benefit from a medication reduction. Nor is it of any use to the many who, for one reason or another, will simply ignore it (treatment compliance is known to be quite poor among those diagnosed with schizophrenia, with surveys indicating that only about 30% to 50% of such people always take their medications exactly as prescribed).[515]

Rational Drug Withdrawal

High non-compliance rates indicate that many diagnosed people do not take their recommended medications at all, or if they do, only take them on an occasional basis, e.g. when they feel they need them. Contemporary psychiatric clinicians, by contrast, are generally inclined to consider neuroleptic medications to be the most important component of effective schizophrenia treatment. Indeed, pharmacological therapies are so heavily emphasised that it has become relatively unusual for non-drug treatments to be considered as a possible option for some people. It seems that many clinicians would now prefer to engage in a process of prolonged experimentation – administering various drugs, dosages, and drug combinations (a practice known as "neuroleptic augmentation") in an attempt to find an effective therapeutic regime – rather than consider the simple possibility that drug-free treatment may be a viable option in some instances. One important consequence of this attitude is that little attention has been devoted to understanding the process of withdrawing (i.e. reducing or stopping) neuroleptic medications. David Cohen, a professor of social work and astute critic of contemporary clinical practice, has summarised the present state of affairs thus:

> Although theoretical, clinical, practical, and ethical justifications for discontinuing or withdrawing neuroleptic drug treatment abound, and although the issue of withdrawal has enormous importance for consumers, *rational drug withdrawal may be the least studied topic in clinical psychopharmacology and the one about which clinicians are most ignorant* ... There are many ways to conduct a study to investigate the potential advantages of neuroleptic withdrawal and substitution of non-drug supports ... Despite the hundreds of different interventions that have been tested for schizophrenia, the author is not aware of a single such study in nearly 50 years of neuroleptic therapy.[516]

The ensuing discussion is based on the assumption that there are a number of legitimate reasons for diagnosed people to reduce their medication. Among them are the following:

1. To establish the lowest effective neuroleptic dose
2. To minimise problematic medication side effects
3. Prior to switching to a different neuroleptic drug
4. Prior to commencing intermittent treatment
5. In the process of stopping neuroleptic therapy

It must be acknowledged that, just as there are various risks associated with prolonged neuroleptic treatment (e.g. short- and long-term side effects), so too are there possible risks associated with reducing or stopping it (e.g. the possibility of symptom exacerbation or an increased likelihood of relapse). Experience teaches that medication reduction can be undertaken in a cautious way or a more risky way. *Anybody who tries to reduce or stop their medication without taking appropriate precautions could experience untoward consequences ranging from severe withdrawal symptoms to another psychotic episode.* Sadly, people who are impatient to get off medication sometimes act in ways that actually *increase* their likelihood of finding themselves back on it! Failure to approach this matter with due care could even result in the imposition of involuntary treatment, e.g. closely supervised depot medication, and other restrictive measures. On the other hand, by observing a few simple precautions it is possible for any diagnosed person to greatly reduce the likelihood that they will end up back at square one. The guidelines outlined in this chapter are based on the principles of risk-minimisation and have been validated by extensive clinical experience.

Before discussing specific practical guidelines it is especially important for all concerned to be aware of the possible consequences, both positive and negative, of changing long-standing treatment regimes. In particular, it is vital to appreciate and make proper allowance for the various contingencies that may arise when people diagnosed with schizophrenia substantially reduce their neuroleptic dosage or stop taking these drugs altogether. Acquiring such an understanding *before* making any alterations to medication regimes provides a sound basis for informed decision-making and forward planning, both of which will help increase the likelihood of being able to successfully negotiate the various changes that accompany medication reduction. *It is vital to understand that medication adjustment is a complex matter which should not be approached in an ill-informed, wilful, or cavalier manner, but rather with intelligence, honesty, and due caution.* Particular care must be exercised when altering the established medication regime of anyone with a demonstrated tendency to relapse rapidly with an accompanying loss of insight. Similar precautions apply if the individual concerned has a recent history of destructive or self-harming behaviour, or if they have engaged in serious anti-social, violent, or aggressive acts in the past.

The Withdrawal Process

To better appreciate what medication reduction entails it is helpful to have a basic understanding of some of the changes that occur in the brain during treatment and as drugs are withdrawn. Far from being a passive organ, the human brain is now known to be a complex, highly dynamic system with a remarkable capacity to alter both its structure and functioning in response to inner and outer stimuli. When psychoactive drugs are ingested, the presence of these foreign chemical substances elicits various changes in the brain. The brain's billions of neuroreceptors are in a state of constant flux and psychoactive drugs are now known to affect their number and configuration within half an hour to an hour of being ingested.[517] (Such changes also occur in response to non-prescribed drugs like alcohol, nicotine, caffeine, and street drugs.) The resulting neurological changes sometimes have various *desirable* consequences, e.g. anxiety reduction with anxiolytic drugs, or mood elevation with antidepressants.

Prolonged and continuous exposure to neuroleptics or other drugs which have powerful effects on the central nervous system causes the brain to adapt to their constant presence. When the drugs are stopped or the dose is substantially reduced, the brain's equilibrium is temporarily upset and a process of readjustment must occur as the brain gradually gets used to functioning without them. Since the initial adaptation may have taken many weeks or months, the readjustment process may require a similar length of time, possibly even longer. Especially if the dosage of a neuroleptic (or other psychoactive drug) is reduced *rapidly*, the ensuing state of temporary disequilibrium may give rise to a set of physical and mental symptoms known collectively as a "withdrawal syndrome". (As well as occurring when medication doses are being lowered, withdrawal syndromes of various kinds can also occur when a person is switched from one of the older conventional neuroleptics to one of the newer atypical ones.[518])

Most people are familiar with the withdrawal syndromes that can accompany a substantial reduction in the consumption of social drugs such as caffeine, nicotine, and alcohol. The various symptoms that occur when withdrawing from these potent psychoactive substances are generally only severe if the level of consumption has been high, has continued over a long time, or intake is stopped or reduced abruptly. Neuroleptic withdrawal symptoms are also likely to be most severe if a person who has been taking large amounts of medication for a long time attempts to reduce the dosage too quickly. Rapid reduction in neuroleptic intake can induce *pharmacological stress* which causes severe shock to the nervous system. Psychiatrist Edward Podvoll makes these observations regarding withdrawal of long-standing neuroleptic medication:

> Patients and doctors seem to generally agree that abrupt withdrawal from long-term medications is ignorant and dangerous; the shock to the nervous system that has been habituated to them is too great, and the whiplash can be overwhelming. Even the graduated withdrawal of medications can be a difficult process ... When a doctor and a patient agree to the withdrawal of anti-psychotic medications they should have a common understanding of what they are doing.[519]

Differences in individual characteristics and circumstances (including genetic factors) play a major role in determining how a given individual will respond to changes in their intake of drugs. For reasons that are not yet fully understood, some people are able to substantially reduce or even cease consumption of social drugs such as caffeine and nicotine with relative ease, while others experience severe and possibly prolonged physiological and psychological withdrawal symptoms. In a similar manner, there can be considerable variation in the way diagnosed people respond to a reduced intake of neuroleptic drugs.

The Neuroleptic Withdrawal Syndrome

Many mental health clinicians continue to deny the reality of a neuroleptic withdrawal syndrome. For example, in his popular book *Surviving Schizophrenia*, psychiatrist E. Fuller Torrey insists: "The person's body does not slowly get used to them [neuroleptics] and therefore require higher and higher doses, and the stopping of these drugs does not usually cause withdrawal symptoms."[520] Despite such claims, a considerable body of evidence attests to the reality of this phenomenon.[521] The existence of a high level of professional denial moved psychopharmacologist David Healy to comment in 2002:

> It should be remembered that, in contrast to dependence on benzodiazepines, dependence on anti-psychotics had been clearly recognised in the mid-1960s but that this recognition was then lost. A series of studies in the mid-1960s demonstrated conclusively that when patients stopped even low doses of anti-psychotics (such as 1 mg haloperidol) taken for brief periods of time (six months), significant withdrawal problems could ensue.[522]

Some of the symptoms commonly associated with neuroleptic withdrawal are described below. It is important to understand that it is not possible to know in advance how a particular individual will respond to a significant reduction in neuroleptic dosage. Furthermore, in practice it is possible that a number of different things could be occurring at the same time, giving rise to a very complex situation. For example, if a person changes more than one prescription medication at a time, or they stop smoking or reduce their consumption of caffeine or street drugs, they could potentially experience a number of different withdrawal effects simultaneously. *As a general rule, any new symptoms which appear within the first few days of stopping a drug, or substantially reducing the dose, are likely to be withdrawal effects.* Since it takes several months for long-acting injectable neuroleptics to be gradually eliminated from the body, any withdrawal effects associated with these drugs may be considerably delayed, compared to those associated with oral medications (tablets) which are likely to become noticeable within a day or two of reducing intake. All of the symptoms listed below can also occur when a person is switching from a conventional neuroleptic (including depot medication) to one of the atypical drugs.[523]

(a) Physical withdrawal symptoms

A number of physical withdrawal symptoms can accompany rapid reduction in neuroleptic dosage. These include anxiety, insomnia, restlessness, and flu-like symptoms such as headache, nausea, aches and pains, malaise, sweating, runny nose, diarrhoea, and vomiting. These symptoms may be quite mild and are invariably transient, though they can sometimes persist for several weeks. Some authorities advise that people who have been taking anti-parkinsonian medications (APs) to control extrapyramidal side effects, should continue these drugs for a short time (at least a few days) *after* they stop neuroleptic treatment. This will prevent the "cholinergic rebound" that is believed to be responsible for physical withdrawal symptoms.[524]

(b) Neurological withdrawal symptoms

Extra-pyramidal symptoms (EPS) such as akathisia and dys-kinesia may appear *for the first time* or become *worse* with neuroleptic dose reduction.[525] EPS that first appear when medication is reduced (*withdrawal-emergent dyskinesias*) are often self-limiting, although it can take several months for them to gradually disappear. On the other hand, EPS such as tardive dyskinesia (TD) may have developed over many years but only become obvious when medication is being reduced or stopped. In such cases, raising the dosage again will often lead to a reduction in the severity of the abnormal movements (this only occurs because the neuroleptic medication masks the underlying problem). Some researchers have suggested that the most severe cases of TD seem to occur when people have stopped neuroleptic medication abruptly.[526] As noted previously, the sudden onset of severe withdrawal-emergent neurological side effects sometimes gives rise to anxiety and distress that is misinterpreted as incipient psychosis.

(c) Psychiatric withdrawal symptoms

Neuroleptic-induced supersensitivity was discussed in *Chapter Two*. Although this phenomenon is poorly recognised, a considerable body of evidence supports the possibility that abrupt withdrawal of neuroleptic medication can itself trigger the onset of acute psychosis (also known as "rebound psychosis") in certain individuals. The observation that relapse is far more likely to occur when neuroleptic drugs are stopped rapidly is consistent with the supersensitivity hypothesis.[527] A severe and florid psychosis characterised by hallucinations, delusions, hostility, and paranoia is known to occur when the atypical neuroleptic clozapine is withdrawn abruptly.[528] In spite of this evidence, clinicians unfamiliar with neuroleptic withdrawal syndromes are unlikely to differentiate between psychotic episodes that are a result of supersensitivity, and those that may involve re-emergence or exacerbation of symptoms that were previously controlled with medication. ("It is interesting to note", psychiatrist Philip Thomas wrote recently, "how the drug withdrawal explanation for 'relapse' has been overwhelmingly neglected in the psychiatric literature."[529]) Researchers who have studied this phenomenon in detail suggest that the supersensitivity psychosis is characterised by the following specific features:[530]

- Psychotic symptoms appear soon – usually within days or weeks of either stopping neuroleptic medication or substantially reducing the dosage
- The psychosis involves positive symptoms (e.g. suspiciousness, hallucinations, delusions) but not negative symptoms (emotional withdrawal, blunted affect)
- The psychosis may be even more severe than it was before treatment and might involve the emergence of some new, previously unreported symptoms
- Signs of growing treatment resistance may have been present prior to stopping medication (i.e. gradually increasing dosages required to control symptoms)
- Symptoms of tardive dyskinesia (TD) are often present and may be severe
- Signs of neuroleptic-induced sexual dysfunction such as reduced sexual drive, loss of libido are often present (due to abnormally elevated prolactin levels)

- Reinstating the neuroleptic that led to the development of supersensitivity provides effective control of the psychotic withdrawal symptoms

The rebound psychosis associated with neuroleptic-induced supersensitivity can vary considerably in duration and intensity. In some instances, the symptoms will abate within a few days without any specific treatment. In more severe cases, in order to alleviate the symptoms it may be necessary to reinstate the neuroleptic which caused the supersensitivity in the first place.* In some cases even this strategy may only be partly effective.[531]

(d) Psychological withdrawal symptoms

In addition to the effects already described, a substantial reduction in neuroleptic dosage can have a range of psychological consequences. An important result of reducing or stopping medication – one that is often overlooked – concerns the changes which may subsequently occur in a diagnosed person's emotional state, motivation, and general level of vitality. If the original medication had a suppressing or dampening effect, reducing the dose may result in a substantial release of physical and mental energy, together with an unmasking of previously attenuated feelings. While this is generally a positive and welcome development, removal of the stress buffer which neuroleptic drugs provide could leave some extremely sensitive

---

* Since olanzapine (Zyprexa) has a similar structure and receptor-blocking profile to clozapine (Clozaril), switching to this drug may help minimise the clozapine-withdrawal syndrome. See: Tollefson, G., et al. (1999) "Controlled Double-Blind Investigation of the Clozapine Discontinuation Symptoms with Conversion to Either Olanzapine or Placebo", *Journal of Clinical Psychopharmacology*, Vol. 19

individuals feeling exposed and vulnerable. This state may be especially anxiety-provoking for those who have experienced an extended period of being "wrapped in cotton wool". Dr Podvoll describes this phenomenon and some of its possible consequences:

> The actual experience of "coming off" [neuroleptic medication] is, of course, very individual ... Fidgeting, leg-swinging, pacing, and agitation are not only signs of being uncomfortable in one's own body, they are also expressions of surges of energy appearing in the mind. For people who have been taking medications for a year or more, sometimes even the slightest reductions can unleash a mental speed that they are unaccustomed to handling ... with this comes an extreme sensitivity to the environment, especially to how one is being treated by others. It is a time when one may no longer feel docile, submissive, or simply submerged in his "own world" ... It is also the time of a generalised awakening to his environment, and to the conditions under which he has suffered.[532]

There is no doubt that some diagnosed people may actually come to *prefer* the protective cocoon of a heavily medicated way of life. For others, the sense of safety provided by medication may even lead to a form of psychological dependency. Learning to accept and feel comfortable with *normal* emotions – including potentially painful or distressing feelings like anxiety, anger, and frustration – is a major challenge for many diagnosed people. Joan Houghton has described how she experienced a veritable awakening when she stopped taking a medication that had caused severe parkinsonian side effects. She soon realised that, in order to maintain her emotional stability without the drugs, she needed to adjust her lifestyle and learn to cope with previously suppressed and denied feelings:

> To maintain a sense of wellbeing I have had to change my lifestyle and my priorities … Once freed from the regulating shackles of medications, I had to substitute their positive effects – a reasonable routine, a slower pace, and a calm atmosphere. I began my new life by setting up a schedule for myself, by providing a structure for everyday living … In the emotional dimensions I have also had many lessons: I have learned to cry … Many emotional lessons in anger have yet to be learned. I often "sit on it". It's there; I feel it; but I don't express it well. All too often it's displaced and misplaced. It's a problem I share with much of our society.[533]

Ironically, if re-awakened feelings are not dealt with constructively, and increased energy is not channelled into some kind of personally meaningful activity, great frustration may result which ultimately leads to despair and demoralisation. In such cases, those concerned may end up feeling even *more* frustrated than they did when they were taking larger amounts of medication.

Guidelines For Reducing Neuroleptic Medication

The onset of withdrawal symptoms, especially if they are severe, persistent, or distressing, is often interpreted by the diagnosed person and others (including those providing treatment) as a sign that reducing the medication has caused the person's illness to worsen. While this may *sometimes* be the case, in many instances the apparent worsening – which could even take the appearance of an imminent relapse – may actually be a manifestation of a process of physical and mental adjustment to the absence or reduced presence of neuroleptic drugs. As in cases where people are withdrawing from nicotine, caffeine, alcohol, or illicit drug addiction, discovering an optimal neuroleptic regime may necessitate a period of getting somewhat worse before starting to get better.

Though withdrawal symptoms are generally transient, they may sometimes cause sufficient distress or discomfort that a decision is made to go back to the former neuroleptic dose. However, simply reinstating the original medication regime for those who are experiencing a withdrawal syndrome could lead to an impasse when what is actually called for is an adequate opportunity to complete the adjustment process. As explained below, rather than simply returning to the *status quo ante*, in some instances the most helpful thing to do may be to take steps to slow the process down, e.g. reducing the dose even more gradually. Because many complex issues are involved, it is most important that everyone concerned approach the task of medication reduction in a careful and methodical fashion. The following guidelines indicate one way this can be done.

(a) Devise and follow a plan

It is very important to adopt a systematic approach to medication reduction. Before doing anything else the person withdrawing should give careful thought to this undertaking so that they are clear in their own mind about their goals and how they intend to go about achieving them. It is most unwise to act in a haphazard or impulsive way, e.g. waking up one morning and simply throwing the pills away. In general, it is not a good idea to make significant decisions about medication (or anything else) when feeling angry, upset, or depressed. Thinking carefully about when would be a good time to begin is a key aspect of forward planning. Clinical experience suggests that reducing or stopping medication relatively soon after a psychotic episode may be significantly more risky than doing so after a reasonable period of stability. Generally speaking, the more recent the episode, the more vulnerable to relapse a person is likely to be.[534] It is highly advisable to choose or arrange a time of low stress (both present and anticipated), and for the withdrawing person not to begin the process of reducing the medication until they feel well and are satisfied all necessary arrangements have been made. A mandatory aspect of planning involves discussing intended goals and strategies with others (see next point).

(b) Seek appropriate guidance and support

The guidance and support of appropriately qualified and experienced people should always be sought when making significant changes to medication regimes. In the case of neuroleptic drugs, this would ideally involve the prescribing psychiatrist or a non-psychiatric medical practitioner working in collaboration with one or more experienced mental health professionals. In the first instance it is essential that diagnosed people discuss the pros and cons of medication reduction with a qualified person who is familiar with their particular circumstances and history. Following such a discussion, some may decide not to alter their medication regime. On the other hand, some people may still wish to proceed even if their doctor is not in favour of them doing so. In such cases it is advisable to seek a second or even third medical opinion before making a final decision. The safest way to proceed is undoubtedly to have the prescribing doctor agree to supervise a gradual dose reduction. In any event, it is highly desirable to have the support of as many people as possible, e.g. trusted friends, family members, and mental health workers who can be relied upon to "be there" if and when their assistance is required. During a period of significant change it can be especially helpful to have regular contact with a trusted helper such as a counsellor or therapist.

(c) Be well prepared

Long before they actually start reducing their medication, diagnosed people should do everything they can to prepare themselves physically, mentally, and spiritually. Anyone hoping to manage on less (or no) medication must be prepared to make an active commitment to doing as much as they possibly can to nurture their health and wellbeing. *It is not simply a matter of taking fewer pills and hoping everything will be all right!* Most people know there are certain aspects of their life they could change or improve, e.g. many people carry considerable emotional baggage (bottled-up feelings, unresolved conflicts) which constitute a significant source of stress. The timely use of supportive counselling can be an invaluable aide in dealing with such issues. An individual's religion or personal spiritual philosophy can be drawn upon in addressing spiritual issues and concerns (which, in some instances, may have come to the fore in the context of a psychotic experience). In the process of making a sincere effort to deal with important personal issues, some people may discover inner resources of which they were previously unaware. Cultivating a positive attitude, working to improve self-confidence and self-esteem, utilising effective stress management skills, and learning non-drug strategies for managing persistent symptoms (such as voices) are among the many tasks people should at least begin as part of their preparations. Adopting a healthy lifestyle involving a balanced diet, regular exercise, adequate rest and sleep, reduced consumption of social drugs, and strict avoidance of all street drugs, will help to restore and strengthen natural self-healing mechanisms, both mental and physical.

(d) Learn to recognise personal warning signals

Diagnosed people who are prone to recurrent episodes of psychosis often experience a range of subtle changes in their feelings and thought processes when they are starting to become psychotic. These changes (sometimes called "prodromal symptoms") can serve as early-warning signals that may indicate an increased likelihood of relapse. With time and experience, many people learn to recognise the characteristic changes that can alert them to the fact that they may need to take steps to avert the development of a full-blown psychotic episode. Familiarity with their own unique pattern of prodromal symptoms can provide diagnosed people and their helpers with an invaluable tool with which to monitor their mental state while reducing their medication. It is important for all concerned to understand that various changes may occur while reducing medication which are *not* indicative of imminent relapse, even though some of them may be quite difficult or distressing, e.g. withdrawal symptoms may occur or painful feelings may emerge that were previously suppressed by medication. The fact that it is sometimes difficult to differentiate between prodromal symptoms and withdrawal effects underscores the importance of maintaining regular contact with people who can help to correctly evaluate what is happening. Remaining open to others and receptive to their feedback and support is crucial to the success of prodromal-symptom monitoring (This important coping skill was discussed in *Chapter Nine* in the context of intermittent treatment.)

(e) Prepare contingency plans

While the process of medication reduction is likely to be relatively uneventful for many people – especially if it is undertaken very gradually – it is not really possible to predict what may occur. Consequently, it is important to be prepared for any eventuality. It can be helpful to draw up a list of all the things that could possibly occur and then write down how they will be dealt with should they eventuate. For example, it is worth thinking about what to do if prodromal symptoms develop, how to deal with withdrawal symptoms, or how to respond should stress, anxiety, or other painful feelings become problematic. Possible coping strategies could be discussed with the treating doctor and other support personnel. It should be remembered that, while increasing the dosage back to its original level is one possible option, there may be others that will allow the medication reduction process to continue – though perhaps at a somewhat slower pace. It is extremely important that contingency plans be formulated *in advance* to avoid disorganised, *ad hoc* responses to crises and other unexpected developments. It is advisable to reach agreement with trusted helpers regarding what they should do if the withdrawing person is temporarily unable to make decisions in his or her own best interest, e.g. a written plan could be prepared spelling out exactly what to do should circumstances arise that involve unacceptable risk or which expose the diagnosed person or others to potential danger.

(f) Reduce medication slowly

Except in the case of people who have only received small amounts of medication for a very short time, neuroleptic dosages should always be reduced slowly. A large body of clinical research has shown that *relapse is much more likely to occur following rapid dose reduction than it is when the medication is reduced very gradually* (a process known as "neuroleptic taper"). Professor Ross Baldessarini has estimated that the proportion of diagnosed people who relapse per month is *three times higher* when treatment is discontinued abruptly rather than being gradually reduced.[535] Other researchers have suggested that rapid reduction is associated with relapse rates more than *six times higher* than occurs when medication is reduced slowly.[536] Severe withdrawal effects are also much more likely with rapid dose reduction due to induction of pharmacological stress. One advantage of gradual reduction is that it leaves open the possibility of temporarily increasing the dosage at any time should the need arise, e.g. if distressing prodromal or other symptoms occur.

Because of the many individual variables involved it is impossible to say at what rate a given person's neuroleptic medication can be safely reduced. Dr Edward Podvoll suggests reducing the medication by 10% of the original dosage in ten consecutive steps, at least one week apart.[537]

After each reduction, the person concerned should remain on the new dose until they feel ready to make the next reduction. If severe withdrawal symptoms or other untoward reactions occur, they should remain at that level – or possibly go back one step – until they feel confident to proceed. It is very important to *take as long as necessary for each step* and to be prepared to make even smaller reductions toward the end. A rather more conservative approach involves reducing the medication in steps no larger than 20% of the original dose at intervals of between three and six months.[538] For those who have been receiving treatment solely in the form of long-acting depot injections, the slow rate at which these drugs are eliminated functions as a kind of automatic neuroleptic taper. Simply having no more medication after receiving a final injection will result in a very gradual reduction in neuroleptic levels over the following 8 to 10 months, since it can take at least this long for depot medications to be entirely eliminated from the body.[539]

It may sometimes be necessary to proceed *extremely* slowly when the medication dosage is very small. This was illustrated in a case reported in the *Canadian Journal of Psychiatry* in 1989, in which a woman receiving just 1 mg per day of oral haloperidol had the dose reduced by 0.25 mg every two weeks. During the final two-week period, she took one 0.25 mg tablet every second day. The treating psychiatrist formed the opinion that this woman had previously experienced a severe rebound psychosis when her medication was reduced slightly more quickly.[540]

While some people may feel comfortable with these recommendations, those in more of a hurry to reduce or stop their medication may be unhappy with the prospect of having to proceed so slowly. While such impatience is understandable, it is worth bearing in mind that trying to change things too quickly can sometimes turn out to be costly in the long run. As frustrating as it might be, when reducing neuroleptic medication, it is generally advisable to err on the side of going a bit too slowly than it is to try to go too quickly. (An exception to this rule would arise if a person develops a severe adverse reaction which necessitates *immediate* discontinuation of neuroleptic treatment. Examples would include side effects such as agranulocytosis and neuroleptic malignant syndrome which require prompt medical attention.)

(g) Change one drug at a time

Many people treated with neuroleptics also take various other psychoactive drugs, including other prescription medications, social drugs (such as alcohol, caffeine, and nicotine), and possibly illicit street drugs. Reducing or stopping more than one potent psychoactive substance at a time can greatly increase the likelihood of complications. For example, quitting cigarette smoking while undertaking neuroleptic reduction may significantly increase the chances of experiencing anxiety, tension, and irritability which could, if severe, compromise the success of *both* endeavours. As a general rule, it is advisable to concentrate on only reducing one drug at a time. Diagnosed persons with substance abuse problems should seek assistance from competent professionals experienced in treating dual diagnosis disorders. Those who have been taking more than one psychiatric drug should seek the advice of the prescribing doctor regarding which medication to reduce first.

(h) Be prepared to increase the dosage if necessary

During the process of gradually reducing neuroleptic medication there may come a point at which it is advisable to stop lowering the dosage or even raise it a little. For example, people who start to experience very mild symptoms as their medication gets to a certain level may decide not to reduce it any further, in the belief that they have reached the minimum effective dose. Some people may choose to remain on that amount of medication indefinitely as their maintenance treatment. Others may decide to remain on it until some time in the future when they may feel ready to try reducing it further. It can sometimes be beneficial to *temporarily* increase the neuroleptic dosage, e.g. some people may find it helpful to increase their medication during an especially stressful or emotionally difficult time. In such cases, it will often be possible to reduce the dosage again when things have settled down. At times it can be hard to know whether to persist with the medication-reduction process or increase the dosage. For example, it can sometimes be difficult to differentiate between withdrawal symptoms – which simply call for patience until they pass – and prodromal symptoms which may indicate a need to increase the medication to reduce the risk of relapse. Experience is undoubtedly the best teacher in this regard. It is most important that the diagnosed person seeks and listens to feedback from others, such as trusted helpers, who are able to provide a relatively objective perspective on developments.

A degree of humility is an invaluable asset to all who want to limit their use of psychiatric medication. Stubborn refusal to accept a temporary increase in medication when it is warranted, due to fear of "giving in", could result in unpleasant consequences for all concerned. Adopting a flexible attitude towards medication can significantly improve any person's chances of eventually achieving the result they desire. It can be helpful to look upon the process of medication reduction as an experiment, and part of a personal learning project, rather than as a desperate struggle whose only possible outcomes are either "success" (getting off medication) or "failure" (staying on it). It is worth remembering that research has shown that some diagnosed people are able to manage well with intermittent treatment, i.e. using medication only when they need it while remaining drug-free the rest of the time (see *Chapter Nine*).

(i) Accept more responsibility
As useful as medication can sometimes be, it should never be seen as excusing diagnosed people from the responsibility of doing everything they can to foster their own healing and recovery. This is true for everybody, and is *especially* pertinent to those who would like to use less medication or who hope to eventually stop taking psychiatric drugs altogether. Such people must be willing to take responsibility for their physical, mental, and spiritual health and wellbeing, and be prepared to work hard to achieve their desired goals. Some of the many things that people with a diagnosis of schizophrenia can do to help reduce, or possibly even eliminate, the need for long-term continuous neuroleptic treatment, were discussed in earlier chapters. Those wishing to reduce their medication must be prepared to approach this challenging task in a responsible and conscientious manner, a point Emma Pierce has strongly emphasised:

Please do not read this, get all enthusiastic and go off your medication. There is a principle of life, a truth that applies here also. No real and lasting change comes overnight. Too fast won't last. If you want to cope without medication, then you must approach the problem sensibly and reasonably. You will not be able to cease medication overnight, unless of course you've been on a small dose a very short time ... What you really need to do is develop the personal resources, the habits for living that will help you cope without the medication. As you slowly develop these resources, you can slowly come off your medication ... You will need to develop understanding, control, courage, confidence, love, acceptance ... you will need to work hard and long at replacing long-established bad habits of thinking and acting and feeling with good ones. It will take time, but take heart, the longest journey begins with the first step ... So remember, it is not realistic to suddenly drop all medication and expect mental health to walk through the door. You must develop it.[541]

Less medication goes hand in hand with increased responsibility. This issue is relevant to all diagnosed persons, *particularly* those who have been required to take psychiatric drugs against their wishes and who believe they no longer need them (some will doubtless insist they never did need them in the first place!). Such people must ask themselves what it was about their behaviour that caused others to feel they required involuntary treatment. Furthermore, in order to reduce the likelihood of finding themselves in a similar situation again, they must be prepared to accept full responsibility for their behaviour and learn to avoid acting in ways that are likely to cause others to feel concerned or afraid. Psychiatrist Ron Leifer has offered the following advice to people in this relatively common situation:

> When somebody comes in to me to get off drugs, the first thing I explain to them is that the basic reason they're on drugs is that their behaviour either doesn't satisfy or disturbs some people around them ... a part of getting off drugs is reducing the demand that other people make that they be on drugs. In order to do that they have to take some increased responsibility for their own behaviour. So getting off drugs goes hand in hand with learning something about oneself so that one becomes more skilled at dealing with people and doesn't get into circumstances where you're being corralled and put on the spot and forced to take drugs basically for other people's benefit ... The first thing they have to understand is that while to them ... their behaviour feels not only appropriate but exhilarating, not everybody may feel that way about their behaviour ... people closest to them may actually be put off by their energy ... [542]

Diagnosed people who are unwilling to accept responsibility for themselves may sooner or later find that others will start making decisions for them, particularly about their treatment. This is especially likely if their behaviour has negative consequences for themselves or for others such as relatives, friends, co-workers, and neighbours.

(j) Don't make medication the centre of your life

Nobody should allow medication to become the central issue in their life, as if it was the only thing upon which their mental health and psychological wellbeing depended. On the other hand, some people become so focussed on *not* being on medication that they make the quest to get off it into an obsessive personal crusade. Neither attitude is helpful to true recovery. Whether or not someone is taking medication, they should be working to improve their life in any and every way they can. Getting the medication right is very important since being on an unsuitable type or dose, or taking drugs that are no longer helpful, can have detrimental consequences. On the other hand, experience has shown that, for some people, being on a suitable type and dosage of neuroleptic medication for the appropriate length of time can be highly beneficial to recovery. In order to help maintain their psychological stability, some people may need to take medication on a regular basis over extended periods. This should not be seen as a sign of weakness or failure on their part, however, nor does it indicate that they are somehow "sicker" than those who may be able to manage without long-term medication.

Relapse Risk Arises Early

When they stop taking neuroleptic medication or substantially reduce the dosage, some diagnosed people *do* become more prone to experiencing relapse (i.e. exacerbation of symptoms or another psychotic episode). However, it is important to remember that this increased risk does *not* apply equally to everyone. As explained earlier, some studies suggest that, within one year of stopping medication, around 54% of diagnosed people may experience relapse.

It can be anticipated that, of those who reduce but do not completely stop the medication, a significantly smaller proportion will relapse. It is also certain that diagnosed individuals can reduce their personal risk substantially by following the guidelines outlined above – particularly the advice regarding the importance of reducing the dosage very slowly and having adequate supports in place.

Researchers who have closely examined what happens when people stop their neuroleptic medication have noted that, if relapse does eventually occur, it is most likely to do so relatively soon after discontinuing treatment. According to the data summarised in *Chapter Six (Table One)*, around 44% of those who stop taking neuroleptic medication may have experienced relapse within three months, while approximately 6% who continue on maintenance treatment may relapse in the same period. Assuming these estimates are correct, people who stop medication are roughly *seven* times more likely to relapse during the first three months than those who stay on it. However, by the end of the first year the estimated rate is 54% for those who stop medica-tion compared to 17% for those still on it, i.e. the relative risk of relapse falls to a little over *three times* greater for those not on medication. After two years, the relative risk for those not on medication is just over *twice* as great as for those receiving maintenance treatment (59% versus 27%). While this data suggests that medication can substantially reduce the likelihood of relapse for some, it also shows that the relative risk of relapse is much greater during the early drug-free period and that during the second year without any medication, the risk of relapsing increases only marginally (from 54% to 59%). As mentioned previously, Professor Baldessarini and his colleagues noted "there were remarkably few additional relapses after the first six months without medication."[543]

An important implication of these findings is that *the first few months after stopping or substantially reducing neuroleptic medication represent a critical period.* This is especially likely to be the case if treatment is terminated abruptly. In order to maximise their chances of surviving this early high-risk period, diagnosed people withdrawing from medication should be protected, as much as possible, from excessive stress, and provided with adequate supports. Despite taking such precautions, some people may experience a relapse within a relatively short time of stopping their medication. It is reassuring to know, therefore, that research has demonstrated that most people who relapse after stopping neuroleptic treatment will regain their stability relatively quickly, often within a few days or weeks of recommencing the medication.[544] This is especially likely if they do so as soon as they start developing schizophrenia symptoms:

> Patients who experienced relapse after neuroleptic withdrawal were usually found to have a rapid return to baseline when neuroleptic therapy was reinstituted. [Stabilisation] was observed within three days to three weeks after neuroleptic treatment was restarted ... This suggests that even when patients experience symptoms after neuroleptic withdrawal, they are generally not subjected to any prolonged exacerbation if neuroleptic therapy is restarted soon.[545]

What is Relapse?

Given that many people will experience a relapse at some time, it is worth taking a closer look at what this phenomenon actually involves. Conventional psychiatry views relapse as a significant worsening of a diagnosed person's "psychotic illness". When people experience relapse, it is often assumed to be directly related to their treatment: either they were not receiving the right kind of medication or they were not taking an adequate amount of it. It is worth noting, however, that despite receiving continuous maintenance medication, a substantial proportion of people will still experience relapse. And, in some instances at least, rather than relapse occurring as a result of non-compliance with medication, the sequence may occur in reverse, i.e. the onset of psychosis leads some people to stop taking their tablets.

In simple lay terms relapse is commonly referred to as "getting sick again". While such terminology is understandable given the pain and distress that is often involved, it nevertheless has the unfortunate effect of focusing almost exclusively on the *negative* aspects of the situation. In fact, there is often a lot more to relapse than meets the eye. For example, studies have shown that hospital readmission often occurs for primarily *social*, rather than specifically psychiatric, reasons. Thus, while the cumulative stress associated with social isolation, loneliness, boredom, unfulfilled ambitions, lack of direction, and a host of other pressing personal concerns may eventually trigger an acute psychotic episode in certain predisposed individuals, in other cases it may simply give rise to behaviours others consider sufficiently maladaptive, disturbing, or bizarre, to justify psychiatric hospital admission. Zan Bockes explains how relapse and subsequent re-hospitalisation provided her with a temporary respite from the demands of everyday life:

As my illness developed, my dependency on psychiatric institutions also escalated since I often responded to real and imagined stressors in my life by entering hospitals. My reasons for becoming "psychotic" again were not just because I'd stopped taking medication, for there was always the enticing possibility of a hospital stay lingering in the back of my mind. And at those points in my life, the safety (albeit restrictive safety) offered by an institution was preferable to the responsibilities I felt I could not handle outside.[546]

Some investigators believe that, in time, certain people (particularly those diagnosed as "chronic schizophrenics") learn to use their symptoms to avoid or control situations or to elicit from others the specific responses they desire. There is no doubt that some individuals do seem to possess an uncanny ability to turn their symptoms on and off at will, though this "talent" can easily escape their control and carry them into chaotic and haphazard mental states. Psychiatrist Arnold Ludwig made the following comments, after observing this process at close quarters:

> In this regard, we have encountered numerous instances where relatively intact chronic schizophrenic patients, in the face of adversity, stress, or the desire for attention, seem to turn on their craziness either to avoid or control the situation. Once their mental ignition switch is turned on, a psychological momentum results, rapidly carrying the patient into the depths of psychological chaos. It is as though the patients' mental brakes have failed or their psychic flywheels have gone awry, and activity that may have started out as purposeful

and volitional may end as fragmented, disorganised, uncontrolled, random behaviour. To analogise further, once the patient opens the floodgates of his mind, he cannot predict with certainty whether a trickle or a flood of craziness will come through. The situation becomes comparable to that of a tail wagging the dog in that patients are no longer in control of the very process they set in motion.[547]

Certain individuals who have become psychotic after refusing medication appear to prefer this state to that of everyday reality. The experience of grandiose delusions, for example, may provide such a profound contrast to the impoverished reality of everyday life that "the wish to be crazy" becomes almost irresistible.[548] For those who *choose* to succumb to the seductive pull of the psychotic dream world, it could reasonably be asked whether any amount or type of neuroleptic medication is likely to be effective.

Because relapse tends to be viewed as an entirely negative occurrence, the possibility is often overlooked that, in some instances, there may be certain positive aspects to this experience. For example, in the course of research conducted by Professor John Strauss and his colleagues, it was noted that schizophrenia symptoms frequently become worse as people move through periods of significant change in their lives.[549] While this type of symptom exacerbation may sometimes result in a temporary setback, some people view such experiences as potentially valuable learning experiences, difficult and painful though they may be:

> I want to emphasise this – I needed to be sick, very sick, before I could heal. I had to be in that pit, struggling.

If all that horror hadn't come up, if I had simply tried to deny all my fear, I would have ended up where I started: feeling like a stone, only able to express myself through rage. By letting myself be sick, by travelling through all that terrible world, those awful delusions, I found my way through it. I needed help, lots of it, no doubt about that. But ultimately I alone had to be the one to discover the pathway out. I had to be inside whoever I was, whatever demented person I had become; I had to be the one at rock bottom.[550]

In situations such as that described above, excessive or injudicious use of medication could have a number of detrimental consequences. On the other hand, the timely administration of small amounts of medication could help facilitate the successful resolution of a psychological crisis by reducing its intensity to a more manageable level. Examples such as this highlight the difference between the indiscriminate use of neuroleptic medication to suppress anxiety-provoking symptoms and experiences, and its skilful use as one way of providing a degree of containment in the context of a therapeutic approach which fosters growth and healing.

Conclusion

It is worth reflecting on the fact that, if sufficiently large amounts of medication were to be used, it would theoretically be possible to prevent virtually *every* diagnosed person from ever experiencing symptoms or relapse. In doing so, however, some people would be exposed to such large dosages that their ability to function would doubtless be severely compromised. Simply preventing relapse should never become the sole aim and purpose of psychiatric treatment. Rather, medication should be used in a way that contributes to an improvement in the diagnosed person's sense of wellbeing and helps enhance their overall quality of life. This way of using medication cannot and should not be expected to make anyone's life completely painless or risk-free.

Much of the discussion in this chapter has focused on the possibility that the risk of relapse may increase for some diagnosed people who reduce or stop neuroleptic treatment. In view of this possibility the importance of adopting strategies designed to minimise risk has been emphasised. In the interest of balance, it is important to point out that the lives of some people doubtless *improve* in various ways as a result of reducing or stopping medication. It has been found that even people with long-standing "chronic" schizophrenia sometimes experience significant enhancement in the quality of their social interactions and a greater sense of satisfaction with life, when their long-term maintenance dosages are reduced.[551] Some people have even experienced substantial improvement in persistent positive symptoms in response to medication reduction.[552] Such facts are a powerful reminder that medication regimes must be tailored to suit the needs and specific circumstances of the individual concerned, and that there are no hard and fast rules when it comes to the treatment of schizophrenia.

Chapter Eleven

TAKING MEDICATION WITH A GRAIN OF SALT

Psychopharmacology is a remarkable enterprise,
full of hope and greed.

Tanya Luhrmann[553]

ANYONE WHO IS SERIOUSLY interested in gaining a truthful understanding of psychiatric drugs must eventually grapple with one of the most complex and urgent issues in modern medicine, namely the consequences of the powerful influence which the pharmaceutical industry has come to exert over biomedical research, clinical education, and health care delivery. It is necessary, in particular, to appreciate the extent to which vested commercial interests shape and control professional and lay knowledge of medicines, the conditions they treat, and doctors' prescribing practices. It must be said, at the outset, that it is difficult to discuss these matters frankly without exposing oneself to the likelihood of being accused of espousing anti-medication, perhaps even anti-psychiatric, views. However, in the interests of truth, these issues are far too important to be allowed to go without comment. The cherished ideal of informed consent is founded, after all, on the assumption that full and truthful information about prescription medications is freely and readily available to doctors, patients, and anybody else who might want it. Many competent authorities believe it is no longer safe to assume that this is the case.[554]

It is beyond the scope of this book to address all of the issues related to the business of developing, manufacturing, and promoting pharmaceutical drugs. However, a number of specific matters will be discussed here which are directly relevant to everyone who takes or prescribes neuroleptic or other psychotropic medications. Just as has occurred over the past two decades with respect to the activities of the tobacco industry, there is growing popular and professional concern about many aspects of the way medical drugs are now marketed. One reflection of this concern can be seen in the fact that the *British Medical Journal* recently devoted an entire issue to discussing some of the many undesirable consequences which result from the complex relationships that have developed between doctors and the pharmaceutical industry.[555] So entangled have these and other industry-driven relationships become, that many believe they now represent a significant threat to public health.

Big Tobacco Revisited

It would be pleasing to be able to rest in the comfortable belief that the major drug firms are benign businesses making a fair profit producing medicines which independent research has proven are both effective and safe. However,

in recent years so much contrary evidence has been provided by authoritative and impartial commentators that
it has become quite clear that such perceptions are naïve
and ill-informed. Complaints are now frequently made
about various aspects of the way the pharmaceutical industry operates. Accusations regarding questionable practices
are nothing new. In the first (1983) edition of *Surviving
Schizophrenia*, vociferously pro-medication psychiatrist
E. Fuller Torrey made the following comments (which,
interestingly enough, are not repeated in any of the later
editions of his popular book):

> Drug companies have a comparatively bad reputa-
> tion among many segments of the American public,
> a reputation which I believe they have earned and
> deserve. Through countless congressional hearings and
> investigations it has become clear that drug companies
> often make excess profits, sometimes falsify test data,
> and frequently put too little money into developing
> new and useful drugs.[556]

Similar views have been expressed by many others both
inside and outside the industry. In 1997 an American pharmaceutical company executive was quoted as estimating
that within twenty years a third of the world's population will be on psychiatric medications of one kind or
another.[557] Schizophrenia alone is usually said to affect
between 1% and 2% of the entire human population. Olanzapine, currently the most frequently prescribed neuroleptic
in Australia, was the world's sixth best-selling drug in 2002
with international sales amounting to $US 3.7 billion in
that year alone.[558] In view of the stupendous profits to be

made, it is not really surprising that the pharmaceutical industry is frequently accused of engaging in deceptive and often ethically dubious practices. One particular issue that has become the subject of acrimonious debate in recent years concerns the way in which drug trials are conducted and their findings reported.

Systematic Bias and Distortion

Experiments aimed at determining whether particular chemical substances (drugs) possess useful therapeutic properties were once carried out primarily in academic settings, such as medical schools, that were largely free of any commercial interest in the outcome of the research. This arrangement has gradually changed and the majority of such research is now sponsored by drug manufacturers. It has recently been estimated that over 60% of biomedical research in the US is now privately funded, and that at least two thirds of academic institutions have financial ties to commercial sponsors. So closely intertwined have academic researchers and industry become that the *British Medical Journal* recently noted how it has become "exceedingly difficult" to find senior medical researchers or clinicians who do not have financial ties to pharmaceutical companies.[559] While such arrangements provide researchers with a welcome source of funding, they raise serious concerns about the potential for bias and distortion. Many commentators – including some senior members of the medical profession – believe that much basic research has been corrupted by the involvement of the pharmaceutical industry. In a contribution to the *British Medical Journal's* 2003 theme issue, Australian investigative journalist Ray Moynihan wrote:

Most scrutinised are the relationships that entail corporate funding of academic research: a recent review of the evidence found financial conflicts of interest to be "pervasive and problematic" in biomedical research, with a quarter of university researchers receiving industry funding and a third having personal financial ties to sponsors. *The concern is that the evidence base of health-care is being distorted fundamentally.* Strong and consistent evidence shows that industry sponsored research tends to draw conclusions favourable to industry and industry sponsored studies were much more likely to reach conclusions that were favourable to the sponsor than were non-industry studies ... The explanations for the "systematic bias" in results is not that sponsored science is bad science but rather that the scientific questions being asked reflect the self-interest of the sponsor.[560]

Abundant evidence has come to light regarding the techniques routinely employed by the pharmaceutical industry in its effort to influence research, control information, and manipulate both the medical profession and general community to suit its own ends. The testing, promotion, and marketing of new drugs are all areas in which vested commercial interests have come to exert an extraordinarily powerful influence.

Evidence-Biased Medicine

Before a pharmaceutical company can begin selling a new product, various trials must be conducted to establish its safety and effectiveness. Such trials eventually involve giving the experimental drug to human beings and observing its effects over a set period. In what are known as "placebo-controlled trials" a similar group of experimental subjects are given an inactive substance (placebo). In order to be considered worthwhile, the drug under investigation must prove more effective than placebo in improving symptoms for which it would eventually be prescribed, while at the same time being shown not to cause unacceptable side effects.* Since the information generated by clinical trials is scrutinised by the regulatory authorities responsible for making the final decision whether or not to approve a new drug's release into the pharmaceutical marketplace, trial results can make or break a potentially lucrative new product's commercial prospects. As substantial amounts of money (often amounting to many millions of dollars) are already likely to have been invested just getting a new drug to the trial stage, unscrupulous manufacturers may experience an irresistible temptation to do all they can to ensure they get a favourable outcome. The pharmaceutical industry has been known to employ a range of sophisticated techniques to achieve these ends, the following being among the most common:

(a) Sponsoring trials

Industry-sponsored trials may be conducted by researchers who are selected, hired, and paid by the drug's manufacturer. Up to 70% of trials are now carried out under conditions which substantially increase the likelihood

---

* Some experts believe the use of placebos in such trials is appealing to manufacturers, since the drug under investigation is almost invariably likely to appear therapeutically superior to an inert substance. Trials which involve comparing a new drug with an older one with proven efficacy may tell a less promising story. See Garratini, S. et al. (2003) "How Can Research Ethics Committees Protect Patients Better?" *British Medical Journal*, Vol. 326

that results could be subjected to systematic manipulation and distortion. "Much research in psychopharmacology is funded by the pharmaceutical industry, whose primary motivation is profit", the editor of the *Journal of Clinical Psychiatry* noted recently. "This raises the potential for bias", he added, as "a pharmaceutical company goes to great pains to construct studies that are likely to turn out in its favour".[561] Trials which involve comparing the effectiveness of a new drug with that of an established medication (referred to as the "comparator drug"), can be carried out in ways which artificially enhance the apparent superiority of the sponsoring company's drug. Comparing the effects of a new drug against an excessively low (i.e. sub-therapeutic) dose of the comparator will invariably favour the drug being tested. On the other hand, using excessively high doses of the comparator, so that its side effects become problematic, will also tend to favour the experimental drug.[562] Some observers believe this technique has been widely employed in an effort to enhance the apparent superiority of the atypical neuroleptics (see discussion below). Independent research has shown that industry-sponsored trials are *four times* more likely to produce results favourable to the manufacturer than are trials without such sponsorship.[563] An investigator with first-hand experience in the way sponsored clinical trials are conducted recently explained how "when results favour the company, everything is great. But when results are disappointing, there is commonly an effort to spin, down-play, or change findings"[564] Researchers who do not produce results acceptable to the manufacturer who hired them to conduct the trials sometimes find they receive no further work from that particular company.

(b) Controlling information

Pharmaceutical companies often demand that all data generated by the clinical trials they sponsor be submitted directly to them for "analysis". This has led to accusations that the data is sometimes "massaged" in various ways, before being released, so that it better suits the sponsor's purposes. Cases are known in which reports have been produced that were created by pooling data from unrelated studies, i.e. favourable pieces of information were selected from a number of different drug trials, but made to look as though they came from a single study. Another way in which drug companies often attempt to censor information, involves the systematic failure to disclose negative findings, so that unfavourable results may simply disappear from view.[565] As a result, the fact that a particular drug has been shown to be ineffective, or has been found to cause unacceptable side effects, may never be revealed. Researchers privately contracted to carry out clinical trials are sometimes required to sign formal confidentiality agreements with the manufacturer, in which they agree not to publish or otherwise disclose information that does not meet the sponsor company's approval.

(c) Limiting the duration of trials

Human trials of new drugs typically last no more than about six or eight weeks. (Though common, this practice has been severely criticised by eminent research psychopharmacologist Roland Kuhn who believes "observations of less than three months are so subject to misinterpretation as to be valueless"[566]). It is now routine for regulatory bodies to approve the release of new drugs that have only been tested on human beings for a period widely considered too short to allow observation of anything but their very short-term effects and side effects. Furthermore, drug companies have been known to examine data collected at different points in a relatively short study, e.g. at the second, fourth, and sixth week, and to then only publish the findings which most favour their product.[567] Psychiatrist Peter Breggin has pointed out the danger inherent in approving new drugs that have only been tested on small numbers of people for a relatively brief period:

> The scientifically controlled pre-marketing studies, averaging four to six weeks, are much too short to pick up most risks. The individual studies at specific sites typically involve fewer than one hundred patients, so that even serious effects that occur at a rate of one in one hundred are likely to be missed. Yet once the drug is marketed to the public, a rate of one in one hundred adverse reactions adds up to ten thousand victims among the first one million patients ... Many serious side effects are not discovered until after the marketing of a drug has begun.[568]

As explained in *Chapter Two*, once a new medication is in general use, its side effects are monitored via an informal system whereby the onus is on individual doctors to report any concerns to regulatory authorities. Many experts believe this *ad hoc*, voluntary approach leads to systematic under-reporting of side effects. People diagnosed with schizophrenia are often given neuroleptic medications for years at a time, perhaps indefinitely. Given the brief period of testing most drugs have undergone before release, it is no exaggeration to say that anyone taking a new medication for more than six or eight weeks is conducting their own research into its long-term effects.

(d) Selective publishing

Since peer-reviewed professional journals are one of the principal means by which information is disseminated within the medical community, receiving favourable reports in such publications is an extremely important component in the process of having a new drug accepted and prescribed. For this reason, pharmaceutical companies go to great lengths to have their products shown in a positive light in such publications. As well as endeavouring to ensure that negative findings are not reported (or if they are, that they only appear in obscure journals which nobody reads), some drug makers may try to maximise the impact of a positive report about a new drug by having different versions of the same test results published in as many journals as possible (a practice referred to as "redundant publishing"). In order to create the most favourable impression possible, companies often employ professional medical writers to produce articles suitable for publication. It has become common for such "ghostwriters" to receive raw data from the researchers who actually conducted the trials and for them to exercise their creative skills turning it into an article acceptable to the manufacturer. A recent report in the *New England Journal of Medicine* described how medical ghostwriters "typically receive a packet of materials from which they write the article; they may be instructed to insert a key paragraph favourable to the company's product."[569]

Publish or Perish

Since they know that having a favourable report published in a prestigious professional journal is a significant
step toward ensuring a new drug's ultimate financial success, pharmaceutical companies frequently use professional
writers to concoct articles extolling the virtues of their
latest offerings. As a drug-industry employee explained in
a 1961 US Senate subcommittee report on this and other
potentially misleading and deceptive practices, the very
fact that an article appears in print lends its contents an air
of credibility it may not really deserve:

> A substantial number of the so-called medical scientific
> papers that are published on behalf of these drugs are
> written within the confines of the pharmaceutical houses
> concerned. Frequently the physician involved merely
> makes the observations and his data, which sometimes
> are sketchy and uncritical, are submitted to a medical
> writer employed by the company. The writer prepares
> the article which is returned to the physician who makes
> the overt effort to submit it for publication. The article
> is frequently sent to one of the journals which looks to
> the pharmaceutical company for advertising and rarely is
> publication refused. The particular journal is of little inter-
> est as the primary concern is to have the article published
> ... There is a rather remarkable attitude prevalent that if a
> paper is published then its contents become authoritative,
> even though before publication the same contents may
> have been considered nonsense.[570]

Pharmaceutical companies go to considerable trouble
to present advertisements in medical journals as though

they were purely objective and unbiased reports. While professional journals purport to be "scientific" and thus free of the potential biasing influence of commercial motives, much of the information they now contain is not as impartial as it is made to appear. For example, independent research has revealed that medical-journal advertisements frequently exaggerate the benefits of new medications, while at the same time obscuring their potential risks.[571] In what has been described as "the confession that created headlines around the world", the prestigious *New England Journal of Medicine* admitted, in February 2000, that it had failed to disclose to its readers the fact that 19 of the 40 drug reviews it published since 1997 were written by researchers funded by the companies marketing the medications.[572] Later that year, the editors acknowledged that the journal was having difficulty complying with its own stated policy of alerting readers to potential conflicts of interest related to published articles. As an example, they cited an article on the treatment of chronic depression published in the May 18th issue: "The author's ties with companies that make antidepressants were so extensive that it would have used too much space to disclose them fully in the *Journal*. We decided merely to summarise them and to provide the details on our Web site."[573]

In 2003 the editors of the *British Medical Journal* summarised the present state of affairs thus: "Journals are caught between publishing the most relevant and valid research and being used as vehicles for drug company propaganda".[574] It is an unfortunate fact, they added, that medical journals now contain some information of doubtful merit:

Something's wrong, and medical journals are part of what's wrong ... We have good evidence to show that much drug advertising is misleading ... In many cases companies [have] over-stated the effectiveness of the drug or minimised its risks ... A 1992 study, which included all 109 full page advertisements from 10 leading medical journals, found many more problems ... In 40% of advertisements the reviewers thought that information on efficacy was not balanced with that on side effects and contraindications. Overall, reviewers would not have recommended publication of 28% of the advertisements and would have required major revisions in a third ... As advertisements influence prescribing yet are often misleading, the question arises whether medical journals should publish them ... Few editors (and fewer owners) refuse advertisements ... The major journals try to counterbalance the might of the pharmaceutical industry, but it is an unequal battle – not least because journals themselves profit from publishing studies funded by the industry ... In one sense, all journals are bought – or at least cleverly used – by the pharmaceutical industry.[575]

In addition to perusing professional journals, doctors and other clinical health care workers often refer to special compendiums when seeking information about the effects and side effects of prescription medications. While it is often assumed that these handbooks contain totally impartial factual information, there is little doubt that drug manufacturers sometimes attempt to manipulate their contents, just as occurs with medical journals. The *MIMS Annual*, a widely used Australian reference commonly referred to as the "medication bible", acknowledges that all of the information contained in both its text and advertising is provided by drug manufacturers:

> The publisher would like to express thanks to those pharmaceutical companies whose advertisements appear within the pages of this publication, and without whose support production ... would not have been possible ... MIMS Annual has been made editorially possible by the co-operation of the pharmaceutical manufacturers who have supplied the information. Editorial details published in the index are based on information supplied by the manufacturer.[576]

The predominant written source of prescription-drug information for doctors in the United States is the *Physicians' Desk Reference,* commonly known as the *PDR.* As with the Australian *MIMS Annual,* all of the information contained within the *PDR* is provided by the pharmaceutical companies whose products are listed therein.

Opinion Leaders

Concern has been growing among both professional and lay commentators regarding the extent to which certain respected and extremely influential medical authorities (in both general medicine and psychiatry) have sometimes appeared to be acting as paid promotional agents for drug firms. Indeed, a strategy frequently employed by pharmaceutical companies involves the deliberate targeting for special attention of doctors considered to be opinion leaders in their particular field. By showering such individuals with attention, flattery, gifts, generous "research grants" and – in a number of notorious cases – outright bribes, drug makers sometimes manage to secure favourable reports or personal endorsements from high-profile experts whose views are often accepted, *ipse dixit*, as incontrovertible pronouncements of truth.

It has become common for leading psychiatrists to be engaged by drug manufacturers to act as consultants, advisers, and "peer educators". The fact that such individuals are being paid by drug companies – often very handsomely – cannot help but raise serious questions regarding the impartiality of their views and the reliability of the information they are disseminating:

> Many leading figures in American – and worldwide – psychiatry act as consultants for the pharmaceutical companies, rely upon them for funds for their research, are involved in clinical trials, testing and evaluation of their products, are on the committees responsible for revising and updating diagnostic criteria, advise the licensing authorities on the acceptability and risks of the drugs, and indeed have financial interests and shares in the companies themselves.[577]

Expert clinicians now regularly compile Clinical Practice Guidelines which present an overview of current evidence regarding various health conditions together with a summary of specific treatment recommendations. Recent research has revealed it has become quite common for the authors of such guidelines to maintain close ties with the pharmaceutical industry, including working as employees or consultants for drug manufacturers, though such involvements are often not disclosed.[578] Since the recommendations contained in Clinical Practice Guidelines are intended to inform and guide widely accepted treatment practices, any undue influence experienced by their authors could eventually be transmitted to very large numbers of clinicians.

Dr Fuller Torrey told the 1998 annual meeting of the National Alliance for the Mentally Ill (NAMI – a support and advocacy group for relatives of diagnosed people in the USA) that caution needs to be exercised when considering information about psychiatric medications, even when it comes from seemingly authoritative and reliable sources:

> What gets put out is not necessarily the truth. You'd be surprised at how much money many of my colleagues are regularly taking from the pharmaceutical industry. Ten thousand dollars is not an uncommon amount to be given for giving a talk.[579]

Such activities have sometimes attracted grave criticism from within the profession itself, such as occurred in a disapproving editorial in a recent edition of the prestigious British medical journal, *The Lancet*:

> When should the individual clinician start to worry that he or she has become too deeply involved with the drug industry? The rules here are far from clear … A few weeks ago a doctor in training at a teaching hospital sent to *The Lancet*, anonymously and after a nervous phone call, a dossier recording the travels of the head of his unit. If everything goes as planned this person will have spent about 50 days away in 1998, not through illness, vacation, or involvement with some

official committee, but at the behest of pharmaceutical companies. The list includes the USA, the Middle and Far East, and a dozen European countries … The danger is that the necessary independence of research and opinion is put at risk when commercial involvement reaches this level … It would be embarrassing if David Lodge were to rewrite his novel *Small World*, this time around the antics of academic clinicians with a reputation for being at anyone's call – if the money is right and the venue exotic enough.[580]

It is not only individual opinion leaders that are selected to receive generous financial and other rewards. Even academic researchers, once the unrivalled exemplars of impartial scientific inquiry, are no longer impervious to these developments. As university departments become ever more reliant on private sources of funding, freedom of thought and expression may soon become a luxury few can afford. "The medical profession is being bought by the pharmaceutical industry, not only in terms of the practice of medicine, but also in terms of teaching and research," declared Harvard professor and former editor of the *New England Journal of Medicine,* Arnold Relman, in a recent critique. He went on to say: "The academic institutions of this country are allowing themselves to be paid agents of the pharmaceutical industry. I think it's disgraceful."[581]

In recent decades, powerful and highly influential professional bodies, such as the American Psychiatric Association in the USA, and the Royal College of Psychiatrists in the UK, have become increasingly reliant on funding from the pharmaceutical industry. For example, in its 1995 *Annual Report,* the Royal College of Psychiatrists acknowledged receiving sponsorship for meetings, campaigns, and other activities, from a variety of sources, more than two-thirds of which were drug companies. The fact that such ostensibly autonomous bodies accept substantial amounts of money from sources with obvious commercial motives raises concerns about potential conflicts of interest. Direct and indirect commercial sponsorship of these once proudly independent bodies has recently increased to such an extent that it has become a source of considerable professional embarrassment to many of their members.

Spin Doctors and Continuing Medical Education

Many people assume that, after receiving their initial instruction about drugs in medical school, doctors subsequently keep abreast of the latest developments by perusing scholarly publications such as medical journals and attending educational activities auspiced by the various professional bodies with which they are affiliated. While such activities may account for *some* of their learning, it is now the case that many doctors receive the majority of their information about medications directly from the manufacturers. It was recently estimated that the training of medical students in Australia costs around $25,000 per year. The pharmaceutical industry, by comparison, spends an average of $21,000 every year on every doctor in the country promoting its wares (as noted above, opinion leaders would be expected to receive a substantially greater share of these funds). The potential clinical ramifications of this disparity were recently the subject of scathing comment in an Australian psychiatric journal:

Clearly, the expenditure by government during a few years of medical education is dwarfed by the expenditure by the industry on "re-education" over a medical career. Generally, "medical education" sponsored by pharmaceutical companies favours drug over non-drug treatment.[582]

The pharmaceutical industry employs a wide variety of methods to convey information to doctors, in addition to placing articles and advertisements in medical journals. Thus, doctors are regularly visited in their offices by drug-company "detailers" (sales representatives) who provide written or audiovisual materials ("product profiles") for the doctor's edification, as well as engaging in face-to-face discussion about their products. Studies carried out in several countries indicate that 80%–95% of doctors see drug-company representatives on a regular basis and that an estimated 80,000 such reps visit US doctors every day.[583] The specific purpose of these frequent and regular contact visits is to influence prescribing behaviour and the preferential use of particular drugs:

There is growing evidence that doctors' prescribing habits are influenced by drug companies, either through discussions with sales representatives or through sales drives dressed up as medical education. A British research group finds that doctors who have frequent contact with drug representatives are more willing to prescribe new drugs, do not like ending consultations with advice only, and are more likely to agree to prescribe a drug that is

not clinically indicated. It is hard not to be per-
suaded by a warm smile, a free meal, and a touch of
flattery ... There is danger too in the glossy reprint
from a prestigious journal that the drug company
representative brings. Unsurprisingly, the representatives do not bring reprints that are unfavourable
to their products.[584]

As a condition of their registration, practicing doctors
are required to participate in a certain number of hours
of accredited continuing medical education (CME) each
year. Much of this is now provided in the form of seminars,
conferences, workshops and training programmes sponsored wholly or in part by the pharmaceutical industry.
It is estimated that, in the United States, drug companies
now sponsor 300,000 such events every year as part of
their on-going promotional activities.[585] Keynote speakers
invited to address doctors who attend forums packaged as
"medical education" are very often opinion leaders paid by
the drug companies sponsoring the event. In such cases,
an informed critic noted, "accredited events in continuing
medical education seem little more than an opportunity for
speakers paid by sponsors to speak about their drugs".[586]
The mere fact that information conveyed by these means
is provided and paid for by a company with an obvious
commercial interest in promoting its wares inevitably raises
questions about its impartiality. Would drug companies
pay for doctors to attend lavish conferences at which their
products were criticised and their claims challenged?

In 2001, the journal *Australasian Psychiatry* published
an article which asked "Does Drug Promotion Adversely
Influence Doctors' Abilities to Make the Best Decisions for

Patients?" The authors opined that psychiatrists as a group "are regarded somewhat cynically" by drug companies, which routinely target them in various ways in an effort to cultivate their loyalty and influence their prescribing practices:

> According to an experienced member of the pharmaceutical industry, a drug company will hand pick doctors to fund for research and "educational" activities specifically for their supportiveness and loyalty to the company, on the basis of analysis of their prescribing habits and profiles. The industry follows the principal that 80% of the market comes from 20% of the prescribers. We are therefore categorised according to how we prescribe, from "A" (high volume prescribers) down to "C" (those not worth targeting). "A"s are well looked after, while "B"s are targeted with a view to converting them to "A"s. Drug detailers profile us during their visits according to our professional and private interests, and also obtain information about our prescribing from local pharmacies. Our names appear in company briefing documents, with notations about who has attended international and other conferences as part of their promotional package, and what the company hoped to achieve from that sponsorship.[587]

Many doctors seem to believe they are not unduly influenced by advertising, direct contact with drug-company sales representatives, and other pharmaceutical-industry promotional activities. Independent research indicates otherwise. Thus, a study published in the *Journal of the American Medical Association* in 2000, found that attending sponsored continuing medical education events and accepting funding for travel or lodging for such events was associated with an increased rate of prescribing of the sponsor's medications.[588] Indeed, there is reason to believe that those who insist they are immune to such influences may, in fact, be *especially* vulnerable to them. As an example, researchers asked a group of hospital doctors if attending an all-expenses-paid drug-company-sponsored seminar would unduly influence them. Most denied it would. However, it was found that, immediately after receiving invitations to the seminar in question, these doctors had started prescribing more of the sponsor's drugs.[589] The pharmaceutical industry's powerful influence on doctors extends well beyond simply affecting the drugs they choose to prescribe. Some critics fear an even more insidious consequence of this unequal relationship concerns the way doctors may become unwilling or unable to consider possibilities other than the ones they have been made familiar with. Professor Jay Cohen has expressed grave concern about this worrying tendency:

... many doctors adopt an attitude of scepticism about anything that doesn't conform to their information, most of which comes from the drug companies ... *Perhaps the most insidious damage caused by doctors' overdependence on drug-company information is that they can become very close-minded about other possibilities.* Many doctors aren't even willing to hear about better, safer dosages, even if these dosages have been proven medically and make sense logically. Thus, doctors unwittingly align themselves with the drug companies, becoming the purveyors and defenders of drug-company methods.[590]

Gilding The Lilly

While the pharmaceutical industry once directed its advertising almost exclusively at the medical profession, its influence is now increasingly felt far beyond these relatively narrow confines. Major drug companies now have huge public-relations departments to help them achieve their objectives. Dedicated pharmaceutical marketing consultants now devise extremely sophisticated strategies to create a favourable impression of their various products. The complex marketing machinery of the pharmaceutical industry is demonstrably capable of shaping what physicians and the lay public believe about the latest medications. An increasingly common ploy involves freelance journalists being hired by a public-relations firm acting on behalf of a drug company. Such journalists may be invited to attend pharmaceutical-industry-sponsored conferences and other events and encouraged to produce up-beat reports concerning the latest "breakthrough" medications. As well as finding their way into medical publications, the resulting stories are increasingly likely to appear in various popular media. As a result, it has become quite common for pharmaceutical drugs to be mentioned in newspaper and TV news reports and lifestyle television programmes.

Feature articles on mental health issues that now appear regularly in popular magazines and newspapers, often carry tantalising information regarding the most recent developments in medical treatment. While these sources of information seem innocuous and are often presented as though their sole purpose was "community education", such appearances are often misleading. Recent research has shown that media reports on medical drugs often give incomplete information, fail to reveal the fact that the experts quoted often have a vested financial interest in the product concerned, and commonly under-emphasise treatment risks. One recent analysis of 180 newspaper articles and 27 television reports on medical drugs in the USA found that half cited an expert or study with financial ties to the manufacturer. This connection was not revealed in 61% of them, while more than half the items (53%) failed to mention any of the potential risks associated with the drugs in question.[591]*

Recent years have seen an extraordinary proliferation of Internet sites devoted to providing information on health-related matters. While these have the advantage of being extremely easy to access, a great deal of care needs to be exercised when gathering information from these sources. Unlike more traditional media such as television and print, the Internet is largely unregulated and it is now possible for anyone to describe an experience, post an opinion, or table a report and have it presented as fact. Lay people are regularly advised to only trust medical information obtained from "reputable" or "official" Internet sites. However, pharmaceutical companies (and other groups with vested interests) have wasted no time ensuring that they have a powerful and influential presence in cyberspace. Given their clearly demonstrated ability to influence the content of medical journals and other supposedly "scientific" publications, such organizations are bound to engage in similar activities wherever the opportunity arises. *Caveat lector.*

The acclaimed Hollywood film, *A Beautiful Mind*, tells

---

* One of the researchers, Professor David Henry, has said that the problem of misleading media reports was not due to any deliberate intention by reporters to mislead their readers. Rather, he believes, journalists often seem to be less sceptical regarding medical stories than they are when reporting other issues, perhaps because they are inclined to believe that health "experts" would not deliberately attempt to mislead the public.

the intriguing tale of mathematical genius John Forbes Nash, Jr. and his remarkable recovery after nearly three decades struggling with incapacitating psychological problems. Widely praised for its realistic portrayal of psychosis, many believe the film made a significant contribution to improving public awareness of issues related to schizophrenia and its treatment. However, shortly after it was released, claims were made that the producers had allowed a subtle form of "product placement" which distorted the film's ultimate message. In the movie, just before he is awarded the Nobel Prize in Economics, Nash refers to taking "newer medications", thereby implying that these drugs played a key role in his recovery. Sylvia Nasar's fascinating biography, on which the film was based, tells a rather different story. In stark contrast to the Hollywood account, it states quite categorically that Nash's eventual recovery was *not* related to use of neuroleptic medications – atypical or otherwise – and that he had, in fact, stopped taking such drugs as early as 1970:

Nash's refusal to take the anti-psychotic drugs after 1970, and indeed during most of the periods when he wasn't in the hospital in the 1960s, may have been fortuitous. Taken regularly, such drugs, in a high percentage of cases, produce horrible, persistent symptoms like tardive dyskinesia – a stiffening of head and neck muscles and involuntary movements, including of the tongue – and a mental fog, all of which would have made his gentle re-entry into the world of mathematics a near impossibility. Nash's remission did not come about, as many people later assumed, because of some new treatment. "I emerged from irrational thinking", he said in 1996, "ultimately without medicine other than the natural hormonal changes of aging". He described the process as one that involved both a growing awareness of the sterility of his delusional state and a growing capacity for rejecting delusional thought ... He believes, rightly or wrongly, that he willed his own recovery.[592]

Since relatively few of the many millions of people who have seen *A Beautiful Mind* are likely to have also read Sylvia Nasar's book, most will be left with the erroneous impression that neuroleptic drugs – "newer medications" in particular – were responsible for Nash's recovery.

Drugs In The Community

With the tremendous broadening of the pharmaceutical industry's reach that has occurred in recent years, community-based organizations such as voluntary self-help and mutual-support groups have increasingly become the focus of its attention. As a result, many such organizations now receive – and some have come to rely on – the largesse of drug companies. This development is a cause for serious concern. In particular, it raises questions regarding the extent to which such arrangements might unduly influence a supposedly independent organization's philosophy, policies and activities, particularly those of an educational nature. The Australian Consumer's Association has expressed alarm at the extent to which pharmaceutical companies are now able to exert a direct and powerful influence on consumer groups (organizations representing health-service users and their families). Especially worrying is the way drug manufacturers manipulate such groups with selective or biased information in an attempt to create artificial demand for particular drugs.[593] A recent letter in the *British Medical Journal* urged caution and offered sage advice regarding these matters:

> The pharmaceutical industry does not donate money to charities for altruistic reasons. It is not allowed to advertise prescription drugs to consumers, but it knows that patient groups are often a strong lobby and have power to influence government ... Consumers trust medical charities and expect their information to be unbiased and uninfluenced by the charity's funding sources. Charities accepting industry funding should declare it as a conflict of interest to enable consumers to question their independence and that of the information they provide and seek further information from more independent sources.[594]

As well as providing community-based groups with much-needed financial assistance that allows them to run various worthy programmes, pharmaceutical-industry "grants" are also often used to fund a range of educational activities. The question that naturally arises is whether there are any strings attached, visible or otherwise. For example, if a self-help support group publishes booklets or produces audiovisual materials paid for wholly or in part by a drug company, can there be any real certainty that such materials contain unbiased information about medications or the conditions they are used to treat? Are they likely to give adequate consideration to non-medical perspectives and non-drug aspects of care and treatment? In fact, it has become common for the drug companies *themselves* to compile, print, and make available to support groups, free of charge, a range of glossy brochures and booklets for distribution to patients, family members, and the general public (these can often be identified by their prominently embossed company names, logos, and slogans). While these skilfully designed publications supposedly have a purely educational purpose, they provide the manufacturers with a way of delivering carefully selected information about their wares directly to readers who are rarely in a position to critically evaluate its accuracy and balance.

A recent development involves drug-company representatives visiting community-based rehabilitation and support services in person, and generously offering to provide information and educational assistance to mental health workers and other non-medical direct-care staff. While these initiatives are often presented as a form of "community service", they invariably entail the delivery of cleverly packaged information about the sponsoring company's products. Psychiatric nurses are increasingly likely to receive instruction about medications in this fashion. Diagnosed persons, in both inpatient and community settings, who request information about their psychiatric condition and treatment, are now often provided with various drug-company-produced leaflets or booklets, as part of their mental health "education". In some instances, receiving such materials may constitute the *whole* of these educational activities.

The largest and undoubtedly most influential mental health support and lobby group in the United States, the National Alliance for the Mentally Ill (NAMI), received $12 million worth of funding from drug companies between 1996 and 1999.[595] This organization vigorously promotes the notion that schizophrenia is a "brain disease" for which pharmaceutical treatment is mandatory. In 1999, Eli Lilly, the company which makes olanzapine (Zyprexa) "loaned" one of its executives to NAMI to assist it with "strategic planning".[596] In Australia, SANE, the peak national body and operating name of the Schizophrenia Australia Foundation, reportedly receives at least a quarter of its annual budget from drug companies.[597] Should organizations to which many vulnerable people might turn in a desperate search for impartial guidance and advice have relationships such as this with powerful pharmaceutical companies that have an unambiguous interest in selling their wares and maximising their profits? Some argue that as long as community groups retain their autonomy, there is nothing wrong with them accepting drug-company money. But are organizations in receipt of such funding *able* to be truly independent? Are they likely to ask "difficult" questions when they know that to do so could prejudice their chances of continuing to receive much-needed financial support? In the opinion of the Australian Consumer's Association, "There's almost no such thing as clean money for most consumer organizations".[598]

An Antidote For Toxic Psychiatry

A host of factors now conspire to make it difficult to obtain unbiased information about psychiatric medications. This situation is unlikely to change until commercial interests and scientific research are clearly separated. A clinical instructor in psychiatry at the prestigious Harvard Medical School, Dr Joseph Glenmullen, has recently urged that a range of measures be immediately put in place in an effort to stop, or at least slow, some of the worst of the abuses described in this chapter. Mental health professionals, particularly those who function as opinion leaders in the psychiatric field, should be specifically required to conform to these proposals:

We need new curbs on excesses in the way the drugs are promoted ... Psychiatric diagnoses should not be expanded and marketed as part of the efforts to market the drugs. Medical ethics, not business standards, need to prevail in health care. Given the public health issues involved, we need a national database in which health care professionals are required to report any financial ties to pharmaceutical companies. The database should be readily accessible on the Internet, so journalists and the public can easily use the information to put in perspective comments made on behalf of drugs by seemingly independent spokespeople. The information would not just be a list of affiliations with pharmaceutical companies. Rather, the full dollar amounts should be disclosed so that the public is informed of the huge sums of money often involved. The argument that this would be an invasion of the individual's privacy is more than overridden by the public safety issues as stake.[599]

Given the increasingly influential role they play as purveyors of information to diagnosed people, their families, and the general public, such a database should also contain details about the funding arrangements of nominally independent community-based support groups (confidentiality agreements entered into with drug companies notwithstanding).

Questions That Matter

The pharmaceutical industry's tremendous power gives it the potential to do a great deal of good – developing new and more effective medications, for example – but also the ability to act in various ways that are ultimately detrimental to patient welfare and health care generally. The editors of the *British Medical Journal* recently expressed their belief that the medical profession itself must bear collective responsibility for some of the negative consequences of its close involvement with the pharmaceutical industry:

> Free pens and pizza lunches. Sponsored conferences and compromised medical education. Courtesy golf and unaffordable holidays. Thought leaders and ghost writers. These are the trappings of doctors and drug companies being entwined in an embrace of avarice and excess, an embrace that distorts medical information and patient care ... How did we reach the point where doctors expect their information, research, education, professional organisations, and attendance at conferences to be underwritten by drug companies? Both doctors and drug companies know there is something unhealthy in this relationship, but seem unable to stop themselves ... The pharmaceutical industry is immensely powerful. It is one of the most profitable industries, truly global, and closely connected to politicians, particularly in the United States. Compared with it, medicine is a disorganised mess. Doctors have become dependent on the industry in a way that undermines their independence and ability to do their best by patients.[600]

There is reason to believe that this state of affairs has become especially problematic in the mental health field. Indeed, the editor of the *New England Journal of Medicine*, Dr Marcia Angell, recently observed that "You are seeing played out in psychiatry the extremes of what is happening elsewhere in medicine"[601] Evidence of this is not difficult to find. A visit to a modern psychiatric facility, such as a hospital ward or community mental health clinic, is an instructive experience in this regard. Noticeable, amid the typically bland furnishings and décor, are ubiquitous forms of advertising: pens, drinking mugs, writing pads, paper weights, post-it notes, patient information booklets, mouse mats, and more, all prominently embossed with the name of a particular drug, its manufacturer's distinctive logo and, inevitably, a pithy slogan extolling the drug's unparalleled virtues. It is now common for doctors, psychiatric nurses, and other mental health professionals to return from conferences and seminars laden with complimentary satchels overflowing with logo-bearing trinkets, colour-coded product profiles, and assorted "educational" materials generously supplied by the drug companies that sponsor the meetings. While constant exposure to this kind of pharmaceutical paraphernalia causes its presence to go largely unnoticed by most staff members, its omnipresent subliminal influence is nevertheless extremely powerful.*At the very least, these talismans, cleverly designed by specialist advertising agencies, serve to declare and reinforce

---

* One can imagine a very different use of simple words and images to convey powerful therapeutic messages. Picture a treatment setting in which words such as "Relax", "Hope", "Trust", and "Try" are placed in strategic locations to act as gentle reminders and sources of subtle affirmation and inspiration. Staff as well as patients would undoubtedly benefit from the influence of such benevolent subliminal advertising!

the chauvinistically drug-oriented nature of the dominant treatment culture.

On a broader level, it is certain that the multiple, often quite subtle, influences associated with the pharmaceutical industry's ubiquitous presence in both clinical and community settings has helped shape a particular way of thinking about mental illness. As Professor David Cohen notes, "The idea that the distress and disorders we refer to as mental illness are genuine physical diseases completely pervades our culture."[602] In recent years catchy phrases such as "chemical imbalance", "genetic predisposition", and "psychotic illness" have gradually found their way into common use and are now uttered with nonchalant ease by lay-person and professional alike. So familiar have such expressions become that they are now widely assumed to be statements of fact. Only rarely are they seen for what they really are: grossly oversimplified shorthand for complex, scientifically unproven hypotheses. Psychopharmacologist David Healy sees the hand of advertising agencies at work:

> The advent of the psychotropic drugs has also given rise to a new biological language in psychiatry. The extent to which this has come to be part of popular culture is in many ways astonishing ... This triumph, however, is not without its ambiguities. It can reasonably be asked whether biological language offers more in the line of marketing copy than it offers in terms of clinical meaning.[603]

Schizophrenia, in particular, has come to be seen almost exclusively in terms of biological malfunction, the unfortunate result of a "chemical imbalance" in the diagnosed person's brain, for which neuroleptic medications are the natural and legitimate response. While there are many who believe this conceptualisation is evidence of psychiatry's recent scientific progress, sceptics may be more inclined to see it is a dream come true for the pharmaceutical industry.

The Psycho-Pharmaceutical Complex

The pharmaceutical industry's strategic agendas determine which issues it considers are worthy of investigation, who it believes should investigate them, and what should be done with the results. Thus, while it may be only too willing to make available virtually unlimited financial resources to study potentially lucrative new drugs, it is unlikely to be as generous to researchers whose interest lies in investigating the effectiveness of *non-drug* coping strategies. Likewise, it is hard to imagine the industry being enthusiastic about sponsoring research into the viability of medication-reduction strategies, such as low-dose or intermittent treatment. As important as these issues are, it is clear the pharmaceutical industry's reach extends well beyond its ability to selectively support certain kinds of research. Indeed, it has come to exert an extraordinarily powerful influence over the way psychiatry as a whole now functions, and not simply by virtue of the fact that it provides the broad and seemingly ever-expanding range of psychotropic medications that many clinicians have come to depend upon.*

---

* To gain an appreciation of the extent to which most psychiatrists have come to depend upon psychotropic drugs, it is instructive to consider what might occur if they were required to go without their prescription pads for a trial period, say twelve months. During such an experiment, some would doubtless be made starkly aware of the extent to which they had allowed their interpersonal therapeutic skills to take second place to those associated with diagnosing, prescribing, and monitoring the effects of medication.

Significant political connections the industry has culti-
vated, combined with the enormous financial resources it
has at its disposal, allow it to influence key areas of mental
health policy and service delivery. Dr Peter Breggin believes
an alliance has evolved between the pharmaceutical industry and mainstream psychiatry which compromises the
independence of the profession and, ultimately, the welfare
of its patients. This "psycho-pharmaceutical complex", as
he terms it, is the result of an insidious intertwining of the
commercial interests of the pharmaceutical industry and
the collective ambitions of the psychiatric profession.[604]
Because the power and resources of this juggernaut are
so great, individual practitioners who do not share its
motives or methods can easily find themselves ostracised
and ignored within their own profession. Some believe
this self-serving alliance has conspired to suppress entire
bodies of important psychiatric knowledge. The fate of the
Soteria Project may be a case in point.

As discussed in *Chapter Five*, research carried out in
the 1970s and early 1980s, under the direction of psychiatrist Loren Mosher, demonstrated that many acutely
psychotic individuals can be successfully treated with
little or no neuroleptic medication, if they are provided
with adequate support in the context of a low-stimulus,
home-like therapeutic environment. Despite the fact
that contemporary studies conducted by Professor Luc
Ciompi and his colleagues in Switzerland have confirmed
the essential validity of Dr Mosher's findings, they have
been ignored by mainstream psychiatry. Psychology professor Daniel Burston is not the first to suggest that the
primary reason the Soteria findings have not been enthusiastically embraced, is that they are perceived as a threat

to the shared interests of the pharmaceutical industry and medication-centred psychiatry:

> Using standard quantitative methods and measures, Mosher demonstrated that therapeutic households that make minimal use of medication and extensive use of suitably trained paraprofessionals are just as effective as standard psychiatric facilities – sometimes more effective – and can circumvent the toxic side effects of neuroleptic drugs or electroshock ... If those results are any indication, therapeutic households that manage psychotic regression effectively can operate as relatively free-standing entities, which in their daily operation do little to enhance the status or financial fortunes of psychiatrists. In fact, reading over the literature on the subject, one gets the sharp impression that if facilities like these were to proliferate, the demand for the services of psychiatrists could fall sharply, and the pharmaceutical industry would be adversely affected as well.[605]

Many respected and informed commentators share Professor Burston's unease regarding mainstream psychiatry's collective failure to give serious consideration to the implications of Dr Mosher's ground-breaking research:

> Mosher's [Soteria] experiment ... has been studiously ignored by the psychiatric community. Until Mosher's work is acknowledged in the psychiatric mainstream, little progress can be made in this area. To many thoughtful people the conspiracy of silence that surrounds the Soteria Project has a decidedly ominous feel

to it. If Mosher is right about the efficacy of such house-holds – and I think he is – then it is hard to account for psychiatry's refusal to consider his findings, except by reference to a covert economic agenda, one that is not even admitted by psychiatrists to themselves.[606]

Most people – including many professionals – are totally unaware of the behind-the-scenes machinations that now play such a large part in shaping contemporary approaches to mental health care. Those, such as patients and families, who daily face the onerous task of dealing in a practical way with "mental illness" are often understandably inclined to take a pragmatic view. Whatever its faults and shortcomings, such people may say, the pharmaceutical industry has recently succeeded in creating a range of more effective medications and that is welcome progress indeed. However, as those who are prepared to look more closely soon discover, the advent of atypical neuroleptics is not the tale of unalloyed scientific progress it is often made out to be.

Not An Atypical Story

The pharmaceutical companies concerned have invested a huge amount in promoting the second-generation or atypical neuroleptics as a significant advance in schizophrenia treatment, a view subsequently echoed by numerous psychiatric clinicians and enthusiastically embraced by many diagnosed people and their families. As noted earlier, these medications do appear to have some advantages over the original neuroleptics, most notably a tendency to cause fewer debilitating neuro-logical side effects. Nevertheless, certain aspects of their rapid ascendancy and widespread acceptance are rather unsettling. For instance, many reputable and informed commentators believe that trials involving atypicals have sometimes been set up in a deliberately misleading way, and that certain important facts have been down-played or overlooked in a cynical attempt to protect the image, and thus the marketability, of these extremely lucrative new drugs.

The scientists who compiled the British National Schizophrenia Guidelines (discussed in *Chapter Three*) were not the only ones to conclude that much of the apparent advantage of atypical neuroleptics is a result of the way the trials comparing them with conventional neuroleptics have generally been set up. They noted, for example, that most published trials have used relatively high dosages of haloperidol as the comparator drug. One of the original first-generation neuroleptics, haloperidol (Serenace), has a well-known propensity to cause severe neurological and other side effects, especially when given in doses above 6-12 mg a day. As investigators have noted, trials in which the effects of an atypical neuroleptic are compared with those of excessively high dosages of a particularly "dirty" drug, such as haloperidol, are certain to make the atypical medication appear significantly better than it actually is. These views were summarised in a report published in the *British Medical Journal* in 2000:

> Most trials compared the effectiveness of atypical antipsychotics with haloperidol. Occasionally, chlor-promazine was also used ... The [size of the] dose of haloperidol significantly affected the outcome in the 23 trials in which it was used ... [statistical analysis] iden-tified a significant advantage for atypical antipsychotics

as the dose of haloperidol increased ... The observed advantage in favour of the atypical drug disappeared as the dose of haloperidol decreased. A similar effect was seen for chlorpromazine, which was used in seven trials ... In other words, the advantages of atypical antipsychotics in terms of efficacy and dropout rates are not seen if haloperidol is used at doses of 12mg/ day or less ... when we controlled for the higher than recommended dose of conventional antipsychotics used in some trials, a modest advantage in terms of extrapyramidal side effects remains, but the differences in efficacy and tolerability disappear, suggesting that *many of the perceived benefits of atypical antipsychotics are really due to excessive doses of the comparator drug used in the trials.*[607]

Most people are unaware that several atypical neuroleptics have been released – with much fanfare – but subsequently withdrawn from use, due to growing concerns about potentially serious though previously unreported side effects. In 1994 remoxipride (Roxiam) was withdrawn from the market in Australia, only three months after it was released, due to reports of drug-induced blood disorders (aplastic anaemia).[608] Sertindole (Serlect) was the fourth atypical neuroleptic approved for general use, but reports of cardiac arrhythmia and sudden death associated with its use resulted in its suspension in the UK in 1998.[609] As noted earlier, an inevitable result of the fact that most new medications are only tested on human beings for a few weeks before they are approved for general release is that certain side effects are only likely to become evident well *after* the drugs are already in widespread use.

As noted in *Chapter Three*, studies conducted by independent researchers have revealed that the atypical neuroleptics can cause a wide range of side effects, many of which have not yet been adequately publicised. When Australian researchers recently collected reports from a large group of people treated with various anti-psychotic medications, they were surprised at the high frequency of side effects they had been led to believe were uncommon with atypical neuroleptics. Noting that some form of extrapyramidal side effects were reported by the majority of respondents on both typical and atypical neuroleptics, these researchers commented: "We draw attention to aspects of the patient-reported profile of side-effects that are somewhat at odds with data from clinical trials."[610] Findings such as these have prompted critics to point out that what happens in the real world of everyday medication use may differ quite substantially from what has reportedly occurred in the highly artificial environment of controlled clinical trials.

Kept In the Dark

Award-winning medical journalist Robert Whitaker recently carried out a critical appraisal of the research used to support claims regarding the superiority of atypical neuroleptics. He concluded that one of the unfortunate legacies of the promotional trickery that has been employed in an effort to ensure the commercial success of these drugs, is that everyone concerned is left with a great deal of uncertainty about what to believe:

> One of the saddest aspects of this "research" process, and the story-telling that accompanies it, is how it has left everyone in the dark about the real merits

of the atypicals. There are certainly many anecdotal accounts of patients who are doing well on them, and so perhaps in some ways they truly are superior to the old drugs. Yet anecdotes do not make for good science, and the testing process was such that little can be known for certain.[611]

Many important questions are yet to be answered regarding the efficacy and relative merits of the atypical neuroleptics and about their long-term effects in particular:

Are the atypicals, for instance, even any better than placebo at knocking down psychosis? If patients suffering a first episode of psychosis were separated into two groups and one group were given a placebo and the other olanzapine, what would the results be at the end of six weeks? Or perhaps more to the point, if a sedative were compared to olanzapine or risperidone, what would be the results? No one knows. As for their comparative merits versus standard neuroleptics – again, who knows? ... The biggest question, of course, is how the new drugs will affect patients' lives over longer periods of time. The old drugs – as shown by the WHO studies – led to an increase in chronic illness and limited the possibility of recovery. They were harmful over the long run. Will the new drugs be equally harmful? Less harmful? Or, in fact, helpful over the long term? No one knows. However, there are already plenty of reasons to worry about their long-term effects. The atypicals – just like standard neuroleptics – cause an abnormal increase in D2 receptors. And while certain side effects, such as the risk of tardive dyskinesia, may be reduced with the atypicals, they also bring their own set of new problems.[612]

Because numerous vested interests are now locked in a fierce struggle for dominance, it is likely to be a very long time before vital questions such as those posed by Robert Whitaker can be answered satisfactorily. If what has occurred with the original neuroleptics is any guide, relevant information will only come to light very slowly, and decades could well pass before a truthful and balanced perspective on the atypical neuroleptics becomes possible.

The 10-20-30-Year Pattern

Over the past two decades or so the mental health field has evolved into a highly competitive commercial battlefield in which individuals and groups, both lay and professional, have become the constant targets of sophisticated (and often cleverly disguised) marketing techniques. In distinct contrast to the relatively innocent circumstances which prevailed when the first neuroleptics were introduced to psychiatry in the early 1950s, a vast and powerful machinery now exists whose sole purpose is to foster the use of psychotropic drugs. In Australia, the pharmaceutical industry now spends over one million dollars every day on a wide range of promotional activities. The fact that questionable methods are now often used to test and promote new medications, means that a great deal of the information furnished to mental health clinicians and the general public can no longer safely be taken at face value. In an arena in which conflicts of interest abound, it behoves those who seek truth to exercise an appropriately high level of discernment.

Aspects of the way the second-generation neuroleptics have been marketed epitomise these issues and highlight a range of other concerns. Dr Joseph Glenmullen has recently described the "10-20-30-year pattern" which he believes characterises the rise and eventual fall from grace of many once popular psychiatric drugs. "Reviewing the history of these drugs", he notes, "one finds a strikingly similar pattern." Thus, upon release, new medications are marketed aggressively with exuberant claims to the effect that they represent "revolutionary breakthroughs" and "remarkable scientific advances over their predecessors". Their relative freedom from the kinds of side effects that detracted from the acceptability of earlier drugs is invariably emphasised as a major selling point. As contrary evidence slowly accumulates these claims begin to look hollow, but it can take many years before growing awareness of the real shortcomings of the drugs leads to them being discredited — at which point the cycle begins again:

> In the typical life span of the drugs, the earliest signs of problems appear about ten years after introduction. Pharmaceutical companies and drug proponents deny the problems, adopting the strategy of defending the medication to the last. As we lack serious long-term monitoring of drug side effects and rely almost entirely on spontaneous, voluntary reporting by doctors, it is typically only at the twenty-year mark that enough data has accrued for the problems to be undeniable and for a significant number of physicians to be sounding the alarm. Still another ten years or more

elapse before professional organisations and regulatory agencies actively take steps to curtail over-prescribing. Thus, the cycle from miracle to disaster typically takes thirty years or more. By then, even the most popular drugs are no longer covered by their patent and even their manufacturers have an incentive to abandon medications that have become passé and disreputable. Typically their energies are then focused on the next breakthrough: newly patented, more profitable agents, which can be promoted as "safer" because their hazards are not yet known.[613]

As Dr Glenmullen points out, evidence is gathered slowly and takes time to filter through to the front-line clinicians responsible for prescribing and monitoring the drugs. Undoubtedly some of the information that eventually emerges will not be viewed favourably by those whose interests are primarily commercial. Given this, the process of developing a more complete picture of the benefits and liabilities of various psychiatric drugs is critically dependent on the availability of the findings of genuinely independent research. For reasons outlined in this chapter, such research is now increasingly rare. As things stand at present, and until such time as adequate steps are taken to ensure that doctors, patients, and others have full and unfettered access to truthful information, everyone concerned would be well advised to proceed with caution, and to take what they are told about neuroleptics and other psychiatric medications with a grain of salt.

Epilogue

THE MOST POWERFUL DRUG THERE IS

Recovery from psychosis is possible [and] is much more likely to come about through the catalyst of human intimacy. There is no medicine that can ever substitute for it.

Edward Podvoll[614]

NEUROLEPTICS AND OTHER PSYCHOTROPIC drugs provide psychiatrists with powerful tools. Indeed, some believe the day is not far distant when it will be possible to banish human misery altogether with the mere stroke of a doctor's pen on a prescription pad. While awaiting this pharmaceutical utopia, most psychiatric patients seem to be seeking something rather simple: acceptance, understanding, reassurance, respect, love. Providing such intangibles was once considered the very essence of the soul-doctor's art. Faced with the tremendous personal and professional challenges that accompany psychosis, there is an understandable tendency for clinicians to utilise whatever therapeutic tools are most readily available. Nevertheless, over a quarter century ago a group of psychiatrists who were regarded as leading lights in their field, warned about the danger of allowing the treatment of schizophrenia to become excessively one-sided. Drs Carpenter, McGlashan, and Strauss, then all senior researchers with the US National Institute of Mental Health, made the following remarks in an article published in the *American Journal of Psychiatry* in 1977:

> For many understandable and good reasons [the use of psychotropic medication] is now pre-eminent in the treatment of schizophrenic patients ... Pharmacological treatment of schizophrenia is extraordinarily important in psychiatry. We believe, however, that *the treatment of schizophrenia has become so extensively drug oriented that a significant impediment has arisen to the exploration of alternative therapeutic approaches* ... This widespread and premature foreclosure on the optimal treatment of schizophrenia is reflected by the fact that millions of people take neuroleptics as the only important component of their treatment. This narrowing of our clinical approach is especially alarming considering how little we know about schizophrenia.[615]

This prescient warning has gone unheeded. Indeed, in her incisive commentary on recent trends in the mental health field, anthropologist Tanya Luhrman noted how psychopharmacology has become "the great, silent dominatrix of contemporary psychiatry".[616] While the range of drugs from which clinicians can choose grows at a bewildering rate, interest in researching and applying non-drug treatment strategies has waned dramatically. Evidence of this trend is not difficult to find. Thus, for example, in a recent (1999) psychiatric text, a leading international authority offered these recommendations to his colleagues regarding the correct approach to treating schizophrenia:

> If patients have not shown at least partial response to an adequate dose of a traditional anti-psychotic after two or three weeks, compliance and plasma levels should be checked ... If these modifications do not yield relevant results within the next two to three weeks, switching to clozapine (or maybe to another of the novel antipsychotics) is indicated. This new treatment trial should last at least two to three months. If response remains unsatisfactory, various options should be considered [including] concomitant administration of lithium, or carbamazepine, as well as, alternatively, the use of benzodiazepines, SSRIs [antidepressants], or serotonin antagonists. ECT [shock treatment] also still has its place in these last resort treatment trials.[617]

Among the various options recommended by this expert, no mention whatsoever is made of anything other than medication (or ECT as a "last resort"). Could it not be that skilful provision of some of the intangible therapeutic factors mentioned above is often what is needed rather than simply another type or combination of pills? Many feel that such factors constitute the appropriate foundations for humane treatment, to which neuroleptics may be added if required. Firing "magic bullets" is far easier, but drugs are no substitute for the comfort and support of human intimacy. In reflecting on the philosophy that guided the

Soteria therapeutic community, founder and director Dr Loren Mosher commented: "I thought that sincere human involvement and understanding were critical to healing interactions ... The idea was to treat people as people, as human beings, with dignity and respect."[618]

Therapeutic Aggression

As drugs have come to be increasingly relied upon, care of diagnosed people has tended to become ever more impersonal. Indeed, as Dr Edward Podvoll has recently noted, with psychiatry and allied health disciplines now focusing almost exclusively on biological theories of schizophrenia and the use of assertive "interventions" and medication-based "management" strategies, diagnosed people are ever more likely to be subjected to *therapeutic aggression*, in the form of over-use of drugs and other physical methods of treatment. Of great concern, in his view, are the inevitable consequences of a lack of professional interest in the human mind and its care. As the "industrialisation of mental health" continues apace, it has become exceedingly rare for clinicians to now receive professional training of a kind that adequately equips them with the knowledge, skills, and understanding a truly holistic approach requires:

An almost exclusive focus of interest on the biological and chemical origins of mental derangement has developed over the past ten years. Government and private funding have become devoted to the so-called medical model, leaving other areas of clinical study in danger of atrophy ... [With] wholesale and gullible acceptance of the "medical model", people have abandoned all the traditional wisdom of caring for themselves and other ill persons. The healing professionals as well have become ignorant of the skills to be learned and practiced in order to care for their own mental health properly … Timeless healing wisdom and simple common sense are now called "anachronistic" – outmoded and no longer useful in the modern era … Almost as distressing as the ill effects of modern mental treatment is that the training for people working with patients who are in extreme mental states has been grossly neglected … The study of mind and its functions has virtually ceased within medical, psychiatric, and most psychological curricula. Training in the psychotherapy of highly disturbed people, or in the disciplines of interpersonal healing in general, is becoming increasingly rare in academic realms – already, nearly all the chairmen of psychiatry departments are biochemists or geneticists. *From where will the training come that allows one to overcome the fear and helplessness one experiences in confronting a mind that has become psychotic?* [619]

An unfortunate legacy of psychiatry's current obsession with "diagnostic precision" is that highly distressed individuals can now find themselves being admitted, examined, and assessed by harried clinicians so intent on making a diagnosis and instigating treatment (starting medication) that they fail to connect with their patients on anything more than a superficial level. In such cases the arduous task of listening to the diagnosed individual's personal story and empathising with his or her emotional concerns may simply never occur.

"You Can't Doctor A Soul With Pills"

In an era of increasing acceptance of "sane-making drugs" some readers are likely to find the views outlined above rather challenging. It is worth pointing out, then, that Professor Manfred Bleuler's intensive, life-long research led him to conclude that the establishment of a supportive relationship is an *indispensable* aspect of effective treatment. He believed, furthermore, that in this respect the physician's role is not necessarily of greater value than that of other helpers:

> It is the physician's first endeavour to make the patient aware that he is accepted in spite of his aberrant behaviour. The patient has to feel his physician's interest and empathy. The right patient-physician relationship might start by listening to the patient and by considering with him his complaints concerning his inner life, to his physical conditions or to his social environment. During such dialogues the therapeutic community is formed and developed and conversely the community opens more and more the way to discussions on what is essential in the patient's former life and in his present situation. The physician has to realise that he has a different role when confronted with the schizophrenic from that of many other medical situations. He cannot be a "healer" prescribing a definite therapy but he can help by being with the patient, by accompanying him for a length of time in his difficult life ... It is evident that the therapeutic role of the nurse in the hospital and of the relatives or helpers who represent the relatives is just as important for the benefit of the schizophrenic as the role of the physician.[620]

Ronald Laing would surely have agreed with these sentiments. Once the *enfant terrible* of orthodox psychiatry, Laing was a strong believer in the importance of what might be termed the psychology of simple human presence. In his view, establishing a feeling connection with another human being provides a vital bridge to those who find themselves alone and adrift in extreme mental states such as psychosis:

> A component in the distress in people who are in a mental state is the feeling of being cut off from ordinary human relationships – a two way chasm or abyss. That in itself is a nightmarish feeling. As time goes on it's rather like blood being cut off. You feel like a hungry ghost. The main factor is presence – making contact – feeling the presence of another human being in itself. If that doesn't happen, nothing does. If that does happen, there's a ground, a basis. But there is no one way for everybody. Other people withdraw from people with extreme or unusual states of mind. To make contact is the most powerful drug there is. That can transform a person's state of mind.[621]

Jungian psychiatrist John Perry has pointed out that being able to talk to someone who will really listen is crucial to those in emotional turmoil. In some instances, judicious use of medication may help to facilitate communication between the diagnosed person and those providing care and treatment. The prescribing of medication may even be perceived as a concrete demonstration of the therapist's concern and willingness to help. On the other hand, however, medication could become a barrier to the establishment of a genuine therapeutic alliance if it is not utilised with great skill and sensitivity. If the administration of drugs takes precedence over simply listening, for example, a message might be given to the diagnosed person that his or her most heart-felt concerns are not going to be taken seriously. In such cases, he or she may feel it is not worth even trying to communicate. As one person in this situation explained, "When my previous therapist took out his prescription pad, I knew I could never tell him anything important".[622]

The Caduceus Has Two Serpents

There is a real danger that the advent of atypical neuroleptics will lead to complacency on the part of many clinicians, diagnosed people, and their families. This is especially likely when these drugs have been heavily promoted as a "major advance" with the implication that they have none of the drawbacks of the earlier drugs. Time will tell to what extent these claims prove to be true. In the meanwhile, it is good to remember that many medications which were at one time seen as virtual cure alls, have later come to be seen in a far more modest light. The large family of drugs known collectively as antibiotics are an example. While their beneficial, at times even life-saving effects are well known, it is now recognised that excessive, unrestrained, and inappropriate use of these powerful medicines has resulted in a range of negative consequences, not the least of which is the rapidly growing problem of antibiotic resistance. An understandable desire for instantaneous and simple solutions to complex human problems is one of the factors driving the current tendency to administer neuroleptics excessively. It is not inconceivable that "too much of a good thing" could eventually result in the creation of significant problems with these drugs, just as has occurred with many others.

In this context, it is interesting to consider modern approaches to the treatment of diabetes, a condition with which schizophrenia is often compared ("You have an illness like diabetes and you will have it all your life. Medication cannot cure your condition but it will help to control the symptoms"). It is now known that a wide range of different treatment strategies are appropriate, and that people with diabetes must adopt an approach that suits their particular circumstances. Thus, while some require regular insulin injections, others only need tablets (oral hypoglycaemic agents). Some do not require medications at all and can manage their condition perfectly well with various lifestyle adjustments that include attending to factors such as diet, weight control, exercise, and stress management. Lifestyle factors are now known to play an extremely important role in many medical conditions, including asthma, hypertension (high blood pressure), heart disease, migraine, and HIV/AIDS. As earlier chapters made clear, lifestyle factors are no less important in regard to schizophrenia. In his popular book, *Surviving Schizophrenia*, psychiatrist Fuller Torrey states that "Antipsychotic drugs for schizophrenia are exactly the same as insulin for diabetes".[623] A different view is expressed by Harvard psychiatrist Joseph Glenmullen, who points out that only around 10% of people with diabetes have a condition severe enough to require insulin, and that the majority can manage well with milder agents, dietary modifications, and other lifestyle changes. Dr Glenmullen asks: "What if doctors tried to make all diabetics dependent on insulin?"[624]

It has become quite clear that people vary tremendously, both in terms of their need for neuroleptic medications and in the ways these drugs affect them. Failure to appreciate and respect this variability has led to a remarkable uniformity in the way those diagnosed with schizophrenia tend to be treated. Thus, psychiatrists such as Dr Torrey confidently assert, "It is not that drugs are the *only* ingredient necessary to treat schizophrenia successfully; they are just the most essential ingredient."[625] Close examination of the facts reveals a far more complex picture, one in which individual variability is the rule. While it may be true that neuroleptic treatment is extremely beneficial for *some* people, it is certainly far less so for others, and for some it may be unnecessary, possibly even harmful. As prominent American consumer activist Judi Chamberlin has pointed out, the appropriate role of medication can only be determined on an individual basis:

> Now I want to make one thing very clear here. I am not advocating that no one should take psychiatric drugs. What I am saying, and I want to make sure this point is understood, is that each individual needs to discover for himself or herself whether or not the drugs are part of the solution or part of the problem. Many people I know and respect tell me that they would not be where they are in their recovery were it not for the particular drugs that they have found work for them. On the other hand, many others, of which I am one, have found that only when we clear ourselves of all psychiatric drugs do we begin to find the road to recovery. We need to respect these choices, and to understand that there is no single path for all of us.[626]

In this context it is instructive to reflect on the symbolism of the caduceus which, with its twin serpents entwined around a winged staff, is the universally recognised emblem of the medical profession. Ancient Greek mythology tells how Asklepius, god of medicine, received his healing powers from Athena, in the form of blood taken from Medusa the Gorgon. According to this story, blood from Medusa's right side had great healing powers – it was even reputed to be able to raise the dead – while blood from the left was believed to be instantly destructive and brought death. Legend has it that, like the Medusa's blood, the bite of one of the snakes depicted on the caduceus is poisonous, while that of the other is healing. A similar dichotomy involving healing and harm is found in the ancient Greek term, *pharmakon*, from which modern words such as "pharmacy" (the science of preparing and dispensing medicinal drugs) are derived. The Greek philosopher Socrates used the word *pharmakon* to refer to both "remedy" and "poison". The renowned Swiss alchemist-physician Paracelsus (1493-1541) also recognised the dual nature of medicines, as expressed in his teaching that the dose determines whether a substance acts as a remedy or a poison. In psychiatry, as in other branches of medicine, we would do well to remember the ancient wisdom reflected in the fact that the caduceus has *two* serpents.

Healing or Harming The Soul?

In a seminal book concerning the psychology of "mental illness" first published in 1908, pioneer psychiatrist Carl Jung pointed out that the ancient Greek word "psyche" originally referred to the human soul or spirit, and that psychiatry itself is properly understood to involve "the art of healing the soul". One of the enduring legacies of Jung's work was his insistence on the vital importance to such healing of attending to the non-physical aspects: "Only beyond the brain", he said, "beyond the anatomical substrate, do we reach what is important for us – the psyche, as indefinable as ever, still eluding all explanation, no matter how ingenious."[627] Because Jungian therapists recognise the centrality of the psyche in human life, they take it for granted that a comprehensive understanding of schizophrenia and other psychotic disorders is impossible without reference to the human soul or spirit. As one eminent Jungian psychiatrist has put it: "Schizophrenia presents us with a problem that leads down to the very roots of the psyche."[628]

Psychiatry today rarely refers to such things, so preoccupied has it become with far more concrete matters, such as identifying the genes believed to be responsible for the predisposition to schizophrenia, or developing ever more effective ways of rectifying the chemical imbalance that is said to occur in the brains of affected individuals. Experience shows that, if used with great skill and sensitivity, neuroleptic and other medications can be enormously helpful at times to many who have been diagnosed with schizophrenia. However, the demonstrated usefulness of psychotropic drugs has helped foster the belief that human beings have acquired the ability to solve complex psychological and spiritual problems by application of a seductively simple notion: "better living through chemistry". The advent of powerful pharmaceutical tools which now make it possible to directly manipulate brain chemistry has led to an enthrallment with neurobiology. This has had the unfortunate effect of leading mainstream psychiatry to the point where it has all but lost sight of the deeper aspects of the human predicaments it professes to treat.

In his thought-provoking book, *Healing the Soul in the Age of the Brain*, psychiatrist and psychotherapist Elio Frattaroli laments the growing tendency of mental health clinicians to neglect the person behind the symptoms. While he acknowledges the potential therapeutic value of modern psychotropic medications, Professor Frattaroli believes that, rather than relying on these powerful tools alone – and then only to suppress symptoms – a more helpful and creative approach would be to use the drugs as an aid to therapies which promote healing on a broader level:

> I am not questioning the therapeutic value of these medications. Used properly, I believe they can be extremely helpful, even life-saving. However, I also want to emphasise that most of the psychiatric medications being prescribed nowadays are not being used properly. They are not being used in the service of healing the soul in the context of a psychotherapeutic process, but rather as a quick, cosmetic fix to produce temporary symptomatic relief. Indeed, most of the psychiatrists who prescribe medications today – especially those trained in the last ten years – know very little about the psychotherapeutic process and so have nothing to offer except a quick fix. Even worse, most of our psychiatric medications are not even being prescribed by psychiatrists. They are being prescribed by general practitioners who have no expertise or interest in treating mental illness … This situation is highly destructive, both to the lives of individual patients and to the humanistic values of our society as a whole.[629]

Skilfully prescribed low-dose atypical neuroleptics are less likely to cause debilitating side effects like sedation, akinesia, and akathisia than are the older drugs. As a result, people receiving such treatment could potentially gain greater benefit from psychotherapy or counselling than may have previously been possible. However, even though the therapeutic value of "talking therapies" has now been clearly established (*Chapter Four*), widespread use of the new drugs has not led to a general increase in the availability of treatments combining medication and psychotherapy.

Beyond the Brain

The potentially harmful effects of therapeutic approaches to psychosis which are based entirely on physical considerations greatly concerned Carl Jung who, in the early 1950s, commented:

> The dogma, or intellectual superstition, that only physical causes are valid still bars the psychiatrist's way to the psyche of his patient and impels him to take the most reckless and incalculable liberties with this most delicate of all organs.[630]

The development and implementation of a truly holistic approach could help redress this tendency. A holistic understanding of life accepts that human beings are multifaceted organisms in whom the social, psychological, spiritual, and biological dimensions are intricately inter-woven to form a unified whole. It takes for granted, furthermore, that it is impossible to fully understand any one of these aspects in isolation from the others. Thus, from a holistic perspective, it makes little sense to speak of schizophrenia as though it involved nothing more than a "biological illness of the brain". In this context, Professor Manfred Bleuler's views represent a refreshing departure from the usual narrow focus. At the end of a very long and productive career largely devoted to the study of schizophrenia, Professor Bleuler stressed the vital importance of non-physical factors: "In my opinion, the schizophrenic happening takes place in the realms of the mind and the emotions, that is, in mental spheres that exist only in man. It is inaccessible to direct influence by elementary physical processes."[631]

It should be emphasised that theories about the cause of schizophrenia do not necessarily have to give precedence to either biological or psychospiritual factors. Indeed, recent developments in neuroscience have made it abundantly clear that a complex *reciprocal* (two-way) relationship exists between mind and brain. The concept of neural plasticity recognises this fact, as psychiatrist John Nelson explains:

Mind and brain operate as a *unitary system* in which changes in one go hand in hand with changes in the other. Within such a unity, cause-and-effect relationships blur beyond distinction, and the best we can say is that any force that changes either brain or mind also changes the other ... Although it is easier to demonstrate that physically altering the brain changes subjective experience, there is mounting evidence that mental events leave their imprints within the brain. The old view that a computer-like brain's hardwiring is fixed at birth, or even at maturity, is now passé. Neuroscience has demonstrated again and again that life experience is at least as powerful as genetic programming in shaping both the cellular architecture and chemical activity of the brain. In other words, plasticity is a fact of brain functioning, even at the relatively coarse level of the cell and synapse.[632]

It is now well known that significant functional and structural changes occur in the human brain in response to psychosocial influences, an understanding that has led to a greater appreciation of the fact that psychological therapies can lead to favourable alterations in brain functioning.[633] It has recently been demonstrated that meditation has tangible effects on brain and immune system functioning and may change them in positive ways.[634] When considering these issues, it is good to remember that, whatever the biological aspects may turn out to be, to those undergoing it psychosis is first and foremost an *experience*. It must be understood and responded to as such. Human beings live in the world of their experiences, after all, not in the world of their brain chemistry!

Psychosis: A Meaningful Disturbance

Because contemporary beliefs about mental illness, both lay and professional, are under the sway of a highly materialistic paradigm (referred to as the "medical model"), many people are not aware that there is a range of alternate views about the nature of psychosis. For example, there is a school of thought which says that, rather than simply being a product of a biochemical imbalance in the brain, symptoms of psychosis may reflect the existence of a deep-seated psychospiritual imbalance in the diagnosed person's life. Professor Frattaroli expresses this notion as follows:

The truth is, we have no scientific evidence that any psychiatric symptom is a disease rather than – like fever, cough, fainting, and physical pain – part of a natural healing process … If we think of psychiatric symptoms as produced by persons in their wholeness rather than brains in their brokenness, then we can see that they are more than disruptions of biological equilibrium. They are adaptive responses to a disruption, not of chemical imbalance in the body, but of the inner harmony of the soul.[635]

As frightening and disconcerting as it may be, psychosis can involve depths of meaning which are lost when the only goal of treatment is to suppress the experience. While there may be times when reducing the intensity and frequency of symptoms is probably in the best interest of all concerned, treatment which fails to pay any heed to the subjective, inner aspects of the diagnosed person's experience may miss the opportunity to promote healing on levels that go far deeper than symptoms. Maryanne Handel explains this point well. As painful as her own experiences were, in the end she felt certain that within them were contained the seeds of change and growth, and that psychosis was for her ultimately a *meaningful* disturbance:

The whole schizophrenic experience means something. It's not just a meaningless chaos that's come to persecute you or to hurt you for no reason. It does mean something. Knowing that was valuable to me. What I experienced was like this inner journey full of temptations and so on. And you are able to come out of it, but come out of it changed on the inside and different. I wanted to have this feeling that I could change through it and that I would be allowed to become normal again. Knowing that was very important to me because it was like a promise that I could. And it gave me hope that I would come out of it. That hope sort of led me on.[636]

These ideas paint a far more hopeful picture than is usually associated with schizophrenia. In particular, they suggest that some who receive this diagnosis may be experiencing a crisis for which psychotropic medication is not required. They also suggest that, with courage, persistent effort, and the right kind of support, many people may eventually be able to grow beyond the need for long-term maintenance treatment.

What Truly Heals?

Despite a huge research effort that has now extended over many decades, there is still so much we do not understand about the condition called "schizophrenia". Some believe its mysteries will soon yield to diligent scientific scrutiny using the new generation of powerful brain-imaging tools and the high-tech methodology of molecular biology. As interesting as the results of such research may be, there is growing suspicion in the minds of many that we have lost sight of something precious along the way. Can we unravel the mysteries of the *Mona Lisa* by analysing the microstructure of the paints Leonardo da Vinci used to portray his subject's enigmatic smile? Or, as Jung suggested long ago, are we just as likely to reach a satisfactory understanding of schizophrenia by focusing exclusively on the physical brain as we are to comprehend the purpose of a majestic cathedral by performing a mineralogical analysis of the stones used in its construction? Would we not learn a great deal more if we set aside our favoured theories and concepts and simply looked with fresh eyes and listened with truly open hearts and minds?

Unanswered questions abound, pointing toward deeper mysteries. How can we account for the fact that some diagnosed people respond well to drug treatment, while others benefit very little or not at all? Concepts such as "treatment resistance" merely beg the question: why do people with the same psychotic illness vary so greatly in terms of their responses to similar drugs? And why do some people remain severely disabled despite intensive treatment with the latest drugs while others prosper without the need for long-term medication? These and many other difficult questions lead to the inevitable conclusion that, while a great deal has been learnt about the medical treatment of schizophrenia during the last fifty years, we still know precious little about the conditions required for true healing. Indeed, we remain profoundly ignorant about the nature of healing, perhaps most particularly in regard to conditions now referred to as "mental illness". What is healing? What can diagnosed people and their helpers do to bring it about?

When they are diagnosed with schizophrenia, people are often told something to the effect that they have a genetically-inherited brain disorder, that they will require medication to correct the abnormal chemical imbalance that is responsible for their symptoms, and that they may need such medication indefinitely, possibly for the rest of their lives, if they wish to retain even a semblance of "normality". Is it really any wonder that many diagnosed people are non-compliant with their medications, and that many become depressed and demoralised? What would happen if they were told a different story, perhaps one like this:

> You are an extremely sensitive person, so sensitive in fact that you sometimes find yourself becoming over-whelmed by feelings that are hard to understand or control because they are so intense. At times your hypersensitivity may cause you to feel you are los-ing control of your thoughts, too, which sometimes dance in your head so vibrantly they seem like living beings alternatively tormenting and enticing you. In time you may learn to handle your sensitivity better so that you are no longer at its mercy. In the mean-while, medication is one of the things that might help you to cope by temporarily reducing the intensity and speed of your feelings and thoughts. Many highly sen-sitive people find that medication can help make their inner world quieter and a little easier to handle so that they have some space to begin sorting things out for themselves.

What would happen if diagnosed people were told something like this? Would they be more willing to cooperate with recommended treatment? Even more importantly, would ideas such as these allow them to feel better about themselves and more hopeful about their future prospects? If so, what beneficial effects might this then have on innate physical, mental, and spiritual heal-ing processes? And what would happen if we encouraged diagnosed people to believe that *they* hold the keys to their own healing? If we acknowledged that medications may be helpful in some ways, but that healing – which literally means "to become whole" – calls for something more, something only the wounded themselves can provide?

The placebo effect points toward the existence of what is sometimes called an "inner healer". Those who are wise in the healing arts invariably acknowledge their indebtedness to this powerful and omnipresent inner resource. In his ground-breaking book, *Anatomy of an Illness,* pioneer holistic healing researcher Norman Cousins relates an anecdote in which the renowned philanthropist/physician, Dr Albert Schweitzer, is reported to have said:

> Each patient carries his own doctor inside him. They come to us not knowing that truth. We are at our best when we give the doctor who resides within each patient a chance to go to work.[637]

Psychiatry is yet to acknowledge this wisdom. Many diagnosed people have already learnt it for themselves. They know this is where their journey of recovery really begins.

APPENDIX A:

OPTIMAL DOSAGE RANGES OF SOME COMMON NEUROLEPTIC DRUGS

WHEN CHLORPROMAZINE (LARGACTIL) was introduced to psychiatry in the early 1950s, it was generally given in maximum dosages of around 200 mg per day. Indeed, doses as low as 50 mg per day were often found to produce what were, at the time, considered miraculous results.[638] Over the following decades dosages gradually rose, until it was not uncommon for people to be receiving 800-1200 mg a day or more by the 1970s and 80s. During this period, haloperidol (Serenace) was also frequently given in large amounts, with many people receiving daily doses of 60-80 mg or more. Long-acting depot neuroleptics such as fluphenazine decanoate (Modecate) were also administered liberally, with dosages of 75-100 mg per fortnight once being common. Contemporary clinical research has shown that, for the vast majority of diagnosed individuals, these doses are seriously excessive and are unlikely to be any more therapeutically beneficial than far smaller ones.[639]

Until relatively recently, clinicians could only determine therapeutic dosages empirically, i.e. by noting the effects, both positive and negative, of different amounts of a drug on those taking it. In the 1970s, it was discovered that neuroleptics work by blocking neuroreceptors in various parts of the brain and, as the range of available medications grew, it was realised that each of them acts on particular receptors. Recent technological advances have made it possible to measure with great precision the extent to which individual neuroleptics block specific receptor sites. As a result, dosage ranges can now be determined on a more objective basis. In particular, pharmacologists are able to work out upper therapeutic limits for individual neuroleptics, this being the dose at which the receptors specifically targeted by that drug are effectively blocked.[640] Increasing the dose above this level cannot produce additional therapeutic benefits, since all of the available receptor sites are already occupied. The only possible consequence of raising the dosage further is to cause more, or increasingly severe, side effects. As an example, research has established that the beneficial effects of chlorpromazine do not increase when the dosage exceeds 375 mg a day. Psychopharmacologist David Healy has pointed out that, while treatment with relatively low doses of chlorpromazine may be helpful, larger amounts are only likely to cause problematic side effects:

> Doses up to this level may bring about a useful increase in feelings of indifference and general calmness. Higher

doses usually will not. They will increasingly tend to make the clinical picture worse by causing side effects – particularly if these higher doses are sustained for a long period of time.[641]

It must be remembered that *individual variability is the rule* when it comes to neuroleptic treatment since people differ greatly regarding the extent and rate at which their bodies absorb and metabolise these drugs. While some diagnosed individuals demonstrate a remarkable sensitivity to the effects and side effects of neuroleptics, others appear to possess a remarkable tolerance to them. Variations in individual physical, psychological, and social circumstances also play a major role. Those exposed to excessive stress and over-stimulation, for example, may have greater need for the protective "stress-buffering" effect of neuroleptics than those who live in calm, low-stress, supportive environments. While it is theoretically possible to specify an "average" dosage for any therapeutic drug, in practice some diagnosed individuals may respond adequately to amounts very much less than this notional average, while others may require substantially more. As emphasised earlier, successful schizophrenia treatment requires that neuroleptic regimes be skilfully tailored to suit the particular needs and circumstances of each diagnosed individual – which may include the possibility of medication-free treatment for some people.

Conventional Neuroleptics

Many of the older neuroleptics are still widely used, especially those administered in the form of long-acting injections. While average dosages can vary widely, the following ranges are common in everyday clinical practice:

Oral medications (tablets):
- chlorpromazine (Largactil) 100-400 mg/day
- trifluoperazine (Stelazine) 5-20 mg/day
- haloperidol (Serenace) 5-20 mg/day
- pericyazine (Neulactil) 25-75 mg/day
- pimozide (Orap) 2-12 mg/day
- thiothixene (Navane) 10-40 mg/day
- zuclopenthixol (Clopixol) 10-75 mg/day

Depot medications (long-acting injections):
- flupenthixol decanoate (Fluanxol) 20-80 mg every 2-4 weeks
- fluphenazine decanoate (Modecate) 12.5-75 mg every 2-4 weeks
- haloperidol decanoate (Haldol) 50-300 mg every 4 weeks
- zuclopenthixol decanoate (Clopixol Depot) 200-400 mg every 2-4 weeks

In regard to both acute treatment and long-term maintenance, research has demonstrated that the optimal medication regime for many people may involve neuroleptic dosages substantially lower than those often used in practice. Professor Ross Baldessarini, a leading international authority on drug treatment of schizophrenia, has concluded that "the majority of chronically psychotic patients can be maintained on doses of neuroleptics as low as one fifth or even a tenth of those commonly employed".[642] In line with these views, the American Psychiatric Association's treatment guidelines for schizophrenia recommend that neuroleptic doses be gradually reduced (by approximately 20% every 6 months) until the minimal effective therapeutic dosage level is reached. For many people, the Association has stated, an effective neuroleptic dose could be as low as the equivalent of 2.5 mg of haloperidol a day or injections of 50 mg haloperidol decanoate (Haldol) per month, while doses of 5–10 mg fluphenazine decanoate (Modecate) a fortnight may be just as therapeutically beneficial as standard dosages which are often many times higher.[643]

Atypical Neuroleptics

These drugs are now widely used and are often prescribed instead of the older neuroleptics because of their generally reduced propensity to cause severe extrapyramidal side effects. Seven atypicals that are now frequently used in Australia are listed below, together with commonly recommended dosage ranges:

Oral medications (tablets):
- clozapine (Clozaril) 300–900 mg/day
- olanzapine (Zyprexa) 10–30 mg/day
- risperidone (Risperdal) 2–6 mg/day
- quetiapine (Seroquel) 300–800 mg/day
- amisulpride (Solian) 50–300 mg/day
- aripiprazole (Abilify) 15–30 mg/day

Depot medications (long-acting injections):
- risperidone (Risperdal Consta) 25 mg every two weeks

Early Psychosis

Young people are often especially sensitive to the effects of psychotropic medications and may respond satisfactorily to dosages far lower than those usually given to older people with a longer psychiatric history. It is now widely accepted that optimal medical treatment of early psychosis (first or second psychotic episode) should generally entail *very low* dosages initially, which are only increased if this is truly necessary. It has become common for such treatment to begin with one of the atypical neuroleptics, the following regimes often being recommended:[644]

- olanzapine (Zyprexa) 2.5-10 mg/day (can be taken once at night)
- risperidone (Risperdal) 1-2 mg/day (can be taken once at night)
- quetiapine (Seroquel) 300-450 mg/day (25 mg twice on the first day, 50 mg twice on day two, 100 mg twice on day three, 150 mg twice on day four)
- amisulpride (Solian) 400 mg per day

In some cases, *extremely low* doses of these drugs may be adequate, e.g. clozapine 12.5 mg/day, olanzapine 2.5 mg/day, risperidone 0.25 mg/day, quetiapine 50 mg/day.[645]

Therapeutic Equivalence

Neuroleptics differ in regard to their relative potencies. As a result, small amounts of high-potency drugs such as haloperidol or risperidone may have therapeutic effects comparable to those of much larger amounts of low potency-drugs like chlorpromazine or quetiapine.

Chlorpromazine 100 mg is generally taken as the basic standard against which other neuroleptics are compared. Approximate therapeutically equivalent doses of some of the most commonly prescribed neuroleptics are shown in *Table Three*. It is important to understand that these values only provide a rough general guide since variations in individual treatment responsiveness could mean that different people will react quite differently to similar dosages of these drugs.

TABLE THREE

NEUROLEPTIC DRUG	DOSE (mg)
Typical Neuroleptics	
Chlorpromazine (Largactil)	100
Thioridazine (Melleril)	100
Trifluoperazine (Stelazine)	5
Thiothixene (Navane)	5
Haloperidol (Serenace)	2
Atypical Neuroleptics	
Clozapine (Clozaril)	50
Quetiapine (Seroquel)	50-100?
Olanzapine (Zyprexa)	2-3?
Risperidone (Risperdal)	1-2

Source: APA, 1997[646]

Guidelines For Establishing Optimal Dosages

The highly idiosyncratic nature of treatment responsiveness makes it impossible to specify optimal dosage ranges precisely. However, those interested in applying the treatment philosophy advocated in this book may find the following general principles helpful:

- If neuroleptic medication is necessary, start with the lowest possible effective dose
- Gradually increase the dose only if absolutely necessary (i.e. "start low and go slow")
- Reduce the medication to the lowest effective dose again as soon as this is feasible
- If the medication does not seem to be helping after an adequate trial, do not continue increasing the dose indefinitely. Consider trying a different neuroleptic. Alternatively, gradually decrease the dosage or consider stopping drug treatment altogether
- Rather than increasing the neuroleptic dosage during periods of severe agitation or psychotic relapse, use a benzodiazepine (Valium-type drug) as a *temporary* measure to help reduce anxiety and dampen down distressing symptoms (e.g. hostile voices)
- Effective non-drug coping strategies will allow medication dosages to be kept to a minimum and may even allow neuroleptic treatment to be avoided altogether
- Using medication on an intermittent basis rather than continuously (i.e. every day), may be a viable option for some people
- Optimal social circumstances (low stress, adequate supports, effective coping skills) can substantially reduce the need for large dosages of neuroleptic medication

Remember that the optimally effective dosage of any drug can only be determined on an individual basis, and that while some people seem to manage well on fairly large neuroleptic dosages, others may experience significant problems on even quite small amounts. The important question, in the end, is whether the medication is helping at the dosages prescribed without causing unacceptable side effects, both immediate and long-term.

APPENDIX B:

MANAGING NEUROLEPTIC SIDE EFFECTS

Whatever their various side effects, neuroleptics should not make someone feel worse. If they do, then too high a dose or the wrong drug is being prescribed.

David Healy[647]

SOME PEOPLE WHO TAKE neuroleptics on a regular basis experience few day-to-day problems related to the side effects of this treatment. On the other hand, these drugs can cause discomfort, distress, or even disability, which in some cases may be severe enough to compromise the treated person's quality of life to a significant degree. Concerns about actual or potential side effects undoubtedly cause some people to become reluctant to cooperate with recommended treatment. Even if they cause no immediate problems, the mere possibility that prolonged neuroleptic treatment could have various delayed adverse effects (e.g. physical health problems, supersensitivity, tardive dyskinesia, memory and cognitive impairment), makes this an issue of vital concern for everyone who takes or prescribes these medications.

People can respond to side effects in a variety of different possible ways. Some responses, while understandable, are inadvisable, since they could lead to even greater problems. Examples of these include unilateral medication refusal (whether openly or in secret), and abuse of social and/or illicit stimulants (e.g. caffeine, amphetamines) in an effort to counter medication-induced sedation or lack of energy. By contrast, there are a wide range of things diagnosed people and their helpers can do to prevent, or at least significantly reduce, problematic side effects, which not only entail few risks, but which are actually likely to be more effective than simply refusing medical treatment or resorting to substance abuse. (Those who refuse medication due to concerns about side effects sometimes find themselves compelled to accept treatment with drugs that may be even *more* likely to cause such problems. As explained earlier, the neurological side effects caused by conventional long-acting depot injections tend to be considerably more severe than those associated with low doses of oral atypical neuroleptics.) Successful management of neuroleptic side effects is based on the following general principles:

(a) Prevention

Severe side effects are not a necessary and inevitable consequence of neuroleptic treatment. In fact, most experts agree that problematic side effects are often a result of too many medications being given at once (a practice referred to as "polypharmacy") or incorrect prescribing, e.g. inappropriate choice of drug, excessive doses, or medication given when it is not necessary. Leaving aside those whose peculiar sensitivity causes them to react adversely even to very small doses of medication, for the majority of diagnosed persons many side effects can be avoided, or at least significantly reduced, if drugs are prescribed skilfully and used wisely. The principle of "harm minimisation" refers to the use of drugs in such a way that the occurrence of undesirable effects is reduced as much as possible. *A range of practical guidelines for using neuroleptic medications wisely were outlined in Chapter Eight.*

(b) Recognition

Actually recognising side effects when they occur is fundamental to managing them successfully. Although this point may seem rather obvious, it needs to be emphasised since correct identification of neuroleptic side effects is *not* always a simple or straightforward matter. While it may be fairly obvious that common side effects such as tremor, blurred vision, dry mouth, and excessive weight gain are due to medication, the cause of others, e.g. lethargy, restlessness, sexual dysfunction, poor concentration, can be more difficult to determine. It must be remembered that such problems *could* be related to factors quite apart from medication, e.g. stress, anxiety, lack of sleep, depression, inactivity, poor diet, and unhealthy lifestyle. Another difficulty is that side effects such as akinesia, parkinsonism, and the Neuroleptic-Induced Deficit Syndrome (NIDS), can so closely resemble the negative symptoms of schizophrenia that even experienced clinicians may fail to tell them apart. Unfortunately, there is still a tendency, in some quarters, to pay inadequate attention to concerns about side effects, or to hastily dismiss them as "part of the illness". To reduce the likelihood of this occurring, all parties concerned should be thoroughly familiar with the wide range of side effects that can occur as a result of neuroleptic treatment (*Chapters Two* and *Three*).

Quite often the only reliable way to work out whether or not a particular problem is in fact a side effect is to alter the medication regime in some way, e.g. reduce the dosage or switch to a different drug, and observe what happens. Adding drugs which counteract side effects can also be useful in this regard, though caution must be exercised as these drugs can have side effects of their own (see below). While some people do *inappropriately* blame medications for all their problems, researchers have found that most diagnosed people are actually quite good at working out whether or not they are experiencing side effects. For example, participants in one recent study were able to correctly attribute their symptoms to medication 69% of the time.[648] It can be extremely beneficial for diagnosed people to have access to others who are able to provide comprehensive information about side effects, and who can also offer accurate feed-back to assist them in correctly evaluating their experiences.

(c) Patience

Just as the human body can develop a tolerance to the effects of social drugs such as alcohol and nicotine, so too can it gradually adjust to some of the effects of neuroleptic medications over time. This is most likely with side effects such as sedation, dry mouth, constipation, and blurred vision, all of which may slowly diminish or even disappear entirely after the first few weeks of treatment (though this is less likely if large amounts of medication are being prescribed). In many instances, having patience and being willing to put up with a degree of discomfort for a little while may be all that is required. It should be noted that extrapyramidal side effects (EPS) and some of the other more serious problems caused by neuroleptic treatment (e.g. metabolic disturbances) are *not* likely to diminish spontaneously with time.

(d) Dosage Reduction

In general, problematic side effects are more likely with higher medication dosages. Consequently, a basic principle for minimising side effects is to always use the lowest effective dose for a given individual. While this may seem rather obvious, it does not always occur in practice. In fact, people diagnosed with "chronic" schizophrenia were once routinely given very large doses of maintenance medication which remained fixed at a high level for years on end with little variation. In the past, concern about possible untoward consequences of lowering the dose led to the common practice of giving diagnosed people *another* drug to counteract side effects, rather than prescribing a smaller amount of neuroleptic medication.[649] Despite this deeply ingrained tendency, there is now a good deal of evidence to show that many diagnosed people do well on much less medication than was once considered necessary. Except in emergency situations, neuroleptic dosages should always be reduced very gradually to avoid severe withdrawal reactions and minimise the likelihood of relapse (see guidelines in *Chapter Ten*).

(e) Responsible Experimentation

The way people respond to neuroleptic medications is notoriously idiosyncratic, both in terms of the therapeutic responses elicited and the side effects caused. In practice, this means that any given individual may react quite differently to drugs that have very similar pharmacological properties. As a result, it is sometimes possible to overcome problematic side effects simply by switching to a different medication. Since it is impossible to predict whether or not a given neuroleptic drug will give rise to troublesome side effects, an empirical approach is necessary, i.e. different medications must be tried until one is found which produces a satisfactory therapeutic response while causing minimal side effects. In general, high-potency neuroleptics (which presently include all long-acting depot preparations) are more likely to cause EPS than are the various low-potency drugs. On the whole, atypical neuroleptics are less likely to cause severe neurological side effects than the older drugs, although various other kinds of adverse reactions are common.

A number of strategies which might help to minimise problematic side effects, while still proving therapeutically effective, were outlined in *Chapter Nine*. These include low-dose regimes, intermittent treatment, and use of non-neuroleptic drugs. The suitability of such strategies for any given individual can only be determined by a process of experimentation.

(f) Healthy Lifestyle

Every drug a person ingests, whether medically prescribed or not, must be metabolised, absorbed, and its by-products eventually excreted. These processes place demands on the body and require a certain amount of energy and the availability of a wide range of naturally occurring biochemical substances including various vitamins, minerals, and enzymes. While being fit and healthy will not necessarily prevent side effects from occurring, it is certain that an optimally-functioning body will be more readily able to cope with the physiological demands drugs make upon it. Older people are more prone to experiencing side effects because their bodies metabolise and excrete drugs rather less efficiently. As a general principle, those who must take neuroleptic or other prescription drugs for extended periods may find that improving their physical health and maintaining a reasonable level of fitness will enhance their body's natural ability to handle these substances. Avoiding illicit drugs entirely, and using social drugs such as alcohol, tobacco, and caffeine in moderation, reduces the overall load of toxic substances the body has to deal with.

As explained in *Chapter Six*, cigarette smoking can reduce the concentration of neuroleptic medications in the bloodstream, with the result that smokers sometimes receive higher dosages of these drugs than do non-smokers, thereby increasing their likelihood of experiencing side effects. In addition to the substantial health benefits associated with giving up smoking, doing so may also indirectly help with side effects by reducing the amount of medication a person is required to take. Learning effective stress-management techniques can help by reducing the need for large dosages of stress-buffering neuroleptic drugs.

(g) Non-Drug Coping Strategies

In addition to effective stress management, it is now clear that many people are able to successfully employ non-drug strategies and techniques to help them deal with various schizophrenia symptoms and with uncomfortable feeling states such as anxiety and depression. A wide variety of simple and easily learnt techniques have been successfully utilised by diagnosed individuals to stop or reduce disturbing "voices" (auditory hallucinations), and to prevent or alleviate intrusive thoughts (some examples were described in *Chapter Four*). People who learn to use such coping strategies may eventually be able to manage on smaller amounts of neuroleptic medication, with a consequent reduction in their risk of experiencing problematic side effects. The sense of mastery and enhanced self-confidence that comes with learning effective coping strategies can have the additional benefit of counteracting the shame and stigma which contribute to the psychological side effects that are often experienced by people who are required to take psychiatric medications.

(h) Once Daily Medication

Although diagnosed people are often instructed to take their medications in divided doses several times a day (e.g. with breakfast, lunch and dinner), many people might actually benefit from taking all of their neuroleptic medication at once, shortly before going to bed at night. There are no good medical reasons against doing this and it may actually have a number of advantages. In particular, taking medication at night can help reduce tiredness or sleepiness during the day if these problems are due to the sedating side effects of the drugs (it may have the additional benefit of reducing the need for sleeping tablets). The following advice pertains to all of the older neuroleptics:

> Every [conventional neuroleptic] can be and has been prescribed once or twice daily without loss of therapeutic efficacy or any significant increase in incidence or severity of side effects compared to equivalent amounts

of the same drug in divided doses ... Once the optimal daily dosage is determined and the patient is stabilised, all the medication should be administered at bedtime or in divided doses after the evening meal and at bedtime ... [this] is advantageous for several reasons ... Usually the patient is asleep and unaware of pharmacologic effects that would be annoying and subjectively distressing during the day. In addition, there is less impairment of mental and physical faculties during the day. This can make the drug more acceptable to the patient ... There is some evidence that a single bedtime dose of a neuroleptic causes less extrapyramidal reaction. This reduces the need for antiparkinson drugs.[650]

Atypical neuroleptics can also be taken in a single daily dose, usually at night shortly before retiring. Quetiapine (Seroquel) is a possible exception to this general recommendation, as it is metabolised and excreted from the body relatively rapidly and therefore may not be suitable for once-daily use (discuss with prescribing physician).

(i) Side-Effect Medications

A range of medications which were once the principal treatment for Parkinson's disease are often used to help alleviate the symptoms of Neuroleptic-Induced Parkinsonism. Sometimes referred to as "side-effect tablets" these anti-parkinsonian drugs (APs) include benztropine (Cogentin) benzhexol (Artane), orphenadrine (Norflex), biperiden (Akineton), procyclidine (Kemadrin), and others. This group of medications are also known as "anticholinergic drugs" since they reduce the activity of the neurotransmitter acetylcholine in the brain and other parts of the body.

It used to be routine practice to prescribe an anti-parkin-sonian drug (AP) concurrently with neuroleptic medication in order to prevent the development of neurological side effects. However, while clinical experience has proven that APs are effective in alleviating some extrapyramidal side effects (EPS), most authorities now consider their routine use to be inadvisable since prolonged or unnecessary exposure to these potent psychoactive drugs can entail a number of potential risks. As a general rule, it is preferable to avoid or minimise EPS by reducing the dosage of the neuroleptic, or by switching to a medication with fewer side effects, than it is to simply give the affected person another drug that is intended to act as an antidote to the first one:

> The first principle of clinical pharmacology is that if a patient develops toxic effects, the offending drug should be stopped if at all possible; alternatively, the drug should be reduced to a minimum dose compatible with clinical needs. Only if these two strategies fail should another drug be prescribed to neutralise the toxic effects.[651]

Anti-parkinsonian drugs are the treatment of choice for severe dystonic reactions (muscular spasms) including oculogyric crises, stiff jaw, and wry neck. In an emergency they can be given by intramuscular injection and will usually provide relief within a few minutes. These drugs can also help to prevent or alleviate symptoms of Neuroleptic-Induced Parkinsonism (e.g. akinesia), akinetic depression, and Neuroleptic-Induced Deficit Syndrome (NIDS). However, since not everyone will develop neurological side effects, it is now considered preferable to refrain from administering AP drugs until it is clear they are actually needed. If required they should only be used for a few weeks at most and then stopped in order to determine whether or not they are still necessary. The advent of atypical neuroleptics, and the general trend toward lower dosages of medication, has meant that long-term administration of APs can often be avoided since diagnosed people are now less likely to experience severe EPS than used to be the case. Most authorities now discourage prophylactic (i.e. preventive) use of anti-parkinsonian (anticholinergic) drugs. A recent consensus statement by the World Health Organisation contained the following advice:

> The prophylactic use of anticholinergics in patients on neuroleptic treatment is not recommended, and may be justified only early in treatment (after which it should be discontinued and its need should be re-evaluated). As a rule these compounds should only be used when Parkinsonism has actually developed, and when other measures, such as the reduction of neuroleptic dosage or the substitution of the administered drug by another less prone to induce Parkinsonism, have proven ineffective.[652]

The following are among a range of factors that have led to greater professional caution regarding routine use of AP drugs for preventing or alleviating extrapyramidal side effects:

- AP drugs are not a panacea. At best they only help to alleviate *some* neurological side effects, particularly muscle spasms (dystonia), muscular stiffness and rigidity, and tremor ("the shakes"). Although sometimes given to people experiencing akathisia (restless agitation), APs are often ineffective against this side effect and may actually cause it to become worse.[653]

- APs have side effects of their own such as dry mouth, blurred vision, urinary retention, and constipation. Since neuroleptic medications can also cause these symptoms, those who take *both* kinds of drugs could potentially develop quite severe problems.

- It is now considered likely that APs contribute to tardive dyskinesia (TD). In addition to causing TD in people who have never taken neuroleptics[654], APs can uncover or aggravate symptoms of neuroleptic-induced TD, possibly to a serious degree.[655]

- APs may reduce the anti-psychotic efficacy of neuroleptic medications and lead to an increase in the severity of psychotic symptoms.[656] Neuroleptic dosages may sometimes need to be increased to compensate for this neuroleptic–anticholinergic antagonism.

- APs can adversely affect memory, making it difficult for people to take in and retain information while under the influence of these drugs (anterograde amnesia).[657] Concurrent use of benzodiazepines ("minor tranquillisers"), alcohol, and "street" drugs could exacerbate this problem.

- Abuse of APs in an attempt to induce a euphoric state (i.e. to get "high") can result in an acute toxic delirium characterised by agitation, disorientation, delusions, and hallucinations.

If anti-parkinsonian "side-effect tablets" are needed, this is most likely to occur during periods when a diagnosed person is receiving relatively large doses of neuroleptic medications (e.g. while being treated for an acute psychotic episode). Later on, during the maintenance phase, when neuroleptic dosages can generally be much lower, the need for APs is likely to be significantly reduced. People who receive neuroleptics in the form of long-acting depot injections may be an exception to this general rule. At the present time, most of the long-acting drugs that are used to treat schizophrenia are neuroleptics of the older type and are more likely to cause EPS than are atypical neuroleptics. Nevertheless, some people on long-acting medication may find they only need to take side-effect tablets for a couple of days immediately after their injection, since adverse effects tend to be most severe when neuroleptic blood levels are at a peak. Use of anti-parkinsonian drugs should be subject to continuous and stringent review. In general, they should be reserved for emergency use only (e.g. acute dystonic reactions), or used as a short-term measure while other options are being investigated, e.g. reducing the medication to the smallest effective dose for the shortest possible time (point (d) above), or switching to a neuroleptic with fewer extrapyramidal side effects (point (e)).

Special Note On Akinesia

A neuroleptic side effect called "akinesia" was described in *Chapter Two*. The characteristic feature of akinesia is a reduction in spontaneity of movement and speech which, in more extreme cases, manifests as apathy, difficulty initiating activities, and a severe impoverishment of thought and feeling. Many authorities believe that akinesia is common among persons receiving neuroleptic treatment – especially with the older drugs – though it is frequently not recognised as a medication side effect since it mimics both depression and negative symptoms of schizophrenia.[658]

It is widely acknowledged that it can be very difficult to differentiate between medication-induced akinesia and loss of spontaneity related to other causes. Indeed, some researchers believe that often the only truly reliable way to identify the presence of neuroleptic-induced akinesia is to observe what happens when one of the following occurs:

- The affected person's neuroleptic dose is reduced or treatment is stopped
- They switch to a neuroleptic drug with fewer extrapyramidal side effects
- They receive sufficient anti-parkinsonian medication to alleviate akinesia

Use of AP medication represents a viable option in cases where reducing the neuroleptic dosage is not considered feasible due to concerns about the possibility that the diagnosed person's symptoms may become worse. If the problem *is* neuroleptic-induced, a noticeable improvement in the treated person's spontaneity and general vitality will often become apparent soon after they commence an anti-parkinsonian drug. An expert committee of psychiatrists has offered the following advice regarding the appropriate management of akinesia:

> To treat patients adequately, clinicians should first be able to recognise the adverse effect and then respond

either by reducing the neuroleptic dosage or by increasing the antiparkinsonian treatment, whichever is more appropriate ... If neuroleptic drugs cannot be further reduced, either because of psychotic symptoms or because of an unacceptable risk of their re-emergence, antiparkinsonian medications should be added in higher dosages to counteract akinesia ... Most patients who are experiencing akinesia will respond rapidly, within a few days to a week, to [such] medication. An ineffective trial of antiparkinsonian medication, therefore, need not be prolonged. Because akinesia is so impairing and so correctable, it is a very unfortunate side effect to leave untreated.[659]

Because use of "side-effect tablets" entails a number of risks (as noted above), due caution must be exercised. In some instances all that may be required to establish the presence of akinesia is a relatively short course of anti-parkinsonian medication. Some researchers have described cases in which complete alleviation of all akinesia symptoms occurred within *one hour* of the affected person being given an AP drug by intramuscular injection.[660] The "diagnostic" use of AP drugs to determine whether or not someone is experiencing akinesia involves few risks, especially when the alternative may be prolonged, unrecognised, and thus unrelieved akinesia. The growing prevalence of substance abuse among diagnosed people, especially when it involves amphetamines ("speed") and other stimulant drugs, suggests that such illicit drug abuse may in some instances constitute a form of "self-medication" resorted to in a desperate effort to alleviate neuroleptic-induced akinesia.

Special Note On Akathisia

As described in *Chapter Two*, a possible adverse consequence of neuroleptic treatment is an extrapyramidal side-effect called "akathisia". Although often characterised by restless physical agitation, akathisia can also take the form of a primarily *subjective sense of inner tension* that may manifest as irritability, impatience, and various kinds of socially destructive acting-out behaviours. While more likely to occur in association with the older drugs, atypical neuroleptics can certainly cause this side effect. Correct diagnosis is vital since people with severe akathisia sometimes have this problem made *worse* as a result of being given more neuroleptic medication in the mistaken belief that the agitation is related to their symptoms, or that it indicates they may be on the verge of psychotic relapse. As noted above, anti-parkinsonian drugs are often ineffective against akathisia and may even cause it to become more severe.

As with most other side effects, the first principle in managing akathisia is to either reduce the dose of the offending neuroleptic or switch to a medication that does not cause this problem. If neither of these strategies is feasible, or they prove ineffective, concurrent administration of other drugs may become necessary. It has been found that drugs belonging to the benzodiazepine family may alleviate neuroleptic-induced extrapyramidal symptoms including akathisia.[661] Propranolol (Inderal), one of a group of drugs known collectively as "beta-blockers", has proven effective in treating some cases of neuroleptic-induced akathisia.[662] (See *Chapter Nine*.)

Complementary Therapies

There is evidence that certain nutritional supplements, vitamins, and herbs may play a valuable role in managing – and possibly preventing – some neuroleptic side effects. This possibility is supported by research which suggests that some neurological side effects may be the result of cellular damage caused by the toxic substances which are produced when dopamine and other neurotransmitters are metabolised (broken down) in the treated person's brain. Referred to as "free radicals", these substances are unstable and highly reactive chemical compounds which are either introduced from the external environment or produced in the body as a result of normal metabolic processes. They are capable of reacting with cells and impairing their ability to function normally. Free-radical-induced cellular damage is now thought to play a key role in the aging process and a wide range of common medical conditions. Some authorities believe that prolonged exposure to neuroleptic drugs generates large numbers of free radicals which can damage synaptic terminals. Tardive dyskinesia and other neurological side effects may be among the various consequences of such damage.[663]

The human body produces a range of enzymes called *antioxidants* which help to protect it from the damaging effects of free radicals. The body's own supply of natural antioxidants can be augmented by those obtained from dietary sources. Nutrients and herbs with antioxidant properties can function as *neuroprotective agents* by helping to reduce neurological damage caused by free radicals. In certain instances it is possible they may also be *neurorestorative*, in the sense that they can sometimes help to undo neuronal damage that has already occurred.

Vitamin E (alpha tocopherol) is a potent antioxidant and powerful free-radical scavenger extensively researched as a treatment for neuroleptic-induced tardive dyskinesia (TD). A number of studies have suggested that vitamin E in doses of 1200 IU to 1600 IU per day can reduce the severity of established tardive dyskinesia symptoms.[664] However, some studies have failed to demonstrate any beneficial effect on long-standing TD symptoms, leading researchers to conclude that vitamin E may only be effective if administered early enough and in sufficient amounts, *before* irreversible neurological damage has occurred. In one ten-year study 11,000 people diagnosed with schizophrenia were given supplementary vitamins (E, B3, B6 and C), in addition to conventional neuroleptic treatment. Significantly, no new cases of TD were observed during the study period, leading the investigators to conclude that these nutritional supplements had helped to *prevent* the development of this potentially irreversible neurological disorder.[665] Interestingly, researchers have noted that some people receiving vitamin E treatment for TD also experienced an improvement in other symptoms such as anxiety, depression, and apathy.[666]

The *American Journal of Psychiatry* recently reported that 400 mg per day of vitamin B6 (pyridoxine) resulted in a significant reduction in extrapyramidal symptoms (EPS), including TD, within three weeks of administration. It was noted that these neurological side effects returned to their pre-treatment level when vitamin supplementation was stopped. The researchers suggested the beneficial effects were probably due to the antioxidant and free-radical scavenging properties of vitamin B6.[667] No side effects were reported in association with this treatment.

Vitamin C (ascorbic acid) is a water-soluble vitamin with powerful antioxidant properties. Some studies have shown that many long-term psychiatric patients may be functionally deficient in vitamin C.[668] Cigarette smoking is known to destroy this vitamin while stress leads to an increase in the body's need for this extremely versatile nutrient. As well as helping to protect against free-radical neuronal damage, vitamin C supplementation may help to lower the risk of agranulocytosis (reduced white blood cell count) in people receiving clozapine.[669]

Important nutrient antioxidants include vitamins E, C, and A, the B group (B2, B3, B6), betacarotene, bioflavanoids, and the minerals manganese, zinc, copper, and selenium. The richest dietary sources of antioxidants include fresh fruits and vegetables, legumes, whole grains, raw nuts (almonds, sunflower seeds), garlic, and seafood (fish, seaweed). Spices such as ginger and turmeric are rich in antioxidants. Many herbs have potent anti-oxidant properties, including ginkgo (*Gingko biloba*), milk thistle (*Silybum marianum*), and St John's Wort (*Hypericum perforatum*). One recent study found that Indian ginseng (*Withania somnifera*) may help prevent the development of tardive dyskinesia, presumably as a result of its antioxidant effects.[670] Green tea (*Camellia sinensis*) is also reputed to be a valuable source of antioxidants.

Prolonged exposure to excessive emotional stress stimulates the production of high levels of adrenal hormones (adrenaline and noradrenaline) which, when metabolised in the human body, generate cell-damaging free radicals in large amounts. Long-term neuroleptic treatment – with both atypical and conventional drugs – adds to the risk of significant free-radical damage (while tardive dyskinesia is an obvious manifestation, in many cases such damage may remain invisible). At the present time it is not clear whether liberal use of antioxidants can provide complete protection, nor whether ordinary dietary sources provide adequate amounts of these beneficial nutrients. In view of this uncertainty, people receiving prolonged neuroleptic treatment should take supplementary antioxidants – especially vitamins E and C – as a precautionary measure, to help counteract the negative effects of their increased exposure to free radicals.*

Metabolic, Endocrine, and Cardiovascular Side Effects

As explained in *Chapter Three*, there is now clear evidence that atypical neuroleptics can cause a wide variety of metabolic side effects including obesity, abnormally elevated levels of blood fats such as cholesterol, and disorders of glucose metabolism including diabetes. Given the potentially serious adverse consequences associated with this treatment, precautions must be taken to reduce the risks as much as possible. An expert panel recently advised that preferably before, or as soon as possible after, commencing any atypical neuroleptic, those receiving treatment should be given a thorough physical assessment and the following information obtained:[671]

---

* In addition to the benefits already noted, there is evidence that supplementary antioxidants may improve therapeutic responses to psychotropic medications. Some researchers recently noted that people receiving conventional medical treatment for schizophrenia with neuroleptic medications fared somewhat better when given supplemental antioxidants than did similar groups who only received drugs. See: Mahadik, S. and Gowda, S. (1996) "Antioxidants in the Treatment of Schizophrenia", *Drugs Today*, Vol. 32.

- Personal and family medical history of obesity, diabetes, hypertension (high blood pressure), elevated blood fats (cholesterol, triglycerides), and cardiovascular disease
- Weight (including waist circumference)
- Fasting blood glucose (blood sugar)
- Fasting lipid profile (blood fats)
- Blood pressure

The panel recommends that people receiving atypical neuroleptics should be closely monitored throughout the course of treatment. Their body weight should be measured at the commencement of treatment and then at 4, 8 and 12 weeks, and every three months thereafter. Anyone who gains 5% or more of their initial weight, at any time, should consider changing medications, preferably to one less likely to promote weight gain. The expert panel advises that the treated person's blood pressure and levels of blood sugar and blood fats should be reassessed after 12 weeks, to determine whether or not they are still within the normal range.

The symptoms of type 2 (adult onset) diabetes include thirst, frequent urination, tiredness or drowsiness, unexplained weight loss, blurred vision, and recurrent infections. This disorder may begin with mildly increased thirst and urinary frequency that gradually becomes more severe over several weeks or months. Prompt referral to an appropriately qualified health care professional for assessment and advice regarding management of diabetes and related medical problems is strongly recommended.

A range of measures may help diagnosed individuals reduce their likelihood of developing neuroleptic-induced metabolic disorders. The following are especially important:

- Weight control (obesity is a major risk factor for diabetes)
- Healthy diet (high in fibre, low in cholesterol and saturated fat)
- Increased intake of fresh fruits and vegetables
- Reduced consumption of refined sugar (e.g. sweet soft drinks)
- Regular exercise (minimum of 10-15 minutes every day)
- Moderate consumption of social drugs (alcohol, caffeine)
- No cigarette smoking or abuse of illicit ("street") drugs
- Effective stress management techniques (e.g. relaxation)
- Adequate dosages of nutritional supplements (see below)

(a) Nutritional Supplements

Despite the fact that some diagnosed people appear to require certain nutrients in unusually large quantities, their dietary intake is often far from adequate. Nutritional supplementation is therefore highly advisable.

1. Antioxidants

Antioxidants can play an important role in protecting against a wide range of medical disorders and conditions.[672] Specific beneficial effects include:

- Protecting the body against the harmful effects of toxic drugs/chemicals
- Raising HDL ("good") cholesterol and reducing the risk of heart disease[673]

- Improving insulin action in non-insulin-dependent diabetic patients[674]
- Strengthening immune system mechanisms responsible for healing

Antioxidant intake can be enhanced by increasing consumption of fresh fruits and vegetables. For additional protection some authorities recommend taking supplements providing 1000 mg vitamin C and 800 IU vitamin E per day.

2. Omega-3 essential fatty acids

Dietary fats belonging to a group known as omega-3 essential fatty acids are now recognised as having a wide range of beneficial effects on both physical and mental health. Numerous scientific studies have shown that adequate intake of these key nutrients may help to prevent or ameliorate a number of medical conditions to which people treated with atypical neuroleptics may be especially vulnerable.[675] Omega-3 fatty acids are especially beneficial in regard to the following conditions:

- Cardiovascular (heart) disease

The cardio-protective effects of omega-3s are well established. These nutrients have a wide range of beneficial effects on the heart and cardiovascular system as a whole. Potential benefits include reduced blood pressure, vasodilation (relaxation of blood vessels, including coronary arteries), reduced serum triglycerides, reduced platelet aggregation (blood less sticky thus reducing the risk of clots), prevention and possible reversal of the build up of arterial plaque (the principal cause of atherosclerosis or "hardening of the arteries"), reduced levels of LDL ("bad") cholesterol, and increased levels HDL ("good") cholesterol. This broad range of beneficial effects can contribute to a significantly reduced risk of coronary artery disease, heart attack, and stroke.

• Diabetes and obesity

Omega-3 fatty acid supplementation can help decrease insulin resistance and may possibly help to prevent the development of diabetes. These nutrients can also help prevent blood-vessel damage, the underlying cause of many of the serious long-term complications of diabetes. Recent studies suggest a link between omega-3 consumption and weight loss, with diets high in these nutrients being associated with loss of fat in specific body regions.

Fish are by far the richest dietary source of omega-3 fatty acids. Oily cold-water species such as Atlantic salmon, ocean trout, tuna, sardines, mackerel, and herring, contain the largest quantities of the omega-3 fats (including EPA and DHA, two of the most important nutrients for optimal brain structure and function). Fish-oil capsules are a convenient and relatively inexpensive source of these nutrients. Psychiatrist Dr Andrew Stoll, an internationally recognised authority in this area, believes a daily intake of 1 to 2 grams (1000-2000 milligrams) of omega-3 fatty acids (EPA plus DHA) is probably adequate for most people to support optimal general health and wellbeing, as well as contributing to enhanced mood and cognitive functioning.[676]

Use of nutritional supplements in combination with

measures that promote good general health (adequate exercise and rest, balanced diet, effective stress management, positive mental attitude), can have numerous beneficial effects on physical and mental health. Potential benefits include detoxifying the body, enhancing energy and vitality, stimulating and strengthening the immune system, reducing anxiety, and helping to alleviate depression. *As a general recommendation, anyone being treated with one of the atypical neuroleptics would be well advised to take nutritional supplements as a preventive measure, especially antioxidants and omega-3 essential fatty acids.* As well as helping to reduce the risk of potentially serious neurological and metabolic side effects, these nutrients may have a wide range of other beneficial effects.

Psychological and Social Side Effects

Although they are quite common, what might be termed the social and psychological side effects of neuroleptics are rarely acknowledged. There is no doubt, however, that some people experience severe embarrassment, shame, guilt, and anger, as a result of having to take neuroleptics and other psychiatric medications. Various simple strategies, e.g. only taking medications in the privacy of one's own home, can help to limit the social embarrassment that may be associated with being seen as a person who needs "psych drugs". Taking measures to prevent or minimise visible side effects which can act as stigma symbols (e.g. tremor, shuffling gait, sedation) will reduce the likelihood of drawing unwanted attention. On a broader level, it is possible to revision the role of medications so that they are less likely to be experienced as an indicator of failure, inadequacy, or dependency. Emphasising the stress-buffering effect of neuroleptics, rather than their supposed "anti-psychotic" effects, may help to reduce the negative connotations so often associated with use of these drugs (this notion was explored in the *Epilogue*).

Diagnosed people who may be prone to feeling inferior or inadequate invariably find that taking an active role in their treatment will help them to feel more confident and less at the mercy of powerful forces beyond their control. Those who accept responsibility for learning about their condition and the medications they take, and who make a decision to become fully involved in their treatment, move from being a passive recipient of the ministrations of others (a "consumer") to being an active participant in their own journey of recovery.

REFERENCES

Chapter One: The Chemistry Of Tranquillity

1   Kramer, P. (1994) *Listening To Prozac*, Harmondsworth: Penguin, p. 290

2   Breggin, P. (1993) *Toxic Psychiatry*, London: HarperCollins; Breggin, P. and Cohen, D. (2000) *Your Drug May Be Your Problem: How And Why To Stop Taking Psychiatric Medication*, Cambridge, MA: Perseus Books

3   Healy, D. (1993) *Psychiatric Drugs Explained*, London: Mosby, pp. 18, 27 (emphasis in original)

4   Anton-Stephens, D. (1954) "Preliminary Observations on the Psychiatric Uses of Chlorpromazine (Largactil)", *Journal of Mental Science*, Vol. 100, p. 550

5   Lehmann, H. and Hanrahan, G. (1954) "Chlorpromazine: New Inhibiting Agent for Psychomotor Excitement and Manic States", *Archives of Neurology and Psychiatry*, Vol. 71, p. 232

6   Klerman, G. (1970) "Clinical Efficacy and Actions of Antipsychotics", in: DiMascio, A. and Schader, R. (eds) *Clinical Handbook of Psychopharmacology*, New York: Jason Aronson

7   Minas, H., Joshua, S., Jackson, H. and Burgess, P. (1988) "Persistent Psychotic Symptoms at Discharge in Patients

with Schizophrenia", *Australian and New Zealand Journal of Psychiatry*,Vol. 22

8   Khan,A., Khan, S., Leventhal, R. and Brown,W. (2001) "Symptom Reduction And Suicide Risk Among Patients Treated With Placebo In Antipsychotic Drug Trials: An Analysis Of The Food And Drug Administration Database", *American Journal of Psychiatry*,Vol. 158, No. 9, p.1454

9   Healy, D. (1989) "Neuroleptics and Psychic Indifference: A Review", *Journal of the Royal Society of Medicine*,Vol. 82

10 Healy, D. (1993) *Psychiatric Drugs Explained*, London: Mosby, p. 15

11 ibid p. 16

12 Falloon, I. (1987) "Cognitive and Behavioural Interventions in the Self Control of Schizophrenia", in: Strauss, J., Böker, W. and Brenner, H. (eds) *Psychosocial Treatment of Schizophrenia*,Toronto: Hans Huber

13 Falloon, I. and Talbot, R. (1981) "Persistent Auditory Hallucinations: Coping Mechanisms and Implications for Management", *Psychological Medicine*,Vol. 11; Nelson, H.,Thrasher, S., and Barnes,T. (1991) "Practical Ways of Alleviating Auditory Hallucinations", *British Medical Journal*,Vol. 302; Watkins, J. (1998) *Hearing Voices: A Common Human Experience*. Melbourne: Hill of Content

14 Coppens, H., Sloof, C., Paans,A.,Wiegman,T.,Vaalburg,W. and Korf, J. (1991) "High Central D2-Dopamine Receptor Occupancy As Assessed With Positron-Emission Tomography in Medicated But Therapy-Resistant Patients", *Biological Psychiatry*,Vol. 29

15 Healy, D. (1991) "D1 and D2 and D3", *British Journal of Psychiatry*,Vol. 159, p. 319

16 Christison, G., Kirch, D., and Wyatt, R. (1991) "When Symptoms Persist: Choosing Among Alternative Somatic Treatments for Schizophrenia", *Schizophrenia Bulletin*,Vol. 17, No. 2

17 Claridge, G. (1985) *Origins of Mental Illness,* Oxford:

Basil Blackwell; Claridge, G. (1987) "Schizophrenia and Individuality", in: Blakemore, C. and Greenfield, S. (eds) *Mindwaves*, Oxford: Basil Blackwell

[18] Kaplan, H. and Sadock, B. (eds) (1981) *Modern Synopsis of Comprehensive Textbook of Psychiatry/III (Third Edition)*. Baltimore: Williams and Wilkins, p. 310

[19] Ciompi, L (1994) "Affect Logic: An Integrative Model of the Psyche and Its Relations to Schizophrenia", *British Journal of Psychiatry*, Vol. 164 (suppl. 23)

[20] Ciompi, L. (1988) *The Psyche and Schizophrenia*, Cambridge, Massachusetts: Harvard University Press, p. 292

[21] Healy, D. (1989) "Neuroleptics and Psychic Indifference: A Review", *Journal of the Royal Society of Medicine*, Vol. 82, p. 618

[22] Bleuler, M. (1986) "Introduction and Overview", in: Burrows, G., Norman, T. and Rubinstein, G. (eds) *Handbook of Studies on Schizophrenia*, Amsterdam: Elsevier, p. 8 (emphasis added)

[23] McGhie, A. and Chapman, J. (1961) "Disorders of Attention and Perception in Early Schizophrenia", *British Journal of Medical Psychology*, Vol. 34, p. 104

[24] Spohn, H., Lacoursiere, R., Thompson, K. and Coyne, L. (1978) "The Effects of Antipsychotic Drug Treatment on Attention and Information Processing in Chronic Schizophrenics", in: Wynne, L., Cromwell, R. and Matthysse, S. (eds.) *The Nature of Schizophrenia: New Approaches to Research and Treatment*. New York: John Wiley and Sons; Spohn, H. and Strauss, M. (1989) "Relation of Neuroleptic and Anticholinergic Medication to Cognitive Functions in Schizophrenia", *Journal of Abnormal Psychology*, Vol. 98

[25] Ciompi, L. (1988) *The Psyche and Schizophrenia*, Cambridge, Massachusetts: Harvard University Press, p. 293

[26] Ciompi, L (1994) "Affect Logic: An Integrative Model of the Psyche and Its Relations to Schizophrenia", *British Journal of Psychiatry*, Vol. 164 (suppl. 23), p. 54

[27] Keck, P., Cohen, B., Baldessarini, R. and McElroy, S. (1989) "Time Course of Antipsychotic Effects of Neuroleptic Drugs", *American Journal of Psychiatry*, Vol. 146, No. 10, pp. 1291-2 (emphasis added)

[28] Chadwick, P. (1997) *Schizophrenia: The Positive Perspective*, London: Routledge, p. 151

[29] Nelson, J. (1990) *Healing the Split*, Los Angeles, CA: Jeremy Tarcher, p. 136

[30] Ciompi, L. (1988) *The Psyche and Schizophrenia*, Cambridge, Massachusetts: Harvard University Press, p. 292

[31] Anton-Stephens, D. (1954) "Preliminary Observations on the Psychiatric Uses of Chlorpromazine (Largactil)", *Journal of Mental Science*, Vol. 100, p. 550 (emphasis added)

[32] Vonnegut, M. (1976) *The Eden Express*, New York: Bantam, p. 253

[33] Nelson, J. (1990) *Healing the Split*, Los Angeles, CA: Jeremy Tarcher. p. 139

[34] ibid p.136.

Chapter Two: Side Effects Of Neuroleptic Medications

[35] Sacks, O. (1991) *Awakenings*, London: Pan Books, p. 262

[36] Van Putten, T., May, P. and Marder, S. (1984) "Response to Antipsychotic Medication: The Doctor's and the Consumer's View", *American Journal of Psychiatry*, Vol. 141, No. 1

[37] Ayd, F. (1973) "Rational Pharmacotherapy: Once-A-Day Drug Dosage", *Diseases of the Nervous System*, Vol. 34, p. 372

[38] Cousins, N. (1981) *Anatomy of an Illness as Perceived by the Patient*, New York: Bantam, p. 52

[39] O'Brien, P. (1978) *The Disordered Mind*. Englewood Cliffs, NJ: Prentice Hall, p. 211

[40] Julien, R. (2000) *A Primer of Drug Action (Ninth Edition)*, New York: Worth Publishers, p. 506

[41] Lader, M. (1979) "Monitoring Plasma Concentrations of Neuroleptics", *Pharmacopsychology*, Vol. 9

[42] Kuehl, P., Zhang, J. et al. (2001) "Sequence Diversity in CYP3A Promoters and Characterisation of the Genetic Basis of Polymorphic CYP3A5 Expression", *Nature Genetics*, Vol. 27, No. 4

[43] Rogers, A., Pilgrim, D. and Lacey, R. (1993) *Experiencing Psychiatry: User's Views of Services*, London: MIND/Macmillan

[44] Wallace, M. (1994) "Schizophrenia – A National Emergency: Preliminary Observations on SANELINE", *Acta Psychiatrica Scandinavica*, Vol. 89, (suppl. 380)

[45] Seltzer, A., Roncari, I. and Garfinkel, P. (1980) "Effect of Patient Education on Medication Compliance", *Canadian Journal of Psychiatry*, Vol. 25

[46] Breggin, P. (1993) *Toxic Psychiatry*, London: HarperCollins, p. 59

[47] Awad, A. and Hogan, T. (1994) "Subjective Response to Neuroleptics and the Quality of Life: Implications for Treatment Outcome", *Acta Psychiatrica Scandinavica*, Vol. 89, (suppl. 380)

[48] Glenmullen, J. (2000) *Prozac Backlash*, New York: Simon and Schuster, p. 21

[49] Sullivan, G. and Lukoff, D. (1990) "Sexual Side Effects of Anti-Psychotic Medications: Evaluation and Interventions", *Hospital and Community Psychiatry*, Vol. 41

[50] Solovitz, B., Fisher, S., Bryant, S., *et al* (1987) "How Well Can Patients Discriminate Drug-Related Side Effects From Extraneous New Symptoms?", *Psychopharmacology Bulletin*, Vol. 23

[51] Group for the Advancement of Psychiatry (1992) *Beyond Symptom Suppression: Improving Long-Term Outcomes of Schizophrenia* (Report No. 134), Washington, DC: American Psychiatric Press, p. 41 (emphasis added)

[52] Krausz, M., Moritz, S., Naber, D., Lambert, M. and Andresen, B. (1999) "Neuroleptic-Induced Extrapyramidal Symptoms Are Accompanied by Cognitive Dysfunction in Schizophrenia", *European Psychiatry*, Vol. 14

[53] Van Putten, T. and Marder, S. (1987) "Behavioural Toxicity of Antipsychotic Drugs", *Journal of Clinical Psychiatry*, Vol. 48 (suppl. 9), pp. 13-19

[54] Kane, J. and Freeman, H. (1994) "Towards More Effective Antipsychotic Treatment", *British Journal of Psychiatry*, Vol. 165 (suppl. 25), p. 27

[55] Arya, D. (1994) "Extrapyramidal Symptoms With Selective Serotonin Reuptake Inhibitors", *British Journal of Psychiatry*, Vol. 165

[56] Healy, D. (1993) *Psychiatric Drugs Explained*, London: Mosby, p. 49

[57] Lindström, L. (1994) "Long-Term Clinical and Social Outcome Studies in Schizophrenia in Relation to the Cognitive and Emotional Side Effects of Antipsychotic Drugs", *Acta Psychiatrica Scandinavica*, Vol. 89 (Suppl. 380)

[58] Bleuler, M. (1978) *The Schizophrenic Disorders: Long-Term Patient and Family Studies*, Newhaven: Yale University Press, p. 301

[59] ibid p. 443

[60] Weiden, P., Mann, J., Haas, G., Mattson, M. and Frances, A. (1987) "Clinical Non-Recognition of Neuroleptic-Induced Movement Disorders: A Cautionary Study", *American Journal of Psychiatry*, Vol. 144

[61] American Psychiatric Association (1994) *Diagnostic and Statistical Manual of Mental Disorders - Fourth Edition (DSM-IV)*, Washington, DC: American Psychiatric Association, p. 743

[62] ibid, p. 736

[63] Decina, P., Mukherjee, S., Caracci, G. and Harrison, K. (1992) "Painful Sensory Symptoms in Neuroleptic-Induced Extrapyramidal Syndromes", *American Journal of Psychiatry*, Vol. 149, No. 8

[64] Kaplan, H. and Sadock, B. (eds) (1981) *Modern Synopsis of Comprehensive Textbook of Psychiatry / III (Third Edition)*, Baltimore: Williams and Wilkins, p. 784

[65] Sacks, O. (1991) *Awakenings*, London: Pan Books, p. 8

[66] Lindström, L. (1994) "Long-Term Clinical and Social Outcome Studies in Schizophrenia in Relation to the Cognitive and Emotional Side Effects of Antipsychotic Drugs", *Acta Psychiatrica Scandinavica*,Vol. 89 (suppl. 380)

[67] Thomas, P. (1997) *The Dialectics of Schizophrenia*. London: Free Association Books, p. 107

[68] American Psychiatric Association (1994) *Diagnostic and Statistical Manual of Mental Disorders - Fourth Edition (DSM-IV)*,Washington, DC: American Psychiatric Association, p. 738

[69] Rifkin, A., Quitkin, F. and Klein, D. (1975) "Akinesia: A Poorly-Recognised Drug-Induced Extrapyramidal Behavioural Disorder", *Archives of General Psychiatry*,Vol. 32

[70] Weiden, P., Mann, J., Haas, G., Mattson, M. and Frances, A. (1987) "Clinical Non-recognition of Neuroleptic-Induced Movement Disorders:A Cautionary Study", *American Journal of Psychiatry*,Vol. 144

[71] Lader, M. and Lewander, T. (eds) (1994) "The Neuroleptic-Induced Deficit Syndrome", *Acta Psychiatrica Scandinavica*, Vol. 89 (suppl. 380); Schooler, N. (1994) "Deficit Symptoms of Schizophrenia: Negative Symptoms versus Neuroleptic-Induced Deficits", *Acta Psychiatrica Scandinavica*,Vol. 89 (suppl. 380)

[72] Group for the Advancement of Psychiatry (1992) *Beyond Symptom Suppression: Improving Long-Term Outcomes of Schizophrenia* (Report No. 134).Washington, DC: American Psychiatric Press. p. 42

[73] Bockes, Z. (1985) "First Person Account: Freedom Means Knowing You Have A Choice", *Schizophrenia Bulletin*,Vol. 11, No. 3, p. 488

[74] Healy, D. (1993) *Psychiatric Drugs Explained*, London: Mosby, p. 34

[75] Van Putten, T., Marder, S. and Mintz, J. (1990) "A Controlled Dose Comparison of Haloperidol in Newly

Admitted Schizophrenic Patients", *Archives of General Psychiatry*,Vol. 47, p. 757

[76] Siris, G. (1992) "Adjunctive Medication in the Maintenance Treatment of Schizophrenia and its Conceptual Implications", *British Journal of Psychiatry*,Vol. 163 (suppl. 22)

[77] Van Putten,T. and May, P. (1978) "'Akinetic Depression' in Schizophrenia", *Archives of General Psychiatry*,Vol. 35

[78] American Psychiatric Association (1994) *Diagnostic and Statistical Manual of Mental Disorders - Fourth Edition (DSM-IV)*,Washington, DC:American Psychiatric Association

[79] Rifkin, A., Quitkin, F. and Klein, D. (1975) "Akinesia: A Poorly-Recognised Drug-Induced Extrapyramidal Behavioural Disorder", *Archives of General Psychiatry*,Vol. 32

[80] Van Putten,T. and May, P. (1978) "'Akinetic Depression' in Schizophrenia", *Archives of General Psychiatry*,Vol. 35

[81] Johnson, D. (1984) "Observations on the Use of Long-Acting Depot Neuroleptic Injections in the Maintenance Therapy of Schizophrenia", *Journal of Clinical Psychiatry*,Vol. 45, No. 5

[82] Van Putten,T. and May, P. (1978) "'Akinetic Depression' in Schizophrenia", *Archives of General Psychiatry*,Vol. 35, pp. 1104–1106

[83] American Psychiatric Association (1994) *Diagnostic and Statistical Manual of Mental Disorders - Fourth Edition (DSM-IV)*.Washington, DC:American Psychiatric Association

[84] Glenmullen, J. (2000) *Prozac Backlash*, New York: Simon and Schuster. p. 153

[85] Chadwick, P. (1997) *Schizophrenia:The Positive Perspective*, London: Routledge, p. 50

[86] Van Putten,T., Marder, S. and Mintz, J. (1990) "A Controlled Dose Comparison of Haloperidol in Newly Admitted Schizophrenic Patients", *Archives of General Psychiatry*,Vol. 47, p. 757

[87] North, C. (1989) *Welcome, Silence*, New York: Avon Books, pp. 86–89

[88] American Psychiatric Association (1994) *Diagnostic and Statistical Manual of Mental Disorders - Fourth Edition (DSM-IV)*, Washington, DC: American Psychiatric Association, p. 745

[89] Halstead, S., Barnes, T. and Speller, J. (1994) "Akathisia: Prevalence and Associated Dysphoria in an In-Patient Population With Chronic Schizophrenia", *British Journal of Psychiatry*, Vol. 164

[90] Group for the Advancement of Psychiatry (1992) *Beyond Symptom Suppression: Improving Long-Term Outcomes of Schizophrenia* (Report No. 134), Washington, DC: American Psychiatric Press, p. 44

[91] Andreasen, N. (1985) *The Broken Brain: The Biological Revolution in Psychiatry*. New York: Harper and Row, p. 210

[92] Wirshing, W., Van Putten, T., Rosenberg, J., Marder, S., Ames, D. and Hicks-Gray, T. (1992) "Fluoxetine, Akathisia and Suicidality: Is There a Causal Connection?", *Archives of General Psychiatry*, Vol. 49

[93] Shear, M., Frances, A. and Weiden, P. (1983) "Suicide Associated with Akathisia and Depot Fluphenazine Treatment", *Journal of Clinical Psychopharmacology*, Vol. 3; Drake, R. and Erlich, J. (1985) "Suicide Attempts Associated with Akathisia", *American Journal of Psychiatry*, Vol. 142

[94] Healy, D. (1993) *Psychiatric Drugs Explained*, London: Mosby

[95] Dufresne, R. and Wagner, R. (1988) "Antipsychotic Withdrawal Akathisia Versus Antipsychotic Induced Akathisia: Further Evidence for the Existence of Tardive Akathisia", *Journal of Clinical Psychiatry*, Vol. 49

[96] Gardos, G. and Cole, J. (1978) "Maintenance Antipsychotic Therapy: Is the Cure Worse than the Disease?", *American Journal of Psychiatry*, Vol. 133, No. 1, p. 35

[97]   Castle, D., Morgan, V. and Jablensky, A. (2001) "Antipsychotic
        Use In Australia: The Patients' Perspective", *Australian and New
        Zealand Journal of Psychiatry*, Vol. 36
[98]   Collinson, S., Pantelis, C. and Barnes, T. (1996) "Abnormal
        Involuntary Movements in Schizophrenia and their
        Association with Cognitive Impairment", In Pantelis, C.,
        Nelson, H. and Barnes, T. *Schizophrenia: A Neuropsychological
        Perspective*, New York: John Wiley and Sons; Waddington, J.
        (1996) "Cognitive Dysfunction in Chronic Schizophrenia
        Followed Prospectively Over Ten Years and Its
        Longitudinal Relationship to the Emergence of Tardive
        Dyskinesia", *Psychological Medicine*, Vol. 26
[99]   Brown, P. and Funk, S. (1986) "Tardive Dyskinesia: Barriers
        to the Professional Recognition of an Iatrogenic Disease",
        Journal of Health and Social Behaviour, Vol. 27
[100]   American Psychiatric Association (1994) *Diagnostic and
        Statistical Manual of Mental Disorders – Fourth Edition
        (DSM-IV)*, Washington, DC: American Psychiatric
        Association, p. 747
[101]   Glazer, W., Morgenstern, H. and Doucette, J. (1993)
        "Predicting the Long-Term Risk of Tardive Dyskinesia
        in Outpatients Maintained on Neuroleptic Medications",
        Journal of Clinical Psychiatry, Vol. 54
[102]   Chouinard, G. (1990) "Early Parkinsonism Vulnerability a
        TD Risk Factor", *Clinical Psychiatry News* (June)
[103]   Dixon, L., Weiden, P., Haas, G., Sweeney, J. and Frances, A.
        (1992) "Increased TD in Alcohol-Abusing Schizophrenia
        Patients", *Comprehensive Psychiatry*, Vol. 33, No. 2
[104]   American Psychiatric Association (1994) *Diagnostic and
        Statistical Manual of Mental Disorders - Fourth Edition (DSM-
        IV)*. Washington, DC: American Psychiatric Association. p.
        748
[105]   Breggin, P. (1993) *Toxic Psychiatry*, London: HarperCollins.
        pp. 69, 72 (emphasis in original)
[106]   Spohn, H. and Strauss, M. (1989) "Relation of Neuroleptic

and Anticholinergic Medication to Cognitive Functions in Schizophrenia", *Journal of Abnormal Psychology*, Vol. 98

[107] Hartlage, L. (1965) "Effects of Chlorpromazine on Learning", *Psychological Bulletin*, Vol. 64, No. 4

[108] King, D. and Green, J. (1996) "Medication and Cognitive Functioning in Schizophrenia", in: Pantelis, C., Nelson, H. and Barnes, T. *Schizophrenia: A Neuropsychological Perspective*, New York: John Wiley and Sons

[109] Goldberg, T. and Weinberger, D. (1996) "Effects of Neuroleptic Medications on the Cognition of Patients with Schizophrenia: A Review of Recent Studies", *Journal of Clinical Psychiatry*, Vol. 57 (suppl. 9); Bilder, R. et al. (2002) "Neurocognitive Effects of Clozapine, Olanzapine, Risperidone, And Haloperidol In Patients With Chronic Schizophrenia Or Schizoaffective Disorder", *American Journal of Psychiatry*, Vol. 159, No. 6

[110] Julien, R. (2000) *A Primer of Drug Action (Ninth Edition)*, New York: Worth Publishers

[111] Calev, A. (1983) "Anticholinergic Drugs and Memory", *British Journal of Psychiatry*, Vol. 143

[112] King, D. and Green, J. (1996) "Medication and Cognitive Functioning in Schizophrenia", in: Pantelis, C., Nelson, H. and Barnes, T. *Schizophrenia: A Neuropsychological Perspective*, New York: John Wiley and Sons, p. 438

[113] Chadwick, P. (1997) *Schizophrenia: The Positive Perspective*, London: Routledge, p. 50

[114] Estroff, S. (1981) *Making It Crazy*, Berkeley: University of California Press, pp. 95 and 109 (emphasis in original)

[115] Group for the Advancement of Psychiatry (1992) *Beyond Symptom Suppression: Improving Long-Term Outcomes of Schizophrenia* (Report No. 134), Washington, DC: American Psychiatric Press, pp. 42–43

[116] Diamond, R. (1985) "Drugs and the Quality of Life: The Patient's Point of View", *Journal of Clinical Psychiatry*, Vol. 46

[117] Anonymous (1983) "First Person Account: A Pharmacy Student's View", *Schizophrenia Bulletin*, Vol. 9, No. 1

[118] Modrow, J. (1992) *How To Become A Schizophrenic*, Washington: Apollyon Press, p. 146

[119] Freed, W. (1988) "Therapeutic Latency Of Neuroleptic Drugs And Nonspecific Postjunctional Supersensitivity", *Schizophrenia Bulletin*, Vol. 14, No. 2

[120] Owen, F., Cross, A., Crow, T., et al. (1978) "Increased Dopamine Receptor Sensitivity in Schizophrenia", *Lancet*, Vol. 2; Davis, K. and Rosenberg, G. (1979) "Is There A Limbic System Equivalent of Tardive Dyskinesia?", *Biological Psychiatry*, Vol. 14; Lee, T. and Seeman, P. (1980) "Elevation of Brain Neuroleptic/Dopamine Receptors in Schizophrenia", *American Journal of Psychiatry*, Vol. 137

[121] Whitaker, R. (2002) *Mad In America: Bad Science, Bad Medicine, and the Enduring Mistreatment of the Mentally Ill.* Cambridge, MA: Perseus Books. p. 184

[122] Warner, R. (1985) *Recovery from Schizophrenia*, London: Routledge and Kegan Paul, p. 244 (emphasis in original)

[123] Asper, H., Baggiolini, M., Burki, H., et al. (1973) "Tolerance Phenomena with Neuroleptics Catalepsy, Apomorphine Stereotypies and Striatal Dopamine Metabolism in the Rat After Single and Repeated Administration of Loxapine and Haloperidol", *European Journal of Pharmacology*, Vol. 22

[124] Chouinard, G., Jones, B. and Annable, L. (1978) "Neuroleptic-Induced Supersensitivity Psychosis", *American Journal of Psychiatry*, Vol. 135

[125] Remington, G., Prendergast, P. and Bezchlibnyk-Butler, K. (1997) "Neuroleptic Dosing In Chronic Schizophrenia: A 10-Year Follow-Up", *Canadian Journal of Psychiatry*, Vol. 42

[126] Hollister, L. (1978) *Clinical Pharmacology of Psychotherapeutic Drugs (Monographs in Clinical Pharmacology, Volume 1)*, New York: Churchill Livingstone, p. 9

[127] Carpenter, W., McGlashan, T. and Strauss, J. (1977) "The

Treatment of Acute Schizophrenia Without Drugs: An Investigation of Some Current Assumptions", *American Journal of Psychiatry*, Vol. 134, No. 1. p. 19 (emphasis in original)

[128] Chouinard, G. and Jones, B. (1980) "Neuroleptic-Induced Supersensitivity Psychosis: Clinical and Pharmacological Characteristics", *American Journal of Psychiatry*, Vol. 137, No. 1

[129] ibid, p. 19

[130] Kahne, G. (1989) "Rebound Psychoses Following the Discontinuation of a High Potency Neuroleptic", *Canadian Journal of Psychiatry*, Vol. 34

[131] Chouinard, G. and Jones, B. (1980) "Neuroleptic-Induced Supersensitivity Psychosis: Clinical and Pharmacological Characteristics", *American Journal of Psychiatry*, Vol. 137, No. 1

[132] Thomas, P. (1997) *The Dialectics of Schizophrenia*, London: Free Association Books, pp. 118-120

[133] Kahne, G. (1989) "Rebound Psychoses Following the Discontinuation of a High Potency Neuroleptic", *Canadian Journal of Psychiatry*, Vol. 34, p. 228

[134] Shiovitz, T., Welke, T., Tigel, P., Anand, R., Hartman, R., Sramek, J., Kurtz, N. and Cutler, N. (1996) "Cholinergic Rebound and Rapid Onset Psychosis Following Abrupt Clozapine Withdrawal", *Schizophrenia Bulletin*, Vol. 22, No. 4. p. 594

[135] Castle, D., Morgan, V. and Jablensky, A. (2001) "Antipsychotic Use In Australia: The Patients' Perspective", *Australian and New Zealand Journal of Psychiatry*, Vol. 36

[136] Robotham, J. (1999) "Australia Lags in Drug Therapy for Mentally Ill", *The Age*, 3/5/99

[137] Lambert, T., Brennan, A. and Castle, D. (2002) "Clinician's Attitudes to Depot Antipsychotics in the Era of the Atypicals", *Schizophrenia Research*, Vol. 53, No. 3 (suppl), p. 173-174

[138] Mond, J., Morice, R., Owen, C. and Korten, A. (2003) "Use of Antipsychotic Medications in Australia Between July 1995 and December 2001", *Australian and New Zealand Journal of Psychiatry*, Vol. 37

Chapter Three: Atypical Neuroleptics: Light At The End Of The Tunnel?

[139] Champ, S. (1999) "A Most Precious Thread", In Barker, P., Campbell, P. and Davidson, B. (eds) *From the Ashes of Experience: Reflections on Madness, Survival and Growth*, London: Whurr Publishers, p. 126

[140] Kane, J., Honigfeld, G., Singer, J. and Meltzer, H. (1988) "Clozapine for the Treatment-Resistant Schizophrenia: A Double-Blind Comparison with Chlorpromazine", *Archives of General Psychiatry*, Vol. 45

[141] Lahti, A., Lahti, R. and Tamminga, C. (1996) "New Neuroleptics and Experimental Antipsychotics: Future Roles", in: Breier, A. (ed) *The New Pharmacotherapy of Schizophrenia*, Washington, DC: American Psychiatric Press

[142] Cromwell, R. (1993) "A Summary View of Schizophrenia", in: Cromwell, R. and Snyder, C. *Schizophrenia: Origins, Processes, Treatment, and Outcome*, New York: Oxford University Press; Johnstone, E., Humphreys, M., Lang, F., Lawrie, S. and Sandler, R. (1999) *Schizophrenia: Concepts and Clinical Management*, Cambridge: Cambridge University Press

[143] Breier, A. and Buchanan, R. (1996) "Clozapine: Current Status and Clinical Applications", in: Breier, A. (ed) *The New Pharmacotherapy of Schizophrenia*, Washington, DC: American Psychiatric Press

[144] Leucht, S., Pitschel-Walz, G., Abraham, D. and Kissling, W. (1999) "Efficacy and Extrapyramidal Side Effects of the New Antipsychotics Olanzapine, Quetiapine, Risperidone, and Sertindole Compared to Conventional Antipsychotics

and Placebo. A Meta-Analysis of Randomised Controlled Trials", *Schizophrenia Research*, Vol. 35, p. 51

[145] Geddes, J., Freemantle, N., Harrison, P. and Bebbington, P. (2000) "Atypical Antipsychotics in the Treatment of Schizophrenia: Systematic Overview and Meta-Regression Analysis", *British Medical Journal*, Vol. 321, p. 1371

[146] ibid

[147] Khan, A., Khan, S., Leventhal, R. and Brown, W. (2001) "Symptom Reduction And Suicide Risk Among Patients Treated With Placebo In Antipsychotic Drug Trials: An Analysis Of The Food And Drug Administration Database", *American Journal of Psychiatry*, Vol. 158, No. 9, p. 1454

[148] Kostakoglu, A., Rezaki, M. and Gögüs, A. (1999) "Early Relapse of Psychotic Symptoms After an Initial Response to Olanzapine", *Acta Psychiatrica Scandinavica*, Vol. 100, No. 4

[149] Stip, E., Tourjman, V., Lew, V., Fabian, J., Cormier, H., Landry, P., Lalonde, P. and Cournoyer, J. (1995) "'Awakenings' Effect With Risperidone", (Letter). *American Journal of Psychiatry*, Vol. 152, No. 12, p. 1833

[150] Mattes, J. (1997) "Risperidone: How Good is the Evidence for Efficacy?", *Schizophrenia Bulletin*, Vol. 23, No. 1, pp. 157-158

[151] Davis, J. and Chen, N. (2002) "Clinical Profile of an Atypical Antipsychotic: Risperidone", *Schizophrenia Bulletin*, Vol. 28, No. 1

[152] Healy, D. (1993) *Psychiatric Drugs Explained*, London: Mosby, p. 24

[153] Lieberman, J., Safferman, A., Pollack, S., Szymanski, S., Johns, C., Kronig, M., Brookstein, P. and Kane, J. (1994) "Clinical Effects of Clozapine in Chronic Schizophrenia: Response to Treatment and Predictors of Outcome", *American Journal of Psychiatry*, Vol. 151

[154] Okasha, A. (1999) "Highlights on the Management of Schizophrenia", in: Maj, M. and Sartorius, N. *Schizophrenia*

(WPA Series, Evidence and Experience in Psychiatry, Volume 2), New York: John Wiley and Sons, p. 142

[155] Geddes, J., Freemantle, N., Harrison, P. and Bebbington, P. (2000) "Atypical Antipsychotics in the Treatment of Schizophrenia: Systematic Overview and Meta-Regression Analysis", *British Medical Journal*, Vol. 321. p. 1374

[156] Castle, D., Morgan, V. and Jablensky, A. (2001) "Antipsychotic Use In Australia: The Patients' Perspective", *Australian and New Zealand Journal of Psychiatry*, Vol. 36, p. 640

[157] Gerlach, J. and Peacock, L. (1994) "Motor and Mental Side Effects of Clozapine", *Journal of Clinical Psychiatry*, Vol. 55 (Suppl. B), pp. 107–109

[158] Cohen, B., Keck, P., Satlin, A. and Cole, J. (1991) "Prevalence and Severity of Akathisia in Patients on Clozapine", *Biological Psychiatry*, Vol. 29, pp. 1215–1218

[159] Jauss, M., Schroder, J., Pantel, J., Bachmann, S., Gersden, I. and Mundt, C. (1998) "Severe Akathisia During Olanzapine Treatment of Acute Schizophrenia", *Pharmacopsychiatry*, 31 (4)

[160] Ahmed, S., Chengappa, K., Naidu, V., Baker, R., Parepally, H. and Schooler, N. (1999) "Clozapine Withdrawal-Emergent Dystonias and Dyskinesias: A Case Series", *Journal of Clinical Psychiatry*, Vol. 59

[161] Ananth, J. and Kenan, J. (1999) "Tardive Dyskinesia Associated with Olanzapine Monotherapy", (Letter). *Journal of Clinical Psychiatry*, Vol. 60, No. 12, p. 870; Spivak, M. and Smart, M. (2000) "Tardive Dyskinesia from Low-Dose Risperidone", (Letter), *Canadian Journal of Psychiatry*, Vol. 45

[162] Modestin, J., Stephan, P., Erni, T. and Umari, T. (2000) "Prevalence of Extrapyramidal Symptoms in Psychiatric Patients and the Relationship of Clozapine Treatment to Tardive Dyskinesia", *Schizophrenia Research*, Vol. 42, pp. 223–228

[163] Marder, S. and Meibach, R. (1994) "Risperidone in the Treatment of Schizophrenia", *American Journal of Psychiatry*, Vol. 151

[164] Rosebush, P. and Mazurek, M. (1999) "Neurologic Side Effects in Neuroleptic-Naïve Patients Treated with Haloperidol or Risperidone", *Neurology*, Vol. 52

[165] Kapur, S. and Remington, G. (2000) "Atypical Antipsychotics: Patients Value The Lower Incidence of EPS", *British Medical Journal*, Vol. 321

[166] McGorry, P. (1999) "Can We Use Pharmacotherapy More Logically in Schizophrenia and Other Psychoses?", in: Maj, M. and Sartorius, N. *Schizophrenia* (WPA Series, Evidence and Experience in Psychiatry, Volume 2), New York: John Wiley and Sons

[167] Bentall, R. (2003) *Madness Explained*, London: Penguin Books, p. 501

[168] Wallis, C. and Willwerth, J. (1992) "Awakenings. Schizophrenia: A New Drug Brings Patients Back to Life", *Time (Australia)*, Vol. 7, No. 27, (July 6th)

[169] Wescott, P. (1979) "One Man's Schizophrenic Illness", *British Medical Journal*, Vol. 1, p. 989

[170] Champ, S. (1999) "A Most Precious Thread", in: Barker, P., Campbell, P. and Davidson, B. (eds) *From the Ashes of Experience: Reflections on Madness, Survival and Growth.* London: Whurr Publishers, p.125

[171] Champ, S. (1999) "A Most Precious Thread", in: Barker, P., Campbell, P. and Davidson, B. (eds) *From the Ashes of Experience: Reflections on Madness, Survival and Growth.* London: Whurr Publishers, pp. 116, 124

[172] Breggin, P. (1993) *Toxic Psychiatry*, London: HarperCollins

[173] Lindström, L. (1994) "Long-Term Clinical and Social Outcome Studies in Schizophrenia in Relation to the Cognitive and Emotional Side Effects of Antipsychotic Drugs", *Acta Psychiatrica Scandinavica*, Vol. 89 (suppl. 380), pp. 74–75 (emphasis added)

[174] Rosenheck, R. et al. (1999) "Impact Of Clozapine On Negative Symptoms And On The Deficit Syndrome In Refractory Schizophrenia", *American Journal of Psychiatry*, Vol. 56, No. 1; Kane, J. et al. (2001) "Clozapine And Haloperidol In Moderately Refractory Schizophrenia", *Archives of General Psychiatry*, Vol. 58, No. 10

[175] Malhotra, A., Pinsky, D. and Breier, A. (1996) "Future Antipsychotic Agents: Clinical Implications", in: Breier, A. (ed) *The New Pharmacotherapy of Schizophrenia*. Washington, DC: American Psychiatric Press, p. 43

[176] Mattes, J. (1997) "Risperidone: How Good is the Evidence for Efficacy?", *Schizophrenia Bulletin*, Vol. 23, No. 1, p. 158

[177] Strauss, J., Rakfeldt, J., Harding, C. and Lieberman, P. (1989) "Psychological and Social Aspects of Negative Symptoms", *British Journal of Psychiatry*, Vol. 155 (suppl.7); Watkins, J. (1996) *Living With Schizophrenia: A Holistic Approach to Understanding, Preventing, and Recovering from Negative Symptoms*, Melbourne: Hill of Content

[178] Umbricht, D. and Kane, J. (1996) "Medical Complications of New Antipsychotic Drugs", *American Journal of Psychiatry*, Vol. 22, No. 3

[179] Abidi, S. and Bhaskara, S. (2003) "From Chlorpromazine To Clozapine – Antipsychotic Adverse Effects And The Clinician's Dilemma", *Canadian Journal of Psychiatry*, Vol. 48, No. 11

[180] Breier, A. and Buchanan, R. (1996) "Clozapine: Current Status and Clinical Applications", in: Breier, A. (ed) *The New Pharmacotherapy of Schizophrenia*, Washington, DC: American Psychiatric Press

[181] ibid

[182] Wieck, A. and Haddad, P. (2002) "Hyperprolactinaemia Caused by Antipsychotic Drugs: This Common Side Effect Needs More Attention", *British Medical Journal*, Vol. 324: 250-252

[183] Zyprexa (Olanzapine) Product Monograph (1997) West

Ryde, NSW: Eli Lilly and Company; Lambert, T. and Castle, D. (2003) "Pharmacological Approaches to the Management of Schizophrenia", *Medical Journal of Australia*, Vol. 178 (supplement)

[184] Healy, D. (1993) *Psychiatric Drugs Explained*, London: Mosby, p. 38

[185] Ziegler, J. and Behar, D. (1992) "Clozapine-Induced Priapism", (Letter), *American Journal of Psychiatry*, Vol. 149, p. 272

[186] Taylor, D. and McAskill, R. (2000) "Atypical Antipsychotics and Weight Gain: A Systematic Review", *Acta Psychiatrica Scandinavica*, Vol. 101

[187] Umbricht, D. and Kane, J. (1996) "Medical Complications of New Antipsychotic Drugs", *American Journal of Psychiatry*, Vol. 22, No. 3

[188] Koro, C., Fedder, D., L'Italien, G., Weiss, S., Magda, L., Kreyenbuhl, J., Revicki, D. and Buchanan, R. (2002) "An Assessment of the Independent Effects of Olanzapine and Risperidone Exposure on the Risk of Hyperlipidemia in Schizophrenic Patients", *Archives of General Psychiatry*, Vol. 59

[189] American Diabetes Association, American Psychiatric Association, American Association of Clinical Endocrinologists, North American Association for the Study of Obesity (2004) "Consensus Development Conference on Antipsychotic Drugs and Obesity and Diabetes", *Diabetes Care*, Vol. 27, No. 2, pp. 596-601

[190] Meyer, J. and Koro, C. (2004) "The Effects Of Antipsychotic Therapy On Serum Lipids: A Review", *Schizophrenia Research*, Vol. 70, Issue 1

[191] Henderson, D., Cagliero, E., Copeland, P. et al. (2005) "Glucose Metabolism in Patients with Schizophrenia Treated with Atypical Antipsychotic Agents", *Archives of General Psychiatry*, Vol. 62

[192] Sernyak, M., Leslie, D., Alarcon, R., Losonczy, M. and Rosenheck, R. (2002) "Association of Diabetes Mellitus

with Use of Atypical Neuroleptics in the Treatment of Schizophrenia", *American Journal of Psychiatry*, Vol. 159, No. 4, pp. 561–566

[193] Henderson, D., Cagliero, E., Gray, C., Nasrallah, R., Hayden, D., Schoenfeld, D. and Goff, D. (2000) "Clozapine, Diabetes Mellitus, Weight Gain, and Lipid Abnormalities: A Five-Year Naturalistic Study", *American Journal of Psychiatry*, Vol. 157, No. 6, pp. 975–981

[194] American Diabetes Association, American Psychiatric Association, American Association of Clinical Endocrinologists, North American Association for the Study of Obesity (2004) "Consensus Development Conference on Antipsychotic Drugs and Obesity and Diabetes", *Diabetes Care*, Vol. 27, No. 2, pp. 596–601

[195] Silvestri, S., Seeman, M., Negrete, J-C., Houle, S., et al. (2000) "Increased Dopamine D2 Receptor Binding After Long-Term Treatment With Antipsychotics in Humans: A Clinical PET Study", *Psychopharmacology*, Vol. 152, No. 2

[196] Ekblom, B. et al. (1984) "Supersensitivity Psychosis in Schizophrenic Patients After Sudden Clozapine Withdrawal", *Psychopharmacology*, Vol. 83; Borison, R. et al. (1988) "Clozapine Withdrawal Rebound Psychosis", *Psychopharmacology Bulletin*, Vol. 24, No. 2: Tollefson, G. et al. (1999) "Controlled, Double-Blind Investigation of the Clozapine Discontinuation Symptoms with Conversion to Either Olanzapine or Placebo", *Journal of Clinical Psychopharmacology*, Vol. 19

[197] Llorca, P., Vaiva, G. and Lancon, C. (2001) "Supersensitivity Psychosis in Patients with Schizophrenia After Sudden Olanzapine Withdrawal", (Letter). *Canadian Journal of Psychiatry*, Vol. 46, p. 87

[198] Baker, R., Chengappa, K., Baird, J., Steingard, S., Christ, M. and Schooler, N. (1992) "Emergence of Obsessive-Compulsive Symptoms During Treatment With Clozapine", *Journal of Clinical Psychiatry*, Vol. 53

[199] Patil, V. (1992) "Development of Transient Obsessive-Compulsive Symptoms During Treatment With Clozapine", (Letter), *American Journal of Psychiatry*, Vol. 149, No. 2, p. 272

[200] Morrison, D., Clark, D., Goldfarb, E. and McCoy, L. (1998) "Worsening of Obsessive-Compulsive Symptoms Following Treatment With Olanzapine", (Letter), *American Journal of Psychiatry*, Vol. 155, No. 6

[201] Abidi, S. and Bhaskara, S. (2003) "From Chlorpromazine To Clozapine – Antipsychotic Adverse Effects And The Clinician's Dilemma", *Canadian Journal of Psychiatry*, Vol. 48, No. 11, p. 749

[202] Rosenheck, R., Doyle, J., Leslie, D. and Fontana, A. (2003) "Changing Environments and Alternative Perspectives in Evaluating the Cost-Effectiveness of New Antipsychotic Drugs", *Schizophrenia Bulletin*, Vol. 29, No. 1, pp. 90-91

[203] Healy, D. (1999) *The Anti-Depressant Era,* Cambridge, Massachusetts: Harvard University Press, p. 304

[204] Valenstein, M., Blow, F., Copeland, L., et al. (2004) "Poor Antipsychotic Adherence Among Patients with Schizophrenia: Medication and Patient Factors", *Schizophrenia Bulletin*, Vol. 30, No. 2, pp. 255-264

[205] Gabbard, G. (1992) "Psychodynamic Psychiatry in the 'Decade of the Brain'", *American Journal of Psychiatry*, Vol. 149, No. 8, p. 997

[206] Baldessarini, R. (1999) "Pharmacotherapy of Psychotic Disorders: A Perspective on Current Developments", in: Maj, M. and Sartorius, N. (eds) *Schizophrenia. Evidence and Experience in Psychiatry*, (World Psychiatric Association Series, Vol. 2) New York: John Wiley and Sons, p. 111

Chapter Four: Treating Schizophrenia Holistically

[207] Sacks, O. (1991) *Awakenings,* London: Pan Books, p. 268

[208] Schachter, M. (ed) (1993) *Psychotherapy and Medication: A Dynamic Integration*, New Jersey: Jason Aronson; Grotstein,

J. (1995) "Orphans of the 'Real': Some Modern and Postmodern Perspectives on the Neurobiological and Psychosocial Dimensions of Psychosis and Other Primitive Mental Disorders", *Bulletin of the Menninger Clinic*, Vol. 59, No. 3

[209] Boisen, A. (1947) "Onset in Acute Schizophrenia", *Psychiatry*, Vol.10; Boisen, A. (1971) *The Exploration of the Inner World*, Philadelphia: University of Philadelphia Press

[210] Rose, S. (1976) *The Conscious Brain*, Harmondsworth: Penguin, pp. 322-323 (emphasis in original)

[211] Falloon, I. and Liberman, R. (1983) "Interactions Between Drug and Psychosocial Therapy in Schizophrenia", *Schizophrenia Bulletin*, Vol. 9, No. 4

[212] Johnson, D. (1984) "Observations on the Use of Long-Acting Depot Neuroleptic Injections in the Maintenance Therapy of Schizophrenia", *Journal of Clinical Psychiatry*, Vol. 45, No. 5, p.13

[213] Surwit, R. et al. (2002) "Stress Management Improves Long-Term Glycemic Control In Type 2 Diabetes', *Diabetes Care*, Vol. 25, pp. 30-34

[214] Wing, J. (1978) "The Social Context of Schizophrenia", *American Journal of Psychiatry*, Vol. 135, p. 1335

[215] Warner, R. (1985) *Recovery from Schizophrenia*, London: Routledge and Kegan Paul. p. 258 (emphasis in original)

[216] Engel, G. (1977) "The Need for a New Medical Model: A Challenge for Biomedicine", *Science*, Vol. 196, No. 4286

[217] May, P. (1976) "Rational Treatment For An Irrational Disorder: What Does The Schizophrenic Patient Need?" *American Journal of Psychiatry*, Vol. 133, No. 9, p. 1010

[218] Frank, A. and Gunderson, J. (1990) "The Role of the Therapeutic Alliance in the Treatment of Schizophrenia", *Archives of General Psychiatry*, Vol. 47; Howgego, I., Yellowlees, P., Owen, C., Meldrum, L. and Dark, F. (2003) "The Therapeutic Alliance: The Key to Effective Patient Outcome? A Descriptive Review of the Evidence in

Community Mental Health Case Management", *Australian and New Zealand Journal of Psychiatry*, Vol. 37

[219] Nuechterlein, K. and Dawson, M. (1984) "A Heuristic Vulnerability/Stress Model of Schizophrenic Episodes", *Schizophrenia Bulletin*, Vol. 10, No. 2

[220] Ciompi, L. (1983) "How to Improve the Treatment of Schizophrenics: A Multicausal Illness Concept and Its Therapeutic Consequences", in: Stierlin, H., Wynne, L. and Wirsching, M. (eds) *Psychosocial Intervention in Schizophrenia: An International View*, Berlin: Springer Verlag

[221] Wing, J. (1978) "Social Influences on the Course of Schizophrenia", in: Wynne, L., Cromwell, R. and Matthysse, S. (eds.) *The Nature of Schizophrenia: New Approaches to Research and Treatment*, New York: John Wiley and Sons, p. 606

[222] Brown, G., Birley, J. and Wing, J. (1972) "Influence of Family Life on the Course of Schizophrenic Disorders: A Replication", *British Journal of Psychiatry*, Vol. 121

[223] Vaughn, C. and Leff, J. (1976) "The Influence of Family and Social Factors on the Course of Psychiatric Illness", *British Journal of Psychiatry*, Vol. 129

[224] McGlashan, T. and Carpenter, W. (1981) "Does Attitude to Psychosis Relate to Outcome?", *American Journal of Psychiatry*, Vol. 138, No. 6

[225] Ciompi, L. (1989) "The Dynamics of Complex Biological-Psychosocial Systems: Four Fundamental Psycho-Biological Mediators in the Long-Term Evolution of Schizophrenia", *British Journal of Psychiatry*, Vol. 155 (suppl. 5), p. 16

[226] Strauss, J. (1989) "Subjective Experiences of Schizophrenia: Toward a New Dynamic Psychiatry – II", *Schizophrenia Bulletin*, Vol. 15, No. 2, p. 184

[227] Tooth, B., Kalyanasundaram, V., Glover, H. and Momenzadah, S, (2003) "Factors Consumers Identify As Important To Recovery From Schizophrenia", *Australasian Psychiatry*, Vol. 11 (supplement)

[228] Leete, E. (1993) "The Interpersonal Environment: A Consumer's Personal Recollection", in: Hatfield, A. and Lefley, H. *Surviving Mental Illness: Stress, Coping and Adaptation,* New York: The Guildford Press, pp. 118, 125, 127

[229] Carr, V. (1988) "Patients' Techniques for Coping with Schizophrenia: An Exploratory Study", *British Journal of Medical Psychology,* Vol. 61; Lee, P., Lieh-Mak, F., Yu, K. and Spinks, J. (1993) "Coping Strategies of Schizophrenic Patients and Their Relationship to Outcome", *British Journal of Psychiatry,* Vol. 163

[230] Watkins, J. (1996) *Living With Schizophrenia: A Holistic Approach to Understanding, Preventing, and Recovering from Negative Symptoms,* Melbourne: Hill of Content; Watkins, J. (1998) *Hearing Voices: A Common Human Experience.* Melbourne: Hill of Content

[231] Weingarten, R. (1994) "The Ongoing Processes of Recovery", *Psychiatry,* Vol. 57, p. 369 (emphasis in original)

[232] ibid, pp. 372-373

[233] Katz, H. (1989) "A New Agenda for Psychotherapy of Schizophrenia: Response to Coursey", *Schizophrenia Bulletin,* Vol. 15, No. 3; Wasylenki, D. (1992) "Psychotherapy of Schizophrenia Revisited", *Hospital and Community Psychiatry,* Vol. 43, No. 2

[234] Wasylenki, D. (1992) "Psychotherapy of Schizophrenia Revisited", *Hospital and Community Psychiatry,* Vol. 43, No. 2

[235] Coursey, R. (1989) "Psychotherapy with Persons Suffering from Schizophrenia: The Need for a New Agenda", *Schizophrenia Bulletin,* Vol. 15, No. 3; Gabbard, G. (1992) "Psychodynamic Psychiatry in the 'Decade of the Brain'", *American Journal of Psychiatry,* Vol. 149, No. 8

[236] A Recovering Patient (1986) "'Can We Talk?' The Schizophrenic Patient in Psychotherapy", *American Journal of Psychiatry,* Vol. 143; Ruocchio, P. (1989) "How Psychotherapy Can Help the Schizophrenic Patient", *Hospital and Community Psychiatry,* Vol. 40, No. 2

[237] Coursey, R., Keller, A. and Farrell, E. (1995) "Individual Psychotherapy and Persons with Serious Mental Illness: The Client's Perspective", *Schizophrenia Bulletin*, Vol. 21, No. 2

[238] McGrath, M. (1984) "First Person Account: Where Did I Go?", *Schizophrenia Bulletin*, Vol. 10. p. 639

[239] Glass, L., Katz, H., Schnitzer, R., Knapp, P., Frank, A., and Gunderson, J. (1989) "Psychotherapy of Schizophrenia: An Empirical Investigation of the Relationship of Process to Outcome", *American Journal of Psychiatry*, Vol. 146, No. 5.

[240] Ciompi, L. (1980) The Natural History of Schizophrenia in the Long-Term, *British Journal of Psychiatry*, Vol. 136. p. 419

[241] Winston, A., Pinsker, H. and McCullough, L. (1986) "A Review of Supportive Psychotherapy", *Hospital and Community Psychiatry*, Vol. 37, No. 11.

[242] Anonymous (1989) "First Person Account: A Delicate Balance", *Schizophrenia Bulletin*, Vol. 15, No. 2

[243] Perry, J. (1989) *The Far Side of Madness,* Dallas, Texas: Spring Publications, p. 2

[244] Rogers, C (1980) *A Way of Being,* Boston: Houghton Mifflin, p. 152

[245] Champ, S. (1999) "A Most Precious Thread", In Barker, P., Campbell, P. and Davidson, B. (eds) *From the Ashes of Experience: Reflections on Madness, Survival and Growth,* London: Whurr Publishers, p. 117

[246] Sarti, P. and Cournos, F. (1990) "Medication and Psychotherapy in the Treatment of Chronic Schizophrenia", *Psychiatric Clinics of North America* Vol. 13, No. 2; Schachter, M. (ed) (1993) *Psychotherapy and Medication: A Dynamic Integration,* New Jersey: Jason Aronson

[247] Coursey, R., Keller, A. and Farrell, E. (1995) "Individual Psychotherapy and Persons with Serious Mental Illness:

The Client's Perspective", *Schizophrenia Bulletin*, Vol. 21, No. 2

[248] Schooler, N. and Keith, S. (1993) "Clinical Research Base for the Treatment of Schizophrenia", *Psychopharmacology Bulletin*, Vol. 29

[249] Nevins, D. (1993) "Adverse Response to Neuroleptics in Schizophrenia" In Schachter, M. (ed) *Psychotherapy and Medication: A Dynamic Integration*, New Jersey: Jason Aronson

[250] Tooth, B., Kalyanasundaram, V., Glover, H. and Momenzadah, S. (2003) "Factors Consumers Identify As Important To Recovery From Schizophrenia", *Australasian Psychiatry*, Vol. 11 (supplement), p. 73

[251] A Recovering Patient (1986) "'Can We Talk?' The Schizophrenic Patient in Psychotherapy", *American Journal of Psychiatry*, Vol. 143, p. 70

[252] Ruocchio, P. (1989) "How Psychotherapy Can Help the Schizophrenic Patient", *Hospital and Community Psychiatry*, Vol. 40, No. 2, pp. 188-190

[253] Schwartz, J. and Begley, S. (2002) *The Mind and The Brain: Neuroplasticity and the Power of Mental Force.* New York: ReganBooks

[254] Gabbard, G. (2000) "A Neurobiologically Informed Perspective on Psychotherapy", *British Journal of Psychiatry*, Vol. 177, p. 119

[255] Gabbard, G. (1992) "Psychodynamic Psychiatry in the 'Decade of the Brain", *American Journal of Psychiatry*, Vol. 149, No. 8

[256] Lambert, T. and Minas, H. (1998) "Transcultural Psychopharmacology and Pharmacotherapy", *Australasian Psychiatry*, Vol. 6, No. 2, p. 62 (emphasis added)

[257] Lewontin, R., Rose, S. and Kamin, L. (1984) *Not In Our Genes,* New York: Pantheon Books, p. 192

[258] Ornstein, R. and Sobel, D. (1999) *The Healing Brain,* Cambridge, MA: Malor Books. p. 86

[259] Julien, R. (2000) *A Primer of Drug Action (Ninth Edition)*, New York: Worth Publishers, pp. 55–56

[260] Lambert, T. and Minas, H. (1998) "Transcultural Psychopharmacology and Pharmacotherapy", *Australasian Psychiatry*, Vol. 6, No. 2

[261] Davis, J. (1978) "Dopamine Theory of Schizophrenia: A Two-Factor Theory". In: Wynne, L., Cromwell, R. and Matthysse, S. (eds) *The Nature of Schizophrenia: New Approaches to Research and Treatment*, New York: John Wiley and Sons

[262] Julien, R. (2000) *A Primer of Drug Action (Ninth Edition)*, New York: Worth Publishers. p. 55

[263] Cousins, N. (1981) *Anatomy of an Illness as Perceived by the Patient*, New York: Bantam, p. 69,

[264] ibid, p. 56

[265] Benson, H. (1996) *Timeless Healing: The Power and Biology of Belief*, Rydalmere, NSW: Hodder and Stoughton

[266] Dallett, J. (1988) *When The Spirits Come Back*, Toronto: Inner City Books, p. 15

[267] Dossey, L. (1993) *Healing Words*, New York: HarperCollins, p.137

[268] Claridge, G. (1972) *Drugs and Human Behaviour*, Harmondsworth: Penguin Books, p. 26

[269] Benson, H. (1996) *Timeless Healing: The Power and Biology of Belief*, Rydalmere, NSW: Hodder and Stoughton

[270] Group for the Advancement of Psychiatry (1992) *Beyond Symptom Suppression: Improving Long-Term Outcomes of Schizophrenia* (Report No.134), Washington, DC: American Psychiatric Press, pp. 35–36 (emphasis added)

[271] Sacks, O. (1991) *Awakenings*, London: Pan Books, p. 272

[272] Falloon, I. and Liberman, R. (1983) "Interactions Between Drug and Psychosocial Therapy in Schizophrenia", *Schizophrenia Bulletin*, Vol. 9, No. 4, p. 550

[273] Menninger, K. (1967) *The Vital Balance*, New York: Viking Press, p. 294

[274] Breggin, P. (1993) *Toxic Psychiatry*, London: HarperCollins, pp. 461-463

Chapter Five: Treating Acute Schizophrenia Without Drugs

[275] Perry, J. (1989) *The Far Side of Madness*, Dallas, Texas: Spring Publications, p. 150

[276] Bentall,R. and Morrison, A. (2002) "More Harm Than Good: The Case Against Using Anti-Psychotic Drugs to Prevent Severe Mental Illness", *Journal of Mental Health*, Vol.11, No. 4

[277] Jablensky, A. (1992) "Schizophrenia: Incidence and Course in Different Countries: A WHO Ten-Country Study", *Psychological Medicine*, Suppl. 20, pp, 1-95

[278] Johnstone, E., Owens, D., Crow, T. and Davis, J. (1999) "Does a Four-Week Delay in the Introduction of Medication Alter the Course of Functional Psychosis?", *Journal of Psychopharmacology*, Vol. 13, No. 3. p. 243 (emphasis added)

[279] Craig, T. et al. (2000) "Is There An Association Between Duration Of Untreated Psychosis And 24-Month Clinical Outcome In A First-Admission Series?", *American Journal of Psychiatry*, Vol. 157, No. 1

[280] Hoff, A. et al. (2000) "Lack Of Association Between Duration Of Untreated Illness And Severity Of Cognitive And Structural Brain Deficits At The First Episode Of Schizophrenia", *American Journal of Psychiatry*, Vol. 157, No. 11

[281] Carpenter, W., McGlashan, T. and Strauss, J. (1977) "The Treatment of Acute Schizophrenia Without Drugs: An Investigation of Some Current Assumptions", *American Journal of Psychiatry*, Vol. 134, No. 1

[282] ibid, p. 18

[283] Rappaport, M., Hopkins, H., Hall, K., et al. (1978) "Are There Schizophrenics For Whom Drugs May Be Unnecessary or Contraindicated?", *International Pharmacopsychiatry*, Vol. 13, p. 107

284 Schooler, N., et al. (1967) "One Year After Discharge: Community Adjustment of Schizophrenic Patients", *American Journal of Psychiatry*, Vol. 123; Buckley, P. (1982) "Identifying Schizophrenic Patients Who Should Not Receive Medication", *Schizophrenia Bulletin*, Vol. 8, No. 3

285 Mosher, L., Reifman, A. and Menn, A. (1973) "Characteristics of Non-Professionals Serving as Primary Therapists for Acute Schizophrenics", *Hospital and Community Psychiatry*, Vol. 24, No. 6

286 Mosher, L. (1991) "Soteria: A Therapeutic Community for Psychotic Persons", *International Journal of Therapeutic Communities*, Vol. 12, No. 1, p. 53

287 Mosher, L. and Menn, A. (1978) "The Surrogate 'Family', An Alternative to Hospitalisation", in: Shershow, J. (ed) *Schizophrenia: Science and Practice*. Cambridge, MA: Harvard University Press, p. 237

288 Warner, R. (1985) *Recovery from Schizophrenia*, London: Routledge and Kegan Paul

289 Ciompi, L. et al. (1992) "The Pilot Project 'Soteria Berne': Clinical Experiences and Results", *British Journal of Psychiatry*, Vol. 161, (suppl.18)

290 ibid, p. 151

291 ibid, p. 152

292 Mosher, L. (1999) "Soteria and Other Alternatives To Acute Psychiatric Hospitalisation: A Personal and Professional Review", *Journal of Nervous and Mental Disease*, Vol. 187, p. 144

293 Bola, J. and Mosher, L. (2003) "Treatment Of Acute Psychosis Without Neuroleptics: Two-Year Outcomes From The Soteria Project", *Journal of Nervous and Mental Disease*, Vol. 191, p. 226

294 Perry, J. (1989) *The Far Side of Madness*, Dallas, Texas: Spring Publications, p. 149

295 ibid, p. 154

296 Miller, J. (1990) "Mental Illness and Spiritual Crisis:

Implications for Psychiatric Rehabilitation", *Psychosocial Rehabilitation Journal*, Vol. 14, No. 2; Sims, A. (1994) "'Psyche' – Spirit As Well As Mind?", *British Journal of Psychiatry*, Vol. 165; Kroll, J. (1995) Religion and Psychiatry. *Current Opinion in Psychiatry*, Vol. 8

[297] Handel, M. (1987) *A Personal Account of Schizophrenia* (Unpublished).

[298] Carpenter, W., McGlashan, T. and Strauss, J. (1977) "The Treatment of Acute Schizophrenia Without Drugs: An Investigation of Some Current Assumptions", *American Journal of Psychiatry*, Vol. 134, No. 1. p. 19

[299] McGlashan, T., Levy, S. and Carpenter, W. (1975) "Integration and Sealing Over: Clinically Distinct Recovery Styles From Schizophrenia", *Archives of General Psychiatry*, Vol. 32

[300] Mosher, L. and Menn, A. (1978) "The Surrogate 'Family', An Alternative to Hospitalisation", in: Shershow, J. (ed) *Schizophrenia: Science and Practice*. Cambridge, MA: Harvard University Press, p. 237

[301] McGlashan, T. and Levy, S. (1977) "Sealing-Over in a Therapeutic Community", *Psychiatry*, Vol. 40

[302] Lucas, R. (2002) "Beyond Medication", In Berke, J. et al. (eds) *Beyond Madness: Psychosocial Interventions In Psychosis*, London: Jessica Kingsley Publishers, p. 48

[303] Buckley, P. (1982) "Identifying Schizophrenic Patients Who Should Not Receive Medication", *Schizophrenia Bulletin*, Vol. 8, No. 3

[304] Warner, R. (1995) *Alternatives to the Mental Hospital for Acute Psychiatric Treatment*, Washington, DC: American Psychiatric Press

[305] Warner, R. (1985) *Recovery from Schizophrenia*, London: Routledge and Kegan Paul, pp. 256-257

[306] Mosher, L. (1999) "Soteria and Other Alternatives to Acute Psychiatric Hospitalisation: A Personal and Professional

Review", *Journal of Nervous and Mental Disease*, Vol. 187, p.143.

[307] McGorry, P., Chanen, A., McCarthy, E., Van Riel, R., McKenzie, D. and Singh, B. (1991) "Posttraumatic Stress Disorder Following Recent Onset Psychosis", *Journal of Nervous and Mental Disease*, Vol. 179, No. 5

[308] Ciompi, L. (1983) "How to Improve the Treatment of Schizophrenics: A Multicausal Illness Concept and Its Therapeutic Consequences", In Stierlin, H., Wynne, L. and Wirsching, M. (eds) *Psychosocial Intervention in Schizophrenia: An International View*, Berlin: Springer Verlag. p. 58

[309] Podvoll, E. (1990) *The Seduction of Madness*, New York: HarperCollins. p. 3

[310] Andreasen, N. (1985) *The Broken Brain: The Biological Revolution in Psychiatry*, New York: Harper and Row

[311] Ross, C. (1989) *Multiple Personality Disorder: Diagnosis, Clinical Features, and Treatment*, New York: John Wiley and Sons, p. 161 (emphasis in original)

[312] Perry, J. (1989) *The Far Side of Madness*, Dallas, Texas: Spring Publications

[313] Perry, J. (1987) *The Self in Psychotic Process*, Dallas, Texas: Spring Publications, p.xvi

[314] Mosher, L. (1999) "Soteria and Other Alternatives To Acute Psychiatric Hospitalisation: A Personal and Professional Review", *Journal of Nervous and Mental Disease*, Vol. 187, p. 148

Chapter Six: Maintenance Neuroleptic Treatment

[315] Birchwood, M., Hallett, S. and Preston, M. (1989) *Schizophrenia: An Integrated Approach to Research and Treatment*. New York: New York University Press, p. 235 (emphasis in original)

[316] Bleuler, M. (1978) *The Schizophrenic Disorders: Long-Term Patient and Family Studies*, Newhaven: Yale University Press

[317] Torrey, E. (1988) *Surviving Schizophrenia: A Family Manual (Revised Edition)*, New York: Harper and Row, p. 192

[318] Crow, T., MacMillan, J., Johnson, A. and Johnstone, E. (1986) "The Northwick Park Study of First Episodes of Schizophrenia, II: A Randomised Control Trial of Prophylactic Neuroleptic Treatment", *British Journal of Psychiatry*, Vol. 148

[319] Johnstone, E., MacMillan, F., Frith, C., Benn, D. and Crow, T. (1990) "Further Investigation of the Predictors of Outcome Following First Schizophrenic Episodes", *British Journal of Psychiatry*, Vol. 157, p. 188

[320] Buckley, P. (1982) "Identifying Schizophrenic Patients Who Should Not Receive Medication", *Schizophrenia Bulletin*, Vol. 8, No. 3; Warner, R. (1985) *Recovery from Schizophrenia*, London: Routledge and Kegan Paul

[321] McGorry, P., Killackey, E., Elkins, K., Lambert, M. and Lambert, T. (2003) "Summary Australian and New Zealand Clinical Practice Guideline for the Treatment of Schizophrenia (2003)", *Australasian Psychiatry*, Vol. 11, No. 2

[322] Strauss, J. et al. (1989) "Psychological and Social Aspects of Negative Symptoms", *British Journal of Psychiatry*, Vol. 155 (suppl. 7); Watkins, J. (1996) *Living With Schizophrenia: A Holistic Approach to Understanding, Preventing, and Recovering from Negative Symptoms*, Melbourne: Hill of Content

[323] Podvoll, E. (1990) *The Seduction of Madness*, New York: HarperCollins

[324] Schooler, N. (1993) "Antipsychotic Medication and Schizophrenia: Effects in Acute and Maintenance Treatment of the Illness", in: Cromwell, R. and Snyder, C. *Schizophrenia: Origins, Processes, Treatment, and Outcome*, New York: Oxford University Press, p. 288

[325] Cromwell, R. (1993) "A Summary View of Schizophrenia", in: Cromwell, R. and Snyder, C. *Schizophrenia: Origins, Processes, Treatment, and Outcome*. New York: Oxford

University Press; Johnstone, E., Humphreys, M., Lang, F., Lawrie, S. and Sandler, R. (1999) *Schizophrenia: Concepts and Clinical Management*, Cambridge: Cambridge University Press

[326] Watkins, J. (1998) *Hearing Voices: A Common Human Experience*. Melbourne: Hill of Content

[327] Watkins, J. (1996) *Living With Schizophrenia: A Holistic Approach to Understanding, Preventing, and Recovering from Negative Symptoms,* Melbourne: Hill of Content

[328] Healy, D. (1990) *The Suspended Revolution*, London: Faber and Faber, p. 218

[329] Gilbert, P., Harris, M., McAdams, L. and Jeste, D. (1995) "Neuroleptic Withdrawal in Schizophrenic Patients: A Review of the Literature", *Archives of General Psychiatry*, Vol. 52

[330] Jeste, D., Gilbert, P., McAdams, L. and Harris, M. (1995) "Considering Neuroleptic Maintenance and Taper on a Continuum", *Archives of General Psychiatry*, Vol. 52. p. 210

[331] Cohen, D. (2002) "Research on the Drug Treatment of Schizophrenia: A Critical Appraisal and Implications for Social Work Education", *Journal of Social Work Education*, Vol. 38, No. 2

[332] Thornley, B. and Adams, C. (1998) "Content and Quality of 2000 Controlled Trials in Schizophrenia Over 50 Years", *British Medical Journal*, Vol. 317, p. 1184

[333] Hogarty, G. (1998) "The Limitations of Antipsychotic Medication on Schizophrenic Relapse and Adjustment and the Contributions of Psychosocial Treatment", *Journal of Psychiatric Research*, Vol. 32

[334] Falloon, I, Boyd, J., McGill, C. et al. (1985) "Family Management in the Prevention of Morbidity in Schizophrenia: Clinical Outcome of a Two-Year Longitudinal Study", *Archives of General Psychiatry*, Vol. 42; Leff, J., Kuipers, L., Berkowitz, R. and Sturgeon, D. (1985) "A Controlled Trial of Social Interventions in the Families

of Schizophrenic Patients: A Two Year Follow-Up", *British Journal of Psychiatry*,Vol. 146

335 Weiden, P. and Olfson, M. (1995) "Cost of Relapse in Schizophrenia", *Schizophrenia Bulletin*,Vol. 21, No. 3

336 Wyatt, J. (1995) "Risks of Withdrawing Antipsychotic Medication", *Archives of General Psychiatry*,Vol. 52. p. 207

337 Baldessarini, R. and Viguera, A. (1995) "Neuroleptic Withdrawal in Schizophrenic Patients", *Archives of General Psychiatry*,Vol. 52

338 Green, A., Faraone,S., Brown,W., Guttierez, J. and Tsuang, M. (1992) "Neuroleptic Dose Reduction Studies: Clinical and Neuroendocrine Effects", presented at the 31st Annual Meeting of the American College of Neuropsychopharmacology, December 14–18, San Juan, Puerto Rico

339 Viguera, A., Baldessarini, R., Hegarty, J., van Kammen, J. and Tohen, M. (1997) "Clinical Risk Following Abrupt and Gradual Withdrawal of Maintenance Neuroleptic Treatment", *Archives of General Psychiatry*,Vol. 54, p. 52

340 World Health Organisation (1979) *Schizophrenia: An International Follow-Up Study*, Chichester, England: Wiley

341 Warner, R. (1985) *Recovery from Schizophrenia*, London: Routledge and Kegan Paul, p.149

342 Viguera, A., Baldessarini, R., Hegarty, J., van Kammen, J. and Tohen, M. (1997) "Clinical Risk Following Abrupt and Gradual Withdrawal of Maintenance Neuroleptic Treatment", *Archives of General Psychiatry*,Vol. 54. p. 53

343 Chouinard, G. and Jones, B. (1980) "Neuroleptic-Induced Supersensitivity Psychosis: Clinical and Pharmacological Characteristics", *American Journal of Psychiatry*,Vol. 137, No. 1; Warner, R. (1985) *Recovery from Schizophrenia*, London: Routledge and Kegan Paul; Thomas, P. (1997) *The Dialectics of Schizophrenia*, London: Free Association Books

344 Fenton, W. and McGlashan, T. (1987) "Sustained Remission

in Drug-Free Schizophrenic Patients", *American Journal of Psychiatry*, Vol. 144, No. 10, p. 1309

345 Hogarty, G. (1998) "The Limitations of Antipsychotic Medication on Schizophrenic Relapse and Adjustment and the Contributions of Psychosocial Treatment", *Journal of Psychiatric Research*, Vol. 32

346 Ciompi, L. (1989) "The Dynamics of Complex Biological-Psychosocial Systems: Four Fundamental Psycho-Biological Mediators in the Long-Term Evolution of Schizophrenia", *British Journal of Psychiatry*, Vol. 155 (suppl. 5)

347 Schooler, N. (1991) "Maintenance Medication for Schizophrenia: Strategies for Dose Reduction", *Schizophrenia Bulletin*, Vol. 17, No. 2, p. 312

348 Paul. G., Tobias, L. and Holly, B. (1972) "Maintenance Psychotropic Drugs in the Presence of Active Treatment Programs", *Archives of General Psychiatry*, Vol. 27, p. 113

349 Fenton, W. and McGlashan, T. (1987) "Sustained Remission in Drug-Free Schizophrenic Patients", *American Journal of Psychiatry*, Vol. 144, No. 10, p. 1309

350 Gardos, G. and Cole, J. (1978) "Maintenance Antipsychotic Therapy: Is the Cure Worse than the Disease?", *American Journal of Psychiatry*, Vol. 133, No. 1, p. 35

351 Dufresne, R. and Wagner, R. (1988) "Antipsychotic-Withdrawal Akathisia Versus Antipsychotic-Induced Akathisia: Further Evidence for the Existence of Tardive Akathisia", *Journal Clinical Psychiatry*, Vol. 49

352 Drake, R. and Wallach, M. (1989) "Substance Abuse Among the Chronic Mentally Ill", *Hospital and Community Psychiatry*, Vol. 40, No. 10

353 Dixon, L., Haas, G., Weiden, P., Sweeney, J. and Frances, A. (1990) "Acute Effects of Drug Abuse in Schizophrenic Patients: Clinical Observations and Patients' Self-Reports", *Schizophrenia Bulletin*, Vol. 16, No. 1

354 Treffert, D. (1978) "Marijuana Use in Schizophrenia: A

Clear Hazard", *American Journal of Psychiatry*,Vol. 135, No. 10

[355] Koczapski, A., Paredes, J., Kogan, C., Ledwidge, B. and Higenbottam, J. (1989) "Effects of Caffeine on Behaviour of Schizophrenic Inpatients", *Schizophrenia Bulletin*,Vol. 15, No. 2

[356] Hyde, A. (1990) "Response to 'Effects of Caffeine on Behaviour of Schizophrenic Inpatients'", *Schizophrenia Bulletin*,Vol. 16, No. 3

[357] Lutz, E. (1976) "Neuroleptic-Induced Akathisia and Dystonia Triggered By Alcohol", *Journal of the American Medical Association*,Vol. 236

[358] Engel, J. and Liljequist, S. (1976) "The Effect of Long-Term Ethanol Treatment on the Sensitivity of the Dopamine Receptors in the Nucleus Accumbens", *Psychopharmacology*,Vol. 49

[359] Glassman, A. (1995) "Cigarette Smoking: Implications for Psychiatric Illness", *American Journal of Psychiatry*,Vol. 150, No. 4

[360] Miller, R. (1977) "Effects of Smoking on Drug Action", *Clinical Pharmacological Therapeutics*,Vol. 22

[361] Kelly, C. and McCreadie, R. (1999) "Smoking Habits, Current Symptoms, and Premorbid Characteristics of Schizophrenic Patients in Nithsdale, Scotland", *American Journal of Psychiatry*,Vol. 156

[362] Eli Lilly and Company (1997) *Zyprexa (Olanzapine) Product Monograph*,West Ryde, NSW: Eli Lilly and Company, p. 85

[363] Goff, D., Henderson, D. and Amico, E. (1992) "Cigarette Smoking in Schizophrenia: Relationship to Psychopathology and Medication Side effects", *American Journal of Psychiatry*,Vol. 149, No. 9

Chapter Seven: "Chronic" Schizophrenia: Treatment and Recovery

[364] Wing, J. (1978) *Reasoning About Madness*, Oxford: Oxford University Press, p. 127

[365] Cohen, P. and Cohen, J. (1984) "The Clinician's Illusion", *Archives of General Psychiatry*, Vol. 41

[366] Harding, C., Zubin, J. and Strauss, J. (1987) "Chronicity in Schizophrenia: Fact, Partial Fact, or Artifact?", *Hospital and Community Psychiatry*, Vol. 38, No. 5, p. 481

[367] Fenton, W. and McGlashan, T. (1987) "Sustained Remission in Drug-Free Schizophrenic Patients", *American Journal of Psychiatry*, Vol. 144, No. 10, p. 1308

[368] Harding, C. and Zahniser. J. (1994) "Empirical Correction of Seven Myths About Schizophrenia with Implications for Treatment", *Acta Psychiatrica Scandinavica*, Vol. 90 (suppl. 384)

[369] Harding, C., Zubin, J. and Strauss, J. (1992) "Chronicity in Schizophrenia: Revisited", *British Journal of Psychiatry*, Vol. 161 (suppl. 18)

[370] ibid

[371] Harding, C., Zubin, J. and Strauss, J. (1987) "Chronicity in Schizophrenia: Fact, Partial Fact, or Artifact?" *Hospital and Community Psychiatry*, Vol. 38, No. 5, p. 483

[372] ibid

[373] Bleuler, M. (1974) "The Long-Term Course of the Schizophrenic Psychoses", *Psychological Medicine*, Vol. 4, p. 245

[374] ibid, p.246 (emphasis added)

[375] Bleuler, M. (1978) "The Long-Term Course of Schizophrenic Psychoses", In: Wynne, L., Cromwell, R. and Matthysse, S. (eds.) *The Nature of Schizophrenia: New Approaches to Research and Treatment.* New York: John Wiley and Sons, p. 634

[376] Bleuler, M. (1983) "Schizophrenic Deterioration" (Discussion)", *British Journal of Psychiatry*, Vol. 143, p. 78

[377] ibid

[378] Bleuler, M. (1978) *The Schizophrenic Disorders: Long-Term Patient and Family Studies*, Newhaven: Yale University Press

[379] Bleuler, M. (1979) "On Schizophrenic Psychoses", *American Journal of Psychiatry*, Vol. 136, No. 11, p. 1404

[380] Bleuler, M. (1979) "My Sixty Years With Schizophrenics", In Bellak, L. (ed) *Disorders of the Schizophrenic Syndrome*, New York: Basic Books, p. vii

[381] Bleuler, M. (1974) "The Long-Term Course of the Schizophrenic Psychoses", *Psychological Medicine*, Vol. 4, p. 247.

[382] Bleuler, M. (1978) "The Long-Term Course of Schizophrenic Psychoses", In: Wynne, L., Cromwell, R. and Matthysse, S. (eds.) *The Nature of Schizophrenia: New Approaches to Research and Treatment*, New York: John Wiley and Sons, p. 635,

[383] Bleuler, M. (1979) "On Schizophrenic Psychoses", *American Journal of Psychiatry*, Vol. 136, No. 11, p. 1408 (emphasis added)

[384] Ciompi, L. (1980) "Catamnestic Long-Term Study on the Course of Life and Aging of Schizophrenics", *Schizophrenia Bulletin*, Vol. 6, No. 4

[385] ibid, p. 616

[386] Ciompi, L. (1980) "The Natural History of Schizophrenia in the Long-Term", *British Journal of Psychiatry*, Vol. 136, p. 420

[387] Teschke, G. (1978) "Die Schizoprenen Geistesstörungen im Lichte Langjähriger Kranken- und Familiengeschichten, by Manfred Bleuler", (Book Review), *Schizophrenia Bulletin*, Vol. 4, No. 1, p. 55

[388] McGorry, P. (1999) "Can We Use Pharmacotherapy More Logically in Schizophrenia and Other Psychoses?" in: Maj, M. and Sartorius, N. (eds) *Schizophrenia. Evidence and Experience in Psychiatry*, (World Psychiatric Association

Series, Volume Two), New York: John Wiley and Sons, p. 127

389 Whitaker, R. (2002) *Mad In America: Bad Science, Bad Medicine, and the Enduring Mistreatment of the Mentally Ill*, Cambridge, MA: Perseus Books, pp. 143-144

390 Van Putten, T., Marder, S. and Mintz, J. (1990) "A Controlled Dose Comparison of Haloperidol in Newly Admitted Schizophrenic Patients", *Archives of General Psychiatry*, Vol. 47

391 Whitaker, R. (2002) *Mad In America: Bad Science, Bad Medicine, and the Enduring Mistreatment of the Mentally Ill*, Cambridge, MA: Perseus Books, p. 210

392 Bentall, R. (2003) *Madness Explained*, London: Penguin Books, p. 501

393 Tooth, B., Kalyanasundaram, V., Glover, H. and Momenzadah, S. (2003) "Factors Consumers Identify As Important To Recovery From Schizophrenia", *Australasian Psychiatry*, Vol. 11 (supplement), p. 73

394 Wallace, M. (1994) "Schizophrenia – A National Emergency: Preliminary Observations on SANELINE", *Acta Psychiatrica Scandinavica*, Vol. 89, (suppl.380), p. 35

395 Ciompi, L. (1989) "The Dynamics of Complex Biological-Psychosocial Systems: Four Fundamental Psycho-Biological Mediators in the Long-Term Evolution of Schizophrenia", *British Journal of Psychiatry*, Vol. 155 (suppl. 5), p. 16

396 Perry, J. (1989) *The Far Side of Madness*, Dallas, Texas: Spring Publications, p. 2

397 Bleuler, M. (1974) "The Long-Term Course of the Schizophrenic Psychoses", *Psychological Medicine*, Vol. 4, pp. 246

398 Bleuler, M. (1978) *The Schizophrenic Disorders: Long-Term Patient and Family Studies,* Newhaven: Yale University Press, p. 300

[399] Bleuler, M. (1983) "Schizophrenic Deterioration (Discussion)", *British Journal of Psychiatry*, Vol. 143, p. 78

[400] Bleuler, M. (1970) "Some Results of Research in Schizophrenia", *Behavioral Science*, Vol. 15, p. 214

[401] Ciompi, L. (1988) "Learning From Outcome Studies: Toward a Comprehensive Biological–Psychosocial Understanding of Schizophrenia", *Schizophrenia Research*, Vol. 1, p. 376

[402] Harding, C., Brooks, G., Ashikaga, T., Strauss, J. and Breier, A. (1987) "The Vermont Longitudinal Study of Persons With Severe Mental Illness, II: Long-Term Outcomes of Subjects Who Retrospectively Met DSM-III Criteria For Schizophrenia", *American Journal of Psychiatry*, Vol. 144, No. 6, p. 730

[403] Bleuler, M. (1978) *The Schizophrenic Disorders: Long-Term Patient and Family Studies*, Newhaven: Yale University Press, p. 215

[404] Ciompi, L. (1980) "The Natural History of Schizophrenia in the Long-Term", *British Journal of Psychiatry*, Vol. 136, p. 419

[405] Torrey, E. (1988) *Surviving Schizophrenia: A Family Manual (Revised Edition)*, New York: Harper and Row, p. 193

[406] Harding, C. (1991) "Aging and Schizophrenia: Plasticity, Reversibility, and/or Compensation", in: Walker, E. (ed) *Schizophrenia: A Life-Course Developmental Perspective*, San Diego: Academic Press, pp. 258, 259, 268

[407] Paul. G., Tobias, L. and Holly, B. (1972) "Maintenance Psychotropic Drugs in the Presence of Active Treatment Programs", *Archives of General Psychiatry*, Vol. 27

[408] Bleuler, M. (1978) *The Schizophrenic Disorders: Long-Term Patient and Family Studies*, Newhaven: Yale University Press, p. 300

[409] Bleuler, M. (1978) "The Long-Term Course of Schizophrenic Psychoses", in: Wynne, L., Cromwell, R. and Matthysse, S. (eds.) *The Nature of Schizophrenia: New*

Approaches to Research and Treatment, New York: John Wiley and Sons, p. 634

[410] Prien, R. and Klett, C. (1972) "An Appraisal of the Long-term Use of Tranquillising Medication with Hospitalised Chronic Schizophrenics: A Review of the Drug-Discontinuation Literature", *Schizophrenia Bulletin*, Vol. 5; Lewander, T. (1994) "Placebo Response in Schizophrenia", *European Psychiatry*, Vol. 9, No. 3

[411] O'Brien, P. (1978) *The Disordered Mind*, Englewood Cliffs, NJ: Prentice Hall, p. 220

[412] Ciompi, L. (1980) "The Natural History of Schizophrenia in the Long-Term", *British Journal of Psychiatry*, Vol. 136, p. 420

[413] Harding, C., Zubin, J. and Strauss, J. (1987) "Chronicity in Schizophrenia: Fact, Partial Fact, or Artifact?", *Hospital and Community Psychiatry*, Vol. 38, No. 5. p. 483

[414] Smith, R. (1994) "Lower-Dose Therapy With Traditional Neuroleptics in Chronically Hospitalised Schizophrenic Patients", (Letter), *Archives of General Psychiatry*, Vol. 51. p. 427

[415] Gardos, G. and Cole, J. (1978) "Maintenance Antipsychotic Therapy: Is the Cure Worse than the Disease?", *American Journal of Psychiatry*, Vol. 133, No. 1, pp. 34, 35, 36 (emphasis in original)

Chapter Eight: Using Medication Wisely

[416] Sacks, O. (1991) *Awakenings*, London: Pan Books, p. 259

[417] May, P. (1976) "Rational Treatment For An Irrational Disorder: What Does The Schizophrenic Patient Need?", *American Journal of Psychiatry*, Vol. 133, No. 9, pp. 1008, 1011

[418] Warner, R. (1985) *Recovery from Schizophrenia*, London: Routledge and Kegan Paul

[419] Blaska, B. (1990) "The Myriad Medication Mistakes in Psychiatry: A Consumer's View", *Hospital and Community Psychiatry*, Vol. 41, No. 9

[420] Bentall, R. (ed) (1990) *Reconstructing Schizophrenia*, London: Routledge

[421] Van Putten, T., May, P. and Marder, S. (1984) "Response to Antipsychotic Medication: The Doctor's and the Consumer's View", *American Journal of Psychiatry*, Vol. 141, No. 1

[422] Van Putten, T. and May, P. (1978) "Subjective Response as a Predictor of Outcome in Pharmacotherapy: The Consumer Has a Point", *Archives of General Psychiatry*, Vol. 35

[423] Healy, D. (1993) *Psychiatric Drugs Explained*, London: Mosby, p. 21

[424] Awad, A. and Hogan, T. (1994) "Subjective Response to Neuroleptics and the Quality of Life: Implications for Treatment Outcome", *Acta Psychiatrica Scandinavica*, Vol. 89 (suppl. 380)

[425] Warner, R. (1985) *Recovery from Schizophrenia*, London: Routledge and Kegan Paul, p. 241

[426] Van Putten, T. and May, P. (1978) "Subjective Response as a Predictor of Outcome in Pharmacotherapy: The Consumer Has a Point", *Archives of General Psychiatry*, Vol. 35; Van Putten, T., May, P. and Marder, S. (1984) "Response to Antipsychotic Medication: The Doctor's and the Consumer's View, *American Journal of Psychiatry*, Vol. 141, No. 1

[427] Horrobin, D. (2002) *The Madness of Adam and Eve*, London: Corgi Books, p. 150

[428] Julien, R. (2000) *A Primer of Drug Action (Ninth Edition)*, New York: Worth Publishers, pp. 51–52

[429] Healy, D. (1993) *Psychiatric Drugs Explained*, London: Mosby, p. 21

[430] Pierce, E. (1988) *Passion for the Possible*, Gladesville, NSW: P. E. Pierce, pp. 122, 123, 127

[431] Champ, S. (1999) "A Most Precious Thread", in Barker, P., Campbell, P. and Davidson, B. (eds) *From the Ashes*

of Experience: Reflections on Madness, Survival and Growth,
London: Whurr Publishers, pp. 114, 123

[432] Moynihan, R. (1998) *Too Much Medicine? The Business of Health – And Its Risks For You,* Sydney, NSW: ABC Books; Hughes, G. and Minchin, L. (2003) "Drug Giants' Big-Money Pitch Exposed", *The Age* (13/12/03)

[433] Awad, A. (1993) "Subjective Response to Neuroleptics in Schizophrenia", *Schizophrenia Bulletin,* Vol. 19, No. 3

[434] Podvoll, E. (1990) *The Seduction of Madness,* New York: HarperCollins, p. 152

[435] ibid, p. 228

[436] ibid

[437] Ciompi, L. (1988) *The Psyche and Schizophrenia,* Cambridge, Massachusetts: Harvard University Press, p. 293

[438] Awad, G. (1992) "Quality of Life of Schizophrenic Patients on Medications and Implications for New Drug Trials", *Hospital and Community Psychiatry,* Vol. 43, No. 3, p. 262

[439] Rappaport, M., Hopkins, H., Hall, K., et al. (1978) "Are There Schizophrenics For Whom Drugs May Be Unnecessary or Contraindicated?", *International Pharmacopsychiatry,* Vol. 13; Buckley, P. (1982) "Identifying Schizophrenic Patients Who Should Not Receive Medication", *Schizophrenia Bulletin,* Vol. 8, No. 3

[440] Gardos, G. and Cole, J. (1978) "Maintenance Antipsychotic Therapy: Is the Cure Worse than the Disease?", *American Journal of Psychiatry,* Vol. 133, No. 1

[441] Grof, C. and Grof, S. (eds) (1989) *Spiritual Emergency: When Personal Transformation Becomes A Crisis,* Los Angeles, CA: Jeremy Tarcher; Grof, C. and Grof, S. (1990) *The Stormy Search For The Self,* Los Angeles, CA: Jeremy Tarcher

[442] Perry, J. (1999) *Trials of the Visionary Mind: Spiritual Emergency and the Renewal Process,* Albany: State University of New York

[443] Carpenter, W., McGlashan, T. and Strauss, J. (1977) "The Treatment of Acute Schizophrenia Without Drugs: An

Investigation of Some Current Assumptions", *American Journal of Psychiatry*, Vol. 134, No. 1, p.19

[444] Boisen, A. (1971) *The Exploration of the Inner World*, Philadelphia: University of Philadelphia Press; Bowers, M. (1974) *Retreat From Sanity: The Structure of Emerging Psychosis*, New York: Human Sciences Press; Epstein, S. (1979) "Natural Healing Processes of the Mind: 1. Acute Schizophrenic Disorganisation", *Schizophrenia Bulletin*, Vol. 5, No. 2; Perry, J. (1989) *The Far Side of Madness*, Dallas, Texas: Spring Publications

[445] Buckley, P. (1982) "Identifying Schizophrenic Patients Who Should Not Receive Medication", *Schizophrenia Bulletin*, Vol. 8, No. 3, p. 431

Chapter Nine: Individualised Medication Strategies

[446] Gilbert, P., Harris, M., McAdams, L. and Jeste, D. (1995) "Neuroleptic Withdrawal in Schizophrenic Patients: A Review of the Literature", *Archives of General Psychiatry*, Vol. 52, p. 209

[447] Schooler, N. (1991) "Maintenance Medication for Schizophrenia: Strategies for Dose Reduction", *Schizophrenia Bulletin*, Vol. 17, No. 2. p. 312

[448] American Psychiatric Association (1997) "Practice Guidelines For The Treatment of Patients With Schizophrenia", *American Journal of Psychiatry*, Vol. 154, No. 4 (suppl), p. 17

[449] Kulkarni, J., Reidel, A., de Castella, A., Fitzgerald, P., Rolfe, T. and Burger, H. (2001) "Oestrogen – A Potential Treatment For Schizophrenia", *Schizophrenia Research*, Vol. 48: 137–144

[450] McEvoy, J., Hogarty, G. and Steingard, S. (1991) "Optimal Dose of Neuroleptic in Acute Schizophrenia: A Controlled Study of the Neuroleptic Threshold and Higher Haloperidol Dose", *Archives of General Psychiatry*, Vol. 48

[451] American Psychiatric Association (1997) "Practice

Guidelines For The Treatment of Patients With Schizophrenia", *American Journal of Psychiatry*, Vol. 154, No. 4 (suppl), p. 17

452 Kane, J., Rifkin, A., Woener, M., et al. (1983) "Low–Dose Neuroleptic Treatment of Outpatient Schizophrenics, I: Preliminary Results for Relapse Rates", *Archives of General Psychiatry*, Vol. 40

453 Bitter, I., Volavka, J. and Scheurer, J. (1991) "The Concept of the Neuroleptic Threshold: An Update", *Journal of Clinical Psychopharmacology*, Vol. 11, No. 1

454 Thompson, C. (1994) "The Use of High–Dose Antipsychotic Medication", *British Journal of Psychiatry*, Vol. 164

455 Coppens, H., Sloof, C., Paans, A. Wiegman, T., Vaalburg, W. and Korf, J. (1991) "High Central D2-Dopamine Receptor Occupancy as Assessed with Positron Emission Tomography in Medicated But Therapy-Resistant Schizophrenic Patients", *Biological Psychiatry*, Vol. 29

456 Farde, L. Wiesel, F-A., Halldin, C. and Sedvall, G. (1988) "Central D2-Dopamine Receptor Occupancy in Schizophrenic Patients Treated with Antipsychotic Drugs", *Archives of General Psychiatry*, Vol. 45

457 Galletly, C. (1992) "Antipsychotic Drug Doses in a Schizophrenia Inpatient Unit", *Australian and New Zealand Journal of Psychiatry*, Vol. 26

458 Liberman, R., Van Putten, T., Marshall, B., et al. (1994) "Optimal Drug and Behaviour Therapy for Treatment-Refractory Schizophrenic Patients", *American Journal of Psychiatry*, Vol. 151; Smith, R. (1994) "Lower-Dose Therapy With Traditional Neuroleptics in Chronically Hospitalised Schizophrenic Patients", *Archives of General Psychiatry*, Vol. 51

459 Faraone, S., Green, A., Brown, W., Yin, P. and Tsuang, M. (1989) "Neuroleptic Dose Reduction in Persistently Psychotic Patients", *Hospital and Community Psychiatry*, Vol. 40, No. 11, p. 1194

[460] Hogarty, G., Goldberg, S. and The Collaborative Study Group (1973) "Drugs and Sociotherapy in the Aftercare of Schizophrenic Patients: One-Year Relapse Rates", *Archives of General Psychiatry*, Vol. 28

[461] Carpenter, W. and Heinrichs, D. (1983) "Early Intervention, Time-Limited, Targeted Pharmacotherapy of Schizophrenia", *Schizophrenia Bulletin*, Vol. 9, No. 4

[462] Docherty, J., Van Kammen, D., Siris, S. and Marder, S. (1978) "Stages of Onset of Schizophrenic Psychosis", *American Journal of Psychiatry*, Vol. 135, No. 4

[463] McCandless-Glimcher, L., McKnight, S., Hamera, E., Smith, B., et al. (1986) "Use of Symptoms by Schizophrenics to Monitor and Regulate Their Illness", *Hospital and Community Psychiatry*, Vol. 37, No. 9; Hamera, E., Peterson, K., Handley, S., Plumlee, A. and Frank-Ragan, E. (1991) "Patient Self-Regulation and Functioning in Schizophrenia", *Hospital and Community Psychiatry*, Vol. 42, No. 6

[464] Herz, M. and Melville, C. (1980) "Relapse in Schizophrenia", *American Journal of Psychiatry*, Vol. 137, No. 7

[465] ibid

[466] Sacks, O. (1991) *Awakenings*, London: Pan Books, p. 249 (emphasis in original)

[467] Birchwood, M. (1992) "Early Intervention in Schizophrenia: Theoretical Background and Clinical Strategies", *British Journal of Clinical Psychology*, Vol. 31, p. 10 (emphasis in original)

[468] Lovejoy, M. (1984) "Recovery From Schizophrenia: A Personal Odyssey", *Hospital and Community Psychiatry*, Vol. 35, No. 8. p. 811

[469] ibid

[470] Carpenter, W. (1999) "Diazepam Treatment for Early Signs of Exacerbation in Schizophrenia", *American Journal of Psychiatry*, Vol. 156, No. 2

[471] Torrey, E. (1988) *Surviving Schizophrenia: A Family Manual (Revised Edition)*, New York: Harper and Row, p.192

[472] Herz, M., Glazer, W., Mirza, M., Mostert, M. and Hafez, H. (1989) "Treating Prodromal Episodes to Prevent Relapse in Schizophrenia", *British Journal of Psychiatry*, Vol. 155 (suppl.5), p. 126

[473] Carpenter, W. and Heinrichs, D. (1983) "Early Intervention, Time-Limited, Targeted Pharmacotherapy of Schizophrenia", *Schizophrenia Bulletin*, Vol. 9, No. 4, p. 538

[474] Karper, L. and Krystal, J. (1996) "Augmenting Antipsychotic Efficacy: New Approaches", in: Breier, A. (ed) *The New Pharmacotherapy of Schizophrenia*, Washington, DC: American Psychiatric Press

[475] Wolkowitz, O. (1996) "Benzodiazepines", in: Breier, A. (ed) *The New Pharmacotherapy of Schizophrenia*, Washington, DC: American Psychiatric Press.

[476] Siris, G. (1992) "Adjunctive Medication in the Maintenance Treatment of Schizophrenia and its Conceptual Implications", *British Journal of Psychiatry*, Vol. 163 (suppl. 22)

[477] Kirkpatrick, B., Buchanan, R., Waltrip, R. et al. (1989) "Diazepam Treatment of Early Symptoms of Schizophrenic Relapse", *Journal of Nervous and Mental Disease*, Vol. 177; Carpenter, W. (1999) "Diazepam Treatment for Early Signs of Exacerbation in Schizophrenia", *American Journal of Psychiatry*, Vol. 156

[478] Arana, G., Ornsteen, M., Kanter, F., et al. (1986) "The Use of Benzodiazepines for Psychotic Disorders: A Literature Review and Preliminary Clinical Findings", *Psychopharmacology Bulletin*, Vol. 22

[479] Keck, P., Cohen, B., Baldessarini, R. and McElroy, S. (1989) "Time Course of Antipsychotic Effects of Neuroleptic Drugs", *American Journal of Psychiatry*, Vol. 146, No. 10

[480] Lingjaerde, O. (1985) "Antipsychotic Effect of

Benzodiazepines", in: Burrows,G., Norman,T. and Davies, B. (eds) *Antipsychotics,* Amsterdam: Elsevier

[481] Nestoros, J. (1980) "Benzodiazepines in Schizophrenia: Need for a Reassessment", *International Pharmacopsychiatry,* Vol. 15

[482] Pato, C.,Wolkowitz, O., Rapaport, M., et al. (1989) "Benzodiazepine Augmentation of Neuroleptic Treatment in Patients With Schizophrenia", *Psychopharmacology Bulletin,*Vol. 25

[483] Csernansky, J., Riney, S., Lombrozo, L., et al. (1988) "Double-Blind Comparison Of Alprazolam, Diazepam, and Placebo for the Treatment of Negative Schizophrenic Symptoms", *Archives of General Psychiatry,*Vol. 45

[484] Menza, M. and Harris, D. (1989) "Benzodiazepines and Catatonia: An Overview", *Biological Psychiatry,*Vol. 26

[485] Watkins, J. (1996) *Living With Schizophrenia: A Holistic Approach to Understanding, Preventing, and Recovering from Negative Symptoms,* Melbourne: Hill of Content

[486] Warner, R. (1985) *Recovery from Schizophrenia,* London: Routledge and Kegan Paul, p. 264

[487] Venables, P. and Wing, J. (1962) "Level of Arousal and Subclassification of Schizophrenia", *Archives of General Psychiatry,*Vol. 7

[488] Kutcher, S.,Williamson, P., MacKenzie, S., et al. (1989) "Successful Clonazepam Treatment of Neuroleptic-Induced Akathisia in Older Adolescents and Young Adults: A Double-Blind, Placebo-Controlled Study", *Journal of Clinical Psychopharmacology,*Vol. 9

[489] Wolkowitz, O.,Turetsky, N., Reus,V., et al. (1992) "Benzodiazepine Augmentation of Neuroleptics in Treatment-Resistant Schizophrenia", *Psychopharmacology Bulletin,*Vol. 28

[490] Turetsky, N.,Wolkowitz, O. and Reus,V. (1993) "Benzodiazepine Maintenance in Schizophrenia", (Paper presented at the Annual Meeting of the American

Psychiatric Association, San Francisco, California, May 1993)

491 Wolkowitz, O. (1996) "Benzodiazepines", in: Breier, A. (ed) *The New Pharmacotherapy of Schizophrenia*, Washington, DC: American Psychiatric Press

492 Delva, N. and Letemendia, F. (1982) "Lithium Treatment in Schizophrenia and Schizoaffective Disorders", *British Journal of Psychiatry*, Vol. 141

493 Small, J., Kellams, J., Milstein, V., et al. (1975) "A Placebo-Controlled Study of Lithium Combined With Neuroleptics in Chronic Schizophrenic Patients", *American Journal of Psychiatry*, Vol. 132

494 Kocis, J. et al. (1993) "Neuropsychological Effects of Lithium Discontinuation", *Journal of Clinical Psychopharmacology*, Vol. 13

495 Silverstone, T. and Romans, S. (1996) "Long-Term Treatment of Bipolar Disorder", *Drugs*, Vol. 51

496 Addonizio, G., Roth, S., Stokes, P. and Stoll, P. (1988) "Increased Extrapyramidal Symptoms With Addition of Lithium to Neuroleptics", *Journal of Nervous and Mental Disease*, Vol. 176

497 Karper, L. and Krystal, J. (1996) "Augmenting Antipsychotic Efficacy: New Approaches", in: Breier, A. (ed) *The New Pharmacotherapy of Schizophrenia*, Washington, DC: American Psychiatric Press

498 Herrera, J., Sramek, J. and Costa, J. (1987) "Efficacy of Adjunctive Carbamazepine in the Treatment of Chronic Schizophrenia", *Drug Intelligence and Clinical Pharmacy*, Vol. 21

499 Dose, M., Apelt, S., Emrich, H. (1987) "Carbamazepine as an Adjunct to Antipsychotic Therapy", *Psychiatry Research*, Vol. 22

500 Kahn, E., Schulz, S., Perel, J., et al. (1990) "Change in Haloperidol Level Due to Carbamazepine – A Complicating Factor in Combined Medication for

Schizophrenia", *Journal of Clinical Psychopharmacology*, Vol. 10

[501] Jann, M., Fidone, G., Hernandez, J., et al. (1989) "Clinical Implications of Increased Antipsychotic Plasma Concentrations Upon Anticonvulsant Cessation", *Psychiatry Research*, Vol. 28

[502] Siris, G. (1992) "Adjunctive Medication in the Maintenance Treatment of Schizophrenia and its Conceptual Implications", *British Journal of Psychiatry*, Vol. 163 (suppl.22)

[503] Siris, S. (1990) "Pharmacological Treatment of Depression in Schizophrenia", in: DeLisi, L. (ed) *Depression in Schizophrenia*, Washington, DC: American Psychiatric Press

[504] Karper, L. and Krystal, J. (1996) "Augmenting Antipsychotic Efficacy: New Approaches", in: Breier, A. (ed) *The New Pharmacotherapy of Schizophrenia*, Washington, DC: American Psychiatric Press

[505] Goff, D., Midha, K., Brotman, A., et al. (1991) "Elevation of Plasma Concentration of Haloperidol After the Addition of Fluoxetine", American Journal of Psychiatry, Vol. 147

[506] Glenmullen, J. (2000) *Prozac Backlash*, New York: Simon and Schuster

[507] Montejo-Gonzalez, A., Llorca, G., Izquierdo, A. et al. (1997) "SSRI-Induced Sexual Dysfunction: Fluoxetine, Paroxetine, Sertraline, and Fluvoxamine in a Prospective, Multicentre, and Descriptive Clinical Study of 344 Patients", *Journal of Sex and Marital Therapy*, Vol. 23

[508] Lipinski, J., Keck, P., McElroy, S. (1988) "Beta-Adrenergic Antagonists in Psychosis: Is Improvement Due To Treatment of Neuroleptic-Induced Akathisia?", *Journal of Clinical Psychopharmacology*, Vol. 8

[509] Ratey, J., Sands, S. and O'Driscoll, G. (1986) "The Phenomenology of Recovery in a Chronic Schizophrenic", *Psychiatry*, Vol. 49

[510] Greendyke, R. and Kanter, D. (1987) "Plasma Propranolol

Levels and Their Effect on Plasma Thioridazine and Haloperidol Concentrations", *Journal of Clinical Psychopharmacology*, Vol. 7

[511] Andreasen, N. (1985) *The Broken Brain: The Biological Revolution in Psychiatry*, New York: Harper and Row, p. 222

[512] Ciompi, L. (1980) "The Natural History of Schizophrenia in the Long-Term", *British Journal of Psychiatry*, Vol. 136, p. 419

[513] Ratey, J., Sands, S. and O'Driscoll, G. (1986) "The Phenomenology of Recovery in a Chronic Schizophrenic", *Psychiatry*, Vol. 49, pp. 286, 288 (emphasis added)

Chapter Ten: Reducing Or Stopping Neuroleptic Medications

[514] Gilbert, P., Harris, M., McAdams, L. and Jeste, D. (1995) "Neuroleptic Withdrawal in Schizophrenic Patients: A Review of the Literature", *Archives of General Psychiatry*, Vol. 52, p. 186

[515] Kane, J. (1985) "Compliance Issues in Outpatient Treatment", *Journal of Clinical Psychopharmacology*, Vol. 5

[516] Cohen, D. (2002) "Research on the Drug Treatment of Schizophrenia: A Critical Appraisal and Implications for Social Work Education", *Journal of Social Work Education*, Vol. 38, No. 2, p. 224 (emphasis added)

[517] Healy, D. (1999) *The Antidepressant Era*, Cambridge, Massachusetts: Harvard University Press

[518] Lambert, T. and Castle, D. (2003) "Pharmacological Approaches to the Management of Schizophrenia", *Medical Journal of Australia*, Vol. 178 (suppl.)

[519] Podvoll, E. (1990) *The Seduction of Madness*, New York: HarperCollins, p. 232

[520] Torrey, E. (1988) *Surviving Schizophrenia: A Family Manual (Revised Edition)*, New York: Harper and Row. p. 193

[521] Gallant, D. et al. (1964) "Withdrawal Symptoms After Abrupt Cessation of Antipsychotic Compounds: Clinical Confirmation in Chronic Schizophrenics", *American*

Journal of Psychiatry, Vol. 121; Gardos, G. et al. (1978) "Withdrawal Syndromes Associated With Antipsychotic Drugs", *American Journal of Psychiatry*, Vol. 135; Tranter, R. and Healy, D. (1998) "Neuroleptic Discontinuation Syndromes", *Journal Of Psychopharmacology*, Vol. 12, No. 4

522 Healy, D. (2002) *The Creation of Psychopharmacology*, Cambridge, MA: Harvard University Press, p. 171

523 Lambert, T. and Castle, D. (2003) "Pharmacological Approaches to the Management of Schizophrenia", *Medical Journal of Australia*, Vol. 178 (suppl.), p. 60

524 Gilbert, P., Harris, M., McAdams, L. and Jeste, D. (1995) "Neuroleptic Withdrawal in Schizophrenic Patients: A Review of the Literature", *Archives of General Psychiatry*, Vol. 52

525 Dufresne, R. and Wagner, R. (1988) "Antipsychotic-Withdrawal Akathisia Versus Antipsychotic-Induced Akathisia: Further Evidence for the Existence of Tardive Akathisia", *Journal of Clinical Psychiatry*, Vol. 49

526 Wyatt, J. (1995) "Risks of Withdrawing Antipsychotic Medication", *Archives of General Psychiatry*, Vol. 52

527 Viguera, A., Baldessarini, R., Hegarty, J., van Kammen, J. and Tohen, M. (1997) "Clinical Risk Following Abrupt and Gradual Withdrawal of Maintenance Neuroleptic Treatment", *Archives of General Psychiatry*, Vol. 54

528 Shiovitz, T., Welke, T., Tigel, P., Anand, R., Hartman, R., Sramek, J., Kurtz, M. and Cutler, N. (1996) "Cholinergic Rebound and Rapid Onset Psychosis Following Abrupt Clozapine Withdrawal", *Schizophrenia Bulletin*, Vol. 22, No. 4

529 Thomas, P. (1997) *The Dialectics of Schizophrenia*, London: Free Association Books, p. 120

530 Chouinard, G. and Jones, B. (1980) "Neuroleptic-Induced Supersensitivity Psychosis: Clinical and Pharmacological Characteristics", *American Journal of Psychiatry*, Vol. 137, No. 1

[531] ibid

[532] Podvoll, E. (1990) *The Seduction of Madness*, New York: HarperCollins, p. 231

[533] Houghton, J. (1982) "First Person Account: Maintaining Mental Health in a Turbulent World", *Schizophrenia Bulletin*, Vol. 8, No. 3, pp. 549, 551

[534] Strauss, J., Hafez, H., Lieberman, P. and Harding, C. (1985) "The Course of Psychiatric Disorder, III: Longitudinal Principles", *American Journal of Psychiatry*, Vol. 142, No. 3

[535] Baldessarini, R. and Viguera, A. (1995) "Neuroleptic Withdrawal in Schizophrenic Patients", *Archives of General Psychiatry*, Vol. 52

[536] Green, A., Faraone, S., Brown, W., Guttierez, J. and Tsuang, M. (1992) "Neuroleptic Dose Reduction Studies: Clinical and Neuroendocrine Effects", presented at the 31st Annual Meeting of the American College of Neuropsychopharmacology, December 14–18, San Juan, Puerto Rico

[537] Podvoll, E. (1990) *The Seduction of Madness*, New York: HarperCollins

[538] Fleischhacker, W. (1999) "Pharmacological Treatment of Schizophrenia: A Review", in: Maj, M. and Sartorius, N. (eds) *Schizophrenia. Evidence and Experience in Psychiatry* (World Psychiatric Association Series, Volume Two), New York: John Wiley and Sons, p. 86

[539] Baldessarini, R. and Viguera, A. (1995) "Neuroleptic Withdrawal in Schizophrenic Patients", *Archives of General Psychiatry*, Vol. 52

[540] Kahne, G. (1989) "Rebound Psychoses Following the Discontinuation of a High Potency Neuroleptic", *Canadian Journal of Psychiatry*, Vol. 34

[541] Pierce, E. (1988) *Passion for the Possible*, Gladesville, NSW: P. E. Pierce, pp. 100, 102

[542] Farber, S. (1993) *Madness, Heresy, and the Rumour of Angels*, Chicago: Open Court, pp. 160-1

543 Viguera, A., Baldessarini, R., Hegarty, J., van Kammen, J. and Tohen, M. (1997) "Clinical Risk Following Abrupt and Gradual Withdrawal of Maintenance Neuroleptic Treatment", *Archives of General Psychiatry*, Vol. 54, p. 51

544 Glovinsky, D., Kirch, D. and Wyatt, R. (1992) "Early Anti-Psychotic Response To Resumption Of Neuroleptics In Drug-Free Chronic Schizophrenic Patients", *Biological Psychiatry*, Vol. 31

545 Gilbert, P., Harris, M., McAdams, L. and Jeste, D. (1995) "Neuroleptic Withdrawal in Schizophrenic Patients: A Review of the Literature", *Archives of General Psychiatry*, Vol. 52, pp. 182, 185

546 Bockes, Z. (1985) "First Person Account: Freedom Means Knowing You Have A Choice", *Schizophrenia Bulletin*, Vol. 11, No. 3, p. 488

547 Ludwig, A. (1971) *Treating The Treatment Failures*, New York: Grune and Stratton, p. 19

548 Van Putten, T., Crumpton, E. and Yale, C. (1976) "Drug Refusal in Schizophrenia and the Wish to be Crazy", *Archives of General Psychiatry*, Vol. 33

549 Strauss, J., Hafez, H., Lieberman, P. and Harding, C. (1985) "The Course of Psychiatric Disorder, III: Longitudinal Principles", *American Journal of Psychiatry*, Vol. 142, No. 3

550 Glass, J. (1989) *Private Terror, Public Life*, New York: Cornell University Press, p. 91

551 Faraone, S., Green, A., Brown, W., Yin, P. and Tsuang, M. (1989) "Neuroleptic Dose Reduction in Persistently Psychotic Patients", *Hospital and Community Psychiatry*, Vol. 40, No. 11

552 Smith, R. (1994) "Lower-Dose Therapy With Traditional Neuroleptics in Chronically Hospitalised Schizophrenic Patients", (Letter) *Archives of General Psychiatry*, Vol. 51, p. 427

Chapter Eleven: Taking Medication With a Grain of Salt

[553] Luhrmann, T. (2000) *Of Two Minds: The Growing Disorder in American Psychiatry*, New York: Alfred Knopf, p. 55

[554] Angell, M. (2005) *The Truth About the Drug Companies: How They Deceive Us and What To Do About It.* Melbourne, Australia: Scribe

[555] Abbasi, K. and Smith, R. (2003) "No More Free Lunches: Patients Will Benefit From Doctors And Drug Companies Disentangling", *British Medical Journal,* Vol. 326, 31 May

[556] Torrey, E. (1983) *Surviving Schizophrenia: A Family Manual,* New York: Harper and Row, p. 115

[557] Luhrmann, T. (2000) *Of Two Minds: The Growing Disorder in American Psychiatry,* New York: Alfred Knopf, p. 287

[558] Barlett, D. and Steele, J. (2004) "Why America Pays So Much For Drugs", *Time* (February 2, 2004, No. 4), pp. 41–48

[559] Moynihan, R. (2003) "Who Pays For The Pizza? Redefining The Relationships Between Doctors and Drug Companies. 1: Entanglement", *British Medical Journal,* Vol. 326

[560] ibid, p. 1190 (emphasis added)

[561] Gelenberg, A. (1999) The Editor Responds, *Journal of Clinical Psychiatry,* Vol. 60, No. 2, p. 122

[562] Safer, D. (2002) "Design and Reporting Modifications in Industry-Sponsored Comparative Psychopharmacology Trials", *Journal of Nervous and Mental Disease,* Vol. 190

[563] Lexchin, J., Bero, L., Djulbegovic, B. and Clark, O. (2003) "Pharmaceutical Industry Sponsorship and Research Outcome and Quality: Systematic Review", *British Medical Journal,* Vol. 326

[564] Bodenheimer, T. (2000) "Uneasy Alliance. Clinical Investigators and the Pharmaceutical Industry", *New England Journal of Medicine,* Vol. 342, No. 20, p. 1542

[565] Melander, H., Ahlqvist-Rastad, J., Meijer, G. and Beermann, B. (2003) "Evidence B(i)ased Medicine - Selective

Reporting from Studies Sponsored by the Pharmaceutical Industry: Review of Studies in New Drug Applications", *British Medical Journal*, Vol. 326

[566] Cited in Healy, D. (1999) *The Antidepressant Era*, Cambridge, Massachusetts: Harvard University Press, p. 140

[567] Bodenheimer, T. (2000) "Uneasy Alliance. Clinical Investigators and the Pharmaceutical Industry", *New England Journal of Medicine*, Vol. 342, No. 20, p. 1541

[568] Breggin, P. and Breggin, G. (1994) *Talking Back To Prozac*, New York: St. Martin's Press, p. 161

[569] Bodenheimer, T. (2000) "Uneasy Alliance. Clinical Investigators and the Pharmaceutical Industry", *New England Journal of Medicine*, Vol. 342, No. 20, p. 1542

[570] Cited in: Whitaker, R. (2002) *Mad In America: Bad Science, Bad Medicine, and the Enduring Mistreatment of the Mentally Ill*, Cambridge, MA: Perseus Books, p.149

[571] Gottlieb, S. (2002) "Congress Criticises Drugs Industry for Misleading Advertising", *British Medical Journal*, Vol. 325

[572] Angell, M., Utiger, R. and Wood, A. (2000) "Disclosure of Authors' Conflict of Interest: A Follow-Up", *New England Journal of Medicine*, Vol. 342, No. 8, February 24, p. 586

[573] Angell, M. (2000) "Is Academic Medicine For Sale?", *New England Journal of Medicine*, Vol. 342, No. 20, May18, p. 1516

[574] Abbasi, K. and Smith, R. (2003) "No More Free Lunches. Patients Will Benefit From Doctors and Drug Companies Disentangling", *British Medical Journal*, Vol. 326, p. 1155

[575] Smith, R. (2003) "Medical Journals and Pharmaceutical Companies: Uneasy Bedfellows", *British Medical Journal*, Vol. 326, pp. 1202-1205

[576] *2000 MIMS Annual* (2000) (Twenty-Fourth Edition), St Leonards, NSW: Havas MediMedia Australia

[577] Rose, N. (2003) "Neurochemical Selves", *Society*, November/December, p. 57

[578] Choudhry, N., Stelfox, H. and Detsky, A. (2002) "Relationships Between Authors of Clinical Practice

Guidelines and the Pharmaceutical Industry", *Journal of the American Medical Association*,Vol. 287, No. 5

[579] Glenmullen, J. (2000) *Prozac Backlash*. New York: Simon and Schuster, p. 225

[580] Editorial (1998) "A Meeting Too Many", *The Lancet*,Vol. 352, October 10th, p. 1161

[581] Moynihan, R. (2003) "Who Pays For The Pizza? Redefining The Relationships Between Doctors and Drug Companies. 1: Entanglement", *British Medical Journal*,Vol. 326, p. 1190

[582] Jureidini, J. and Mansfield, P. (2001) "Does Drug Promotion Adversely Influence Doctors' Abilities to Make the Best Decisions for Patients?", *Australasian Psychiatry*,Vol. 9, No. 2, p. 96

[583] Moynihan, R. (2003) "Who Pays For The Pizza? Redefining The Relationships Between Doctors and Drug Companies. 1: Entanglement", *British Medical Journal*,Vol. 326

[584] Abbasi, K. and Smith, R. (2003) "No More Free Lunches. Patients Will Benefit From Doctors and Drug Companies Disentangling", *British Medical Journal*,Vol. 326, p. 1155

[585] Moynihan, R. (2003) "Who Pays For The Pizza? Redefining The Relationships Between Doctors and Drug Companies. 1: Entanglement", *British Medical Journal*,Vol. 326

[586] ibid, p. 1190

[587] Jureidini, J. and Mansfield, P. (2001) "Does Drug Promotion Adversely Influence Doctors' Abilities to Make the Best Decisions for Patients?", *Australasian Psychiatry*,Vol. 9, No. 2, p. 98

[588] Wazana, A. (2000) "Physicians and the Pharmaceutical Industry: Is a Gift Ever Just a Gift?", *Journal of the American Medical Association*,Vol. 283

[589] Orlowski, J. and Wateska, L. (1992) "The Effects of Pharmaceutical Firm Enticements on Physician

Prescribing Patterns: There's No Such Thing As a Free Lunch", *Chest*, Vol. 102

[590] Cohen, J. (2001) *Over Dose: The Case Against The Drug Companies*, New York: Jeremy Tarcher/Putnam, pp. 215-217 (emphasis added)

[591] Moynihan, R., Bero, L., Ross-Degnan, D., Henry, D., Lee, K., Watkins, J. et al. (2000) "Coverage by the News Media of the Benefits and Risks of Medications", *New England Journal of Medicine*, Vol. 342

[592] Nasar, S. (1998) *A Beautiful Mind*, New York: Simon and Schuster, p. 353

[593] Hughes, G. and Minchin, L. (2003) "Drug Giants' Big-Money Pitch Exposed", *The Age* (13/12/03).

[594] Hirst, J. (2003) "Charities and Patient Groups Should Declare Interests", (Letter), *British Medical Journal*, Vol. 326, p. 1211

[595] Herxheimer, A. (2003) "Relationships Between the Pharmaceutical Industry and Patients' Organisations", *British Medical Journal*, Vol. 326

[596] Whitaker, R. (2002) *Mad In America: Bad Science, Bad Medicine, and the Enduring Mistreatment of the Mentally Ill*, Cambridge, MA: Perseus Books, p. 283 (fn)

[597] Hughes, G. and Minchin, L. (2003) "Drug Giants' Big-Money Pitch Exposed", *The Age* (13/12/03).

[598] Ibid, p.1

[599] Glenmullen, J. (2000) *Prozac Backlash*, New York: Simon and Schuster, p. 336

[600] Abbasi, K. and Smith, R. (2003) "No More Free Lunches. Patients Will Benefit From Doctors and Drug Companies Disentangling", *British Medical Journal*, Vol. 326, p. 1156

[601] Angell, M (2000) "Is Academic Medicine For Sale?" Third National Ethics Conference, November 4th, Baltimore, MD, Cited in: Whitaker, R. (2002) *Mad In America: Bad Science, Bad Medicine, and the Enduring Mistreatment of the Mentally Ill*, Cambridge, MA: Perseus Books, p. 265

[602] Cohen, D. (2002) "Research on the Drug Treatment of Schizophrenia: A Critical Appraisal and Implications for Social Work Education", *Journal of Social Work Education*, Vol.38, No.2. p.230.

[603] Healy, D. (1999) *The Antidepressant Era*, Cambridge, Massachusetts: Harvard University Press. p. 5

[604] Breggin, P. (1993) *Toxic Psychiatry*, London: HarperCollins.

[605] Burston, D. (1996) *The Wing of Madness: The Life and Work of R.D. Laing*, Cambridge, MA: Harvard University Press, p.244.

[606] ibid, p. 245

[607] Geddes, J., Freemantle, N., Harrison, P. and Bebbington, P. (2000) "Atypical Antipsychotics in the Treatment of Schizophrenia: Systematic Overview and Meta-Regression Analysis", *British Medical Journal*, Vol. 321, pp. 1372-1373 (emphasis added)

[608] Kane, J. and Freeman, H. (1994) "Towards More Effective Antipsychotic Treatment", *British Journal of Psychiatry*, Vol. 165 (suppl.25)

[609] Geddes, J., Freemantle, N., Harrison, P. and Bebbington, P. (2000) "Atypical Antipsychotics in the Treatment of Schizophrenia: Systematic Overview and Meta-Regression Analysis", *British Medical Journal*, Vol. 321

[610] Castle, D., Morgan, V. and Jablensky, A. (2001) "Antipsychotic Use In Australia: The Patients' Perspective", *Australian and New Zealand Journal of Psychiatry*, Vol. 36, p. 640

[611] Whitaker, R. (2002) *Mad In America: Bad Science, Bad Medicine, and the Enduring Mistreatment of the Mentally Ill*, Cambridge, MA: Perseus Books, p. 283

[612] ibid, p. 284

[613] Glenmullen, J. (2000) *Prozac Backlash*, New York: Simon and Schuster, p. 12

Epilogue: The Most Powerful Drug There Is

[614] Podvoll, E. (1990) *The Seduction of Madness*, New York: HarperCollins, p. 255

[615] Carpenter, W., McGlashan, T. and Strauss, J. (1977) "The Treatment of Acute Schizophrenia Without Drugs: An Investigation of Some Current Assumptions", *American Journal of Psychiatry*, Vol. 134, No. 1, p. 14 (emphasis added)

[616] Luhrmann, T. (2000) *Of Two Minds: The Growing Disorder in American Psychiatry*, New York: Alfred Knopf, p. 47

[617] Fleischhacker, W. (1999) "Pharmacological Treatment of Schizophrenia: A Review", in: Maj, M. and Sartorius, N. (eds) *Schizophrenia. Evidence and Experience in Psychiatry*, (World Psychiatric Association Series, Volume Two), New York: John Wiley and Sons, p. 81

[618] Cited in: Whitaker, R. (2002) *Mad In America: Bad Science, Bad Medicine, and the Enduring Mistreatment of the Mentally Ill*, Cambridge, MA: Perseus Books, p. 221

[619] Podvoll, E. (1990) *The Seduction of Madness*, New York: HarperCollins, pp. 2-3 (emphasis in original)

[620] Bleuler, M. (1986) "Introduction and Overview", in: Burrows, G., Norman, T. and Rubinstein, G. (eds) *Handbook of Studies on Schizophrenia*, Amsterdam: Elsevier, p. 8

[621] Fields, R. (1986) "R. D. Laing and The Psychology of Simple Presence", *The Vajradhatu Sun*, Vol. 8, No. 5, p. 3

[622] Guthiel, T. (1993) "The Psychology of Psychopharmacology", in: Schachter, M. (ed) *Psychotherapy and Medication: A Dynamic Integration*, New Jersey: Jason Aronson, p. 5

[623] Torrey, E. (1988) *Surviving Schizophrenia: A Family Manual (Revised Edition)*, New York: Harper and Row, p. 193

[624] Glenmullen, J. (2000) *Prozac Backlash*, New York: Simon and Schuster, p. 196

[625] Torrey, E. (1988) *Surviving Schizophrenia: A Family Manual (Revised Edition)*, New York: Harper and Row, p. 189

[626] Chamberlin, J. (1997) "Confessions of a Non-Compliant Patient", *National Empowerment Centre Newsletter*, Lawrence, MA: National Empowerment Centre (Summer/Fall), p. 8

[627] Jung, C.G. (1989) *The Psychogenesis of Mental Disease*, Princeton: Princeton University Press, p. 158

[628] Baynes, H.G. (1969) *Mythology of the Soul*, London: Rider and Company, p. xvii

[629] Frattaroli, E. (2001) *Healing the Soul in the Age of the Brain*, New York: Viking Penguin, p. 368

[630] Jung, C.G. (1952) Foreword, in: Custance, J. *Wisdom, Madness and Folly*, New York: Pellegrini and Cudahy

[631] Bleuler, M. (1978) *The Schizophrenic Disorders: Long-Term Patient and Family Studies*, Newhaven: Yale University Press, p. 500

[632] Nelson, J. (1990) *Healing the Split*, Los Angeles, CA: Jeremy Tarcher, p. 129 (emphasis in original)

[633] Gabbard, G. (1992) "Psychodynamic Psychiatry in the 'Decade of the Brain'", *American Journal of Psychiatry*, Vol. 149, No. 8; Gabbard, G. (2000) "A Neurobiologically Informed Perspective on Psychotherapy", *British Journal of Psychiatry*, Vol. 177

[634] Davidson, R. et al. (2003) "Alterations In Brain And Immune Function Produced By Mindfulness Meditation", *Psychosomatic Medicine*, Vol. 65, 564–570

[635] Frattaroli, E. (2001) *Healing the Soul in the Age of the Brain*, New York: Viking Penguin, p. 281

[636] Handel, M. (1987) *A Personal Account of Schizophrenia* (Unpublished)

[637] Cousins, N. (1981) *Anatomy of an Illness as Perceived by the Patient*, New York: Bantam, p. 69

Appendix A: Optimal Dosage Ranges for Some Common Neuroleptic Drugs

[638] Healy, D. (2002) *The Creation of Psychopharmacology*, Cambridge, MA: Harvard University Press

[639] Bollini, P., Pampallona, S., Orza, M., Adams, M. and Chalmers, T. (1994) "Antipsychotic Drugs: Is More Worse? A Meta-Analysis of Published Randomised Control Trials", *Psychological Medicine*, Vol. 24

[640] Farde, L. Wiesel, F-A., Halldin, C. and Sedvall, G. (1988) "Central D2 Dopamine Receptor Occupancy in Schizophrenic Patients Treated with Antipsychotic Drugs", *Archives of General Psychiatry*, Vol. 45

[641] Healy, D. (1993) *Psychiatric Drugs Explained*, London: Mosby, p.18

[642] Baldessarini, R., Cohen, B. and Teicher, H. (1988) "Significance of Neuroleptic Dose and Plasma Level in Pharmacological Treatment of Psychosis," *Archives of General Psychiatry*, Vol. 45, p. 87

[643] American Psychiatric Association (1997) "Practice Guidelines For The Treatment of Patients With Schizophrenia", *American Journal of Psychiatry*, Vol.154, No. 4 (suppl.)

[644] Bochner, F. et al. (2000) *Therapeutic Guidelines: Psychotropic (Version 4)*, North Melbourne, Victoria: Therapeutic Guidelines Ltd.; McGorry, P., Killackey, E., Elkins, K. et al. (2003) "Summary Australian and New Zealand Clinical Practice Guideline for the Treatment of Schizophrenia (2003)", *Australasian Psychiatry*, Vol. 11, No. 2

[645] Baldessarini, R. (1999) "Pharmacotherapy of Psychotic Disorders: A Perspective on Current Developments", in: Maj, M. and Sartorius, N. (eds) *Schizophrenia. Evidence and Experience in Psychiatry*, (World Psychiatric Association Series, Volume 2), New York: John Wiley and Sons

[646] American Psychiatric Association (1997) "Practice Guidelines For The Treatment of Patients With Schizophrenia", *American Journal of Psychiatry*, Vol. 154, No. 4 (suppl.), p. 10

Appendix B: Managing Neuroleptic Side Effects

[647] Healy, D. (1993) *Psychiatric Drugs Explained*, London: Mosby, p. 21

[648] Solovitz, B., Fisher, S., Bryant, S., *et al.* (1987) "How Well Can Patients Discriminate Drug-Related Side Effects From Extraneous New Symptoms?", *Psychopharmacology Bulletin*, Vol. 23

[649] Weiden, P., Mann, J., Haas, G., Mattson, M. and Frances, A. (1987) "Clinical Non-recognition of Neuroleptic-Induced Movement Disorders: A Cautionary Study", *American Journal of Psychiatry*, Vol. 144

[650] Ayd, F. (1973) "Rational Pharmacotherapy: Once-A-Day Drug Dosage", *Diseases of the Nervous System*, Vol. 34, pp. 374-376

[651] Johnson, D. (1984) "Observations on the Use of Long-Acting Depot Neuroleptic Injections in the Maintenance Therapy of Schizophrenia", *Journal of Clinical Psychiatry*, Vol. 45, No. 5, p. 18

[652] Consensus Statement by World Health Organisation (1990) "Prophylactic Use of Anticholinergics in Patients on Long-Term Neuroleptic Treatment", *British Journal of Psychiatry*, Vol. 156, p. 412

[653] Johnson, D. (1977) "Practical Considerations in the Use of Depot Neuroleptics for the Treatment of Schizophrenia", *British Journal of Hospital Medicine*, Vol. 17

[654] Birkett-Smith, E. (1974) "Abnormal Involuntary Movements Induced by Anticholinergic Therapy", *Acta Neurologica Scandinavica*, Vol. 50

[655] Gerlach, J. (1977) "The Relationship Between Parkinsonism and Tardive Dyskinesia", *American Journal of Psychiatry*, Vol. 134

[656] Johnstone, E., Crow, T., Ferrier, I., Frith, C., Owens, D., Bourne, R. and Gamble, S. (1983) "Adverse Effects of Anticholinergic Medication on Positive Schizophrenic Symptoms", *Psychological Medicine*, Vol. 13

657 Fayen, M., Goldman, M., Moulthrop, M., et al. (1988) "Differential Memory Function with Dopaminergic Versus Anticholinergic Treatment of Drug-Induced Extrapyramidal Symptoms", *American Journal of Psychiatry*, Vol. 145

658 Rifkin, A., Quitkin, F. and Klein, D. (1975) "Akinesia: A Poorly Recognised Drug-Induced Extrapyramidal Behavioural Disorder", *Archives of General Psychiatry*, Vol. 32

659 Group for the Advancement of Psychiatry (1992) *Beyond Symptom Suppression: Improving Long-Term Outcomes of Schizophrenia* (Report No. 134), Washington, DC: American Psychiatric Press, pp. 42–43

660 Rifkin, A., Quitkin, F., Kane, J., Struve, F. and Klein, D. (1978) "Are Prophylactic Antiparkinsonian Drugs Necessary?", *Archives of General Psychiatry*, Vol. 35

661 Kutcher, S., Williamson, P., MacKenzie, S., et al. (1989) "Successful Clonazepam Treatment of Neuroleptic-Induced Akathisia in Older Adolescents and Young Adults: A Double-Blind, Placebo-Controlled Study", *Journal of Clinical Psychopharmacology*, Vol. 9

662 Kramer, M., Gorkin, R., DiJohnson, C., et al. (1988) "Propranolol in the Treatment of Neuroleptic-Induced Akathisia (NIA) in Schizophrenics: A Double-Blind, Placebo-Controlled Study", *Biological Psychiatry*, Vol. 24

663 Shiriqui, C. and Jones, B. (1990) "Free Radicals and Tardive Dyskinesia" (Letter), *Canadian Journal of Psychiatry*, Vol. 35; Tsai, G., Goff, D., Chang, R. et al. (1998) "Markers of Glutamatergic Neurotransmission and Oxidative Stress Associated with Tardive Dyskinesia", *American Journal of Psychiatry*, Vol. 155, No. 9; Zhang, X., Zhou, D., Cao, L. et al (2003) "Blood Superoxide Dismutase in Schizophrenic Patients with Tardive Dyskinesia: Association with Dyskinetic Movements", *Schizophrenia Research*, Vol. 62, No. 3

664 Lohr, J., Cadet, J., Lohr, M. et al. (1988) "Vitamin E in the

Treatment of Tardive Dyskinesia: The Possible Involvement of Free Radical Mechanisms", *Schizophrenia Bulletin*, Vol. 14, No. 2; Adler, L., Peselow, E., Rotrosen, J. et al. (1993) "Vitamin E Treatment of Tardive Dyskinesia", *American Journal of Psychiatry*, Vol. 150

665 Tkacz, C. (1984) "A Preventive Measure for Tardive Dyskinesia", *Journal of the International Academy of Preventive Medicine*, Vol. 8, No. 5

666 Lohr, J., Cadet, J., Lohr, M. et al. (1988) "Vitamin E in the Treatment of Tardive Dyskinesia: The Possible Involvement of Free Radical Mechanisms", *Schizophrenia Bulletin*, Vol. 14, No. 2

667 Lerner, V., Miodownik, C. et al. (2001) "Vitamin B6 in the Treatment of Tardive Dyskinesia: A Double-Blind, Placebo-Controlled, Crossover Study", *American Journal of Psychiatry*, Vol. 158, No. 9.

668 Milner, G. (1963) "Ascorbic Acid in Chronic Psychiatric Patients: A Controlled Trial", *British Journal of Psychiatry*, Vol. 109

669 Fischer, V., Haar, J., Greiner, L., Lloyd, R. and Mason, R. (1991) "Possible Role of Free Radical Formation in Clozapine-Induced Agranulocytosis", *Molecular Pharmacology*, Vol. 40

670 Bhattacharya, S., Bhattacharya, D., Sairam, K. and Ghosal, S. (2002) "Effect of *Withania Somnifera* Glycowithanolides on a Rat Model of Tardive Dyskinesia", *Phytomedicine*, Vol. 9, No. 2

671 American Diabetes Association, American Psychiatric Association, American Association of Clinical Endocrinologists, North American Association for the Study of Obesity (2004) "Consensus Development Conference on Antipsychotic Drugs and Obesity and Diabetes", *Diabetes Care*, Vol. 27, No. 2, pp. 596-601

672 Brighthope, I. (1994) "The Therapeutic Potential of Antioxidants in the Prevention and Treatment of

Degenerative Diseases", *Journal of the Australasian College of Nutritional and Environmental Medicine*, Vol. 13, No. 1

[673] Manson, J. et al. (1993) "Antioxidants and Cardiovascular Disease: A Review", *Journal of the American College of Nutrition*, Vol. 12, No. 4

[674] Paolisso, G. et al. (1993) "Pharmacologic Doses of Vitamin E Improve Insulin Action in Healthy Subjects and Non-Insulin-Dependent Diabetic Patients", *American Journal of Clinical Nutrition*, Vol. 57

[675] Stoll, A. (2002) *The Omega-3 Connection*, London: Simon and Schuster

[676] ibid, p. 209

Index